PHYSIOLOGY SECRETS

Second Edition

HERSHEL RAFF, PhD
Professor, Departments of Medicine and Physiology
Medical College of Wisconsin
Director, Endocrine Research Laboratory
St. Luke's Medical Center
Milwaukee, Wisconsin

HANLEY & BELFUS, INC. / Philadelphia

Publisher: HANLEY & BELFUS, INC.
Medical Publishers
210 South 13th Street
Philadelphia, PA 19107
(215) 546-7293; 800-962-1892
FAX (215) 790-9330
Web site: http://www.hanleyandbelfus.com

Library of Congress Control Number: 2002112871

PHYSIOLOGY SECRETS, 2nd edition ISBN 1-56053-509-1

Last digit is the print number: 9 8 7 6 5 4 3 2 1

CONTENTS

CONTRIBUTORS

Marshall B. Dunning III, Ph.D., M.S.
Associate Professor, Department of Medicine, Medical College of Wisconsin; Director, Pulmonary Diagnostic Laboratory, Froedtert Memorial Lutheran Hospital, Milwaukee, Wisconsin

Lauren Jacobson, Ph.D.
Assistant Professor, Center for Neuropharmacology and Neuroscience, Albany Medical College, Albany, New York

Maureen Keller-Wood, Ph.D.
Professor, Department of Pharmacodynamics, University of Florida College of Pharmacy, Gainesville, Florida

Anne E. Kwitek, Ph.D.
Assistant Professor, Department of Physiology, Human and Molecular Genetics Center, Medical College of Wisconsin, Milwaukee, Wisconsin

Leonard M. Lichtenberger, Ph.D.
Professor, Department of Integrative Biology and Pharmacology, The University of Texas Medical School at Houston, Houston, Texas

Julian H. Lombard, Ph.D.
Professor, Department of Physiology, Medical College of Wisconsin, Milwaukee, Wisconsin

David L. Mattson, Ph.D.
Associate Professor, Department of Physiology, Medical College of Wisconsin, Milwaukee, Wisconsin

Paula E. Papanek, Ph.D., MPT, FACSM
Associate Professor, Department of Physical Therapy; Director of Exercise Sciences and Athletic Training, Marquette University, Milwaukee, Wisconsin

Hershel Raff, Ph.D.
Professor, Departments of Medicine and Physiology, Medical College of Wisconsin; Director, Endocrine Research Laboratory, St. Luke's Medical Center, Milwaukee, Wisconsin

Nancy J. Rusch, Ph.D.
Professor, Department of Pharmacology, Medical College of Wisconsin, Milwaukee, Wisconsin

Willis K. Samson, Ph.D.
Professor, Department of Pharmacologic and Physiologic Science, Saint Louis University School of Medicine, St. Louis, Missouri

Jeanne L. Seagard, Ph.D.
Professor, Departments of Anesthesiology and Physiology, Medical College of Wisconsin; Clement J. Zablocki Veterans Affairs Medical Center, Milwaukee, Wisconsin

Joseph L. Shaker, M.D.
Associate Clinical Professor, Department of Medicine, Medical College of Wisconsin; Endocrine-Diabetes Center, St. Luke's Medical Center, Milwaukee, Wisconsin

Meghan M. Taylor, Ph.D.
Department of Pharmacologic and Physiologic Science, Saint Louis University School of Medicine, St. Louis, Missouri

Charles E. Wood, Ph.D.
Professor, Department of Physiology and Functional Genomics, University of Florida College of Medicine, Gainesville, Florida

PREFACE TO THE SECOND EDITION

Several significant changes and additions have been made in the second edition of this book. All of the chapters have been updated to reflect new information. The "Cardiovascular Physiology" chapter has a new author who has expanded the sections on the electrocardiogram and blood. The "Respiratory Physiology" chapter has been extensively revised to make it more descriptive and less formulaic. The "Cells, Nerves, and Muscles"; "Renal Physiology"; "Gastrointestinal Physiology"; "Endocrine Physiology"; "Maternal-Fetal Physiology"; and "Temperature Regulation" chapters have been updated, although major changes were not necessary. The chapter on exercise physiology has been revised to lessen redundancy with the chapter on cells, nerves, and muscles.

There are several new chapters. "Cell Signaling" extensively covers the myriad of membrane and intracellular pathways by which cells respond to input. "Physiologic Genomics" outlines the next step after the sequencing of the human genome—to establish the function of newly discovered genes and their translated proteins. A chapter briefly covering the physiology of bone has been added. In addition, two chapters have been added to highlight the interaction and integration between metabolism, immunology, and endocrinology. Finally, a chapter on the physiology of aging has been added to explore the increasing importance of understanding changes in control systems in the elderly.

Hershel Raff, Ph.D.

DEDICATION

To my wife, Judy, for her constant support and expert proofreading.
To my son, Jonathan, the ultimate arbiter of syntax, grammar, and punctuation.

To my mentors, Robert S. Fitzgerald at Johns Hopkins, Mary F. Dallman at UCSF, Allen W. Cowley at the Medical College of Wisconsin, and James W. Findling at St. Luke's Medical Center.

HR

PREFACE TO THE FIRST EDITION

The word *physiology* is derived from the Greek words *physis* (nature) and *logos* (study): the study of nature. In its most general terms, physiology is the science of the function of living things—"how things work." *Physiology Secrets* focuses on human "organ systems" physiology as it is routinely taught in medical school curricula in the United States. It is designed to be used as an adjunct to, and not a substitute for, a standard textbook or syllabus.

A noticeable characteristic of this book is that the physiology of the central nervous system and spinal cord does not appear. In the "old days" (i.e., when I was a student), physiology courses included the nervous system. Currently, medical school curricula have a separate course entitled "Neurosciences" that includes neuroanatomy and neurophysiology. For that reason, and taking the example of recent textbooks such as Johnson's *Essential Medical Physiology,* we have omitted neurophysiology except for a section on the basic function of nerves. The publisher is planning a *Neuroscience Secrets* to meet the needs of modern medical school curricula in that area. You may also notice that there are two sections on skeletal muscle. These complementary sections are necessary because one takes the point of view of a cell physiologist while the other takes the point of view of an exercise physiologist.

Any of you who remember the movie *The Paper Chase,* about students at Harvard Law School, will recall the dramatic power of the Socratic method. A question is followed by an answer, which is followed by another question *ad infinitum,* pointing out that one never knows the complete answer. I have found that the best (and perhaps only) way to know if one really knows a subject is to try to teach it to someone else. The intent of this book is to supply the questions and then allow the student to answer, thereby testing her or his knowledge and, in the process, learning the material.

The contributors are grateful to our teachers and students for their time and energy. As editor, I am indebted to my contributors and friends for their diligence in preparing their sections.

Hershel Raff, Ph.D.

I. Cell Physiology

1. CELLS, NERVES, AND MUSCLES

Julian H. Lombard, Ph.D., and Nancy J. Rusch, Ph.D.

CELL MEMBRANE COMPOSITION AND TRANSPORT

1. What are the main components of the cell membrane?

The **lipids** are amphipathic, or two-sided. They have a phosphorylated glycerol backbone with two hydrophobic fatty acid tails attached by ester bonds. The fatty acid tail of each phospholipid molecule is repelled by water but mutually attracted to other fatty acid tails. Hence, the tails face the inside of the membrane and form the membrane core. Each lipid also contains a phospholipid head, which faces outward because it is polar and attracted to the surrounding water.

The **proteins** float in the lipid bilayer. Substances that cannot pass directly through the lipid bilayer move through protein channels or use carrier proteins for facilitated transport across the membrane. Other proteins involved in cell signaling are located on the inner or outer surface of the membrane, such as receptor molecules for neurotransmitters or transducing proteins, which link receptors to cytoplasmic proteins and enzymes.

Cholesterol is interspersed between the phospholipids of mammalian cell membranes. The steroid structure of cholesterol does not permit it to span the membrane. Cholesterol acts to reduce membrane fluidity at physiologic temperatures but increases fluidity at lower temperatures to maintain normal membrane function. The lipid and protein composition of the membrane varies greatly between different cell types.

Carbohydrates bind to external sites of membrane protein and lipid molecules to form glycoproteins and glycolipids. The resulting carbohydrate layer on the outer membrane surface is called the **glycocalyx**. The glycocalyx, which is negatively charged, performs several important functions. It binds extracellular Ca^{2+} to stabilize membrane structures and acts as an attachment matrix for other cells (see figure).

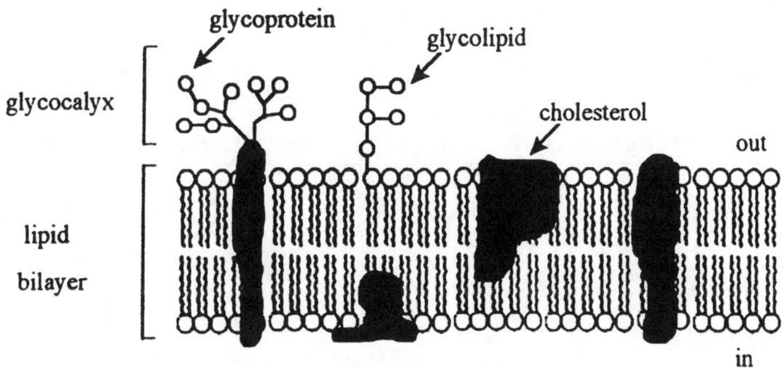

Lipid and protein components of the cell membrane.

2. What is another name for the cell membrane?
Plasma membrane.

3. At what cellular site are membrane lipids and proteins synthesized?
The **endoplasmic reticulum (ER)** of the cell is the site of synthesis. Lipids are synthesized within the ER, whereas proteins are synthesized on the surface of the ER by the interaction of messenger RNA with ribosomes. The Golgi apparatus processes the ER products for final translocation to the plasma membrane.

4. How does the membrane contribute to cell homeostasis?
The main function of the plasma membrane is to maintain cell homeostasis by closely controlling the internal milieu of the cell cytoplasm. The phospholipid bilayer acts as a barrier to insulate the cell cytoplasm from immediate changes in the outside environment and provides a lipid suspension within which membrane proteins can move to enact critical changes in cell function. Normal membrane fluidity is required for cell function and growth and for optimal function of the transport, carrier, and signaling proteins.

5. Where are membrane proteins located?
Proteins may be located at the internal or external surfaces of the cell membrane or span across the entire lipid bilayer.

6. What are the functions of membrane proteins?
- To transport hydrophilic, large polar substances and ions across the membrane
- To act as signaling or transducing sites to conduct messages across the cell membrane (several proteins may interact to process one signal across the membrane)

7. Does the plasma membrane of different kinds of cells express the same types of proteins?
The population profile of membrane proteins varies tremendously among different kinds of cells and is "tailor made" for each cell's function. For example, neurons rely on membrane Na^+ channels for cell excitation and the release of neurotransmitters, whereas smooth muscle cells do not require Na^+ for cell excitation and contraction. Nerve cell membranes are densely populated with Na^+ channels, whereas Na^+ channels are not found in the plasma membrane of smooth muscle cells.

8. How does the composition of the intracellular and extracellular fluid differ?
The extracellular fluid contains high concentrations of sodium (Na^+) and chloride (Cl^-). Hence, from an evolutionary perspective, mammalian cells continue to be surrounded by a solution resembling dilute sea water. In contrast, the intracellular fluid contains a high concentration of the cation, potassium (K^+). The negative charges inside the cell are mainly attributable to negatively charged proteins and phosphates. Other important substances, such as glucose and Ca^{2+},

Composition of Intracellular Fluid Versus Extracellular Fluid

CONSTITUENT	INTRACELLULAR CONCENTRATION	EXTRACELLULAR CONCENTRATION
Na^+	14 mEq/L	140 mEq/L
K^+	140 mEq/L	4 mEq/L
Ca^{2+}	10^{-7} M (ionized)	2.5 mEq/L
Cl^-	10 mEq/L	110 mEq/L
HCO_3^-	10 mEq/L	20 mEq/L
Glucose	100 mg/dL	≈ 10 mEq/L
Osmolarity	295 mOsm/L	295 mOsm/L
pH	≈ 7.1	7.4

also are differentially distributed across the plasma membrane. Knowing the intracellular and extracellular concentrations of ions and other critical substances is essential for predicting in which direction these substances will cross the membrane when transport systems are activated.

9. How do lipophilic (lipid-soluble) and hydrophilic (water-soluble) substances cross the cell membrane?

Uncharged lipophilic substances can cross the plasma membrane by simply passing through its lipid core. Important examples of these substances are the gases oxygen and carbon dioxide, which can readily cross all cell membranes. Some small polar substances, including water, also can easily move across the lipid bilayer through intermolecular pores. Hydrophilic substances or large polar molecules, which are not lipid-soluble and are repelled by the lipid core of the membrane, must interact with a specialized carrier protein or channel protein to cross the cell membrane. Lipid-insoluble substances, which require special transport proteins to permeate the membrane, include glucose and amino acids (large polar substances) and all species of ions (Na^+, K^+, $Cl-$, HCO_3^-).

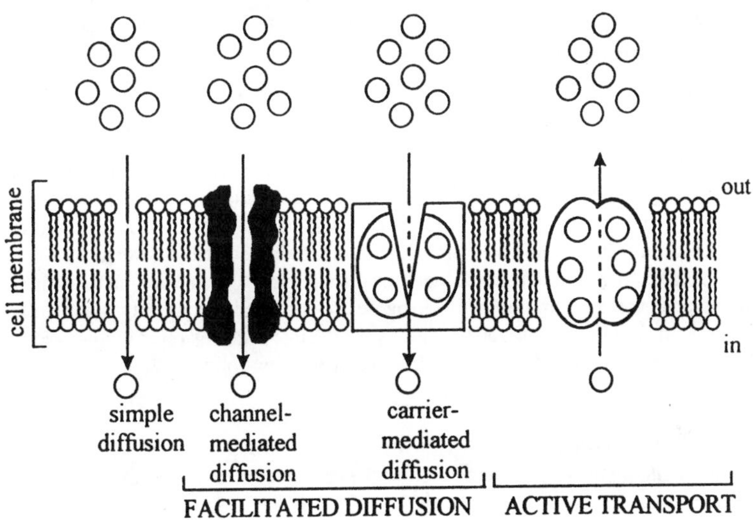

Mechanisms for the movement of substances across the cell membrane.

10. Can the lipid solubility of a single substance change under physiologic conditions?

The lipid solubility of many substances depends on their environment. For example, many molecules can exist in either a protonated (positively charged) form or in an unprotonated (uncharged) form, depending on the surrounding pH. A protonated molecule does not cross the membrane as readily as a neutral, unprotonated molecule.

11. Discuss how lipid solubility is used in drug therapy.

The principle governing lipid solubility is used to advantage in treatments to reduce blood levels of phenobarbital during barbiturate overdose. For example, at the normal blood pH of 7.4, phenobarbital molecules are half-protonated and half-unprotonated. Only the unprotonated form readily crosses membranes from the blood to the urine for removal from the body. Administration of sodium bicarbonate, however, increases the pH of the blood, and some of the protonated phenobarbital molecules lose their proton to the alkaline environment. The resulting increase in unprotonated, membrane-permeable phenobarbital molecules enhances the passing of this drug from the blood to the urine to lower systemic drug levels.

12. List the three main processes by which substances cross cell membranes.

1. Simple diffusion
2. Facilitated diffusion (also called carrier-mediated diffusion)
3. Active transport

13. Define diffusion.

The random motion by which a molecule crosses the cell membrane down its electrochemical gradient.

14. What is a diffusion coefficient?

A diffusion coefficient is a measure of the rate at which a solute can cross a membrane having an area of 1 cm and a thickness of 1 cm, when the concentration difference across the membrane is 1 mol/L. Uncharged, lipophilic substances (oxygen, carbon dioxide) and small polar molecules (water) have high diffusion coefficients because they can quickly cross the cell membrane. Many drugs, such as general anesthetic agents, also are lipophilic and have high diffusion coefficients. These drugs can readily diffuse across cell membranes to exert their effects. Large polar molecules (sugars, amino acids) and ions have low diffusion coefficients. Hence, these substances require transport proteins to cross the cell membrane.

15. Which four factors determine the total amount of uncharged solute that can diffuse across a cell membrane?

Simple diffusion of an uncharged solute is **directly** proportional to (1) the concentration gradient of the solute, (2) the solute's diffusion coefficient, and (3) the membrane area and is **inversely** proportional to (4) the membrane thickness. Changes in the level of these four factors can greatly impact simple diffusion. For example, pulmonary fibrosis reduces the lung membrane area available for gas exchange and hence reduces the diffusion of oxygen from the lung into the blood, which is required for oxygenation of body tissues. During pulmonary infections, inflammation and thickening of the lung membrane may also slow the rate of diffusion of oxygen from the lungs to the pulmonary capillaries. In both cases, these diffusional limitations may result in systemic hypoxia.

16. Define simple diffusion.

During **simple diffusion,** substances cross the cell membrane by simple movement through intermolecular spaces.

17. What are the properties of simple diffusion?

- Diffusion occurs down an electrochemical gradient.
- Diffusion is not rate-limiting but represents a linear function of the concentration gradient.
- The diffusion process is not saturable.
- No energy is required.

18. Define facilitated diffusion.

During **facilitated diffusion,** substances cross the membrane by contacting a transport protein. Large polar molecules are transported by **carrier proteins,** whereas charged ions are transported by **channel proteins**.

19. What are the properties of facilitated diffusion?

- Diffusion occurs down an electrochemical gradient.
- The substance binds to a transport carrier protein, which undergoes a reversible, conformational change to transport the substance across the membrane.*
- The diffusion process is rate-limiting and saturable because it depends on the availability of a finite number of carrier or channel proteins.*
- No energy is required.

* Property is different from simple diffusion.

20. What is osmosis?

Water is a small, polar molecule, which can easily diffuse across cell membranes through intermolecular spaces. This simple diffusion of water down its concentration gradient is called **osmosis**. Osmosis occurs from an area of low solute concentration (where the water concentration is high) to an area of high solute concentration (where the water concentration is low) and results in the displacement of volume. Hence, osmosis provides a mechanism whereby the cells can regulate their volume.

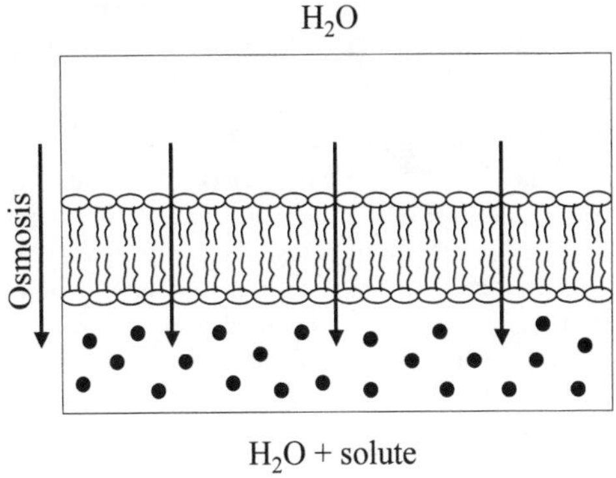

H_2O

Osmosis

H_2O + solute

Diffusion of water across a membrane down its concentration gradient

21. What is osmotic pressure?

The pressure exerted by particles in solution, which provides a concentration gradient for the diffusion of water.

22. How is osmotic pressure determined?

Osmotic pressure is proportional to the number of solute particles per unit volume of fluid and is not determined by the size of the solute particles because the kinetic energy of single solute particles is quite similar regardless of size.

23. How does glucose cross the plasma membrane of muscle cells?

Glucose is a large, polar molecule, which is more concentrated in the extracellular fluid than in the cell cytoplasm. Glucose is transported into the cell down its concentration gradient by facilitated diffusion. Thus, the diffusion of glucose is rate-limiting and saturable but does not require energy.

24. How does insulin enhance the diffusion of glucose across muscle cell membranes?

Insulin, a product of the pancreas, increases the rate of facilitated transport of glucose into muscle cells. Some evidence suggests that this occurs when insulin binds to its receptors on the cell membrane and speeds the translocation of glucose transport proteins from the cytoplasm to the cell membrane. The increased membrane density of glucose transport proteins permits greater glucose entry into the cells.

25. Why is there glucose in the urine in diabetes mellitus?

Glucose in the bloodstream is filtered by the kidney into the urine. Normal levels of glucose in the filtrate can be completely reabsorbed back into the bloodstream by facilitated diffusion in the renal tubules. Thus, no glucose is normally detected in the urine. In diabetes mellitus, blood glucose levels are high, and more glucose is filtered into the urine. The abnormally high levels of glucose in the filtrate saturate the transport proteins in the kidney that are responsible for tubular reabsorption, and a residual level of glucose is detected in urine samples as a hallmark sign of diabetes mellitus.

26. What is active transport?

The movement of substances across the cell membrane **against** an electrochemical gradient.

27. List the characteristics of active transport.

- Substances are moved against their electrochemical gradient.
- The exchange of substances requires a transport protein.
- The process is rate-limiting and saturable.
- The breakdown of adenosine triphosphate (ATP) is required to provide energy.

28. What are the two types of active transport?

- **Primary active transport** requires energy directly derived from the breakdown of ATP or some other high-energy phosphate compound.
- **Secondary active transport** derives energy secondarily from ionic concentration differences across the membrane, which were originally created by primary active transport.

29. Which ion pump is a model of primary active transport?

The Na^+, K^+ pump is often considered the prototype of active transport. The Na^+, K^+ pump is composed of two α-subunit proteins, which constitute the primary transport protein, and two ancillary β-subunit proteins. The cytoplasmic side of the α-subunit binds one ATP molecule and three intracellular Na^+ ions and exchanges them for two external K^+ ions. A single exchange cycle requires the breakdown of one molecule of ATP because energy is required to pump both Na^+ and K^+ against their chemical gradients. The Na^+, K^+ pump is called an **electrogenic** exchange mechanism because the exchange of three internal Na^+ ions for two external K^+ ions generates a net intracellular charge of -1.

30. What are two forms of *secondary* active transport?

- **Cotransport** occurs when two substances are transported unidirectionally across the cell membrane by the same energy-driven transport protein.
- **Countertransport** refers to the coupled exchange by a transport protein of two substances in opposite directions across the cell membrane.

31. Why is cotransport important in the absorption of sugars and amino acids in the gastrointestinal tract?

This secondary active transport mechanism takes advantage of the Na^+ gradient established by the ATP-driven Na^+, K^+ pump, which maintains a high Na^+ concentration (140 mEq/L) in the extracellular fluid and a low Na^+ concentration (14 mEq/L) intracellularly. Because Na^+ concentration is higher outside the cell, the membrane transport protein involved in the cotransport process has a high possibility of binding extracellular Na^+ to its outer face. The subsequent cobinding of either a sugar or an amino acid to the outer face of the same transport protein initiates a conformational change, which provides the outer protein surface accessibility to the inside of the membrane. Hence Na^+ is cotransported with a sugar or amino acid molecule into the epithelial cells. This form of secondary active transport is important for the absorption of sugars and amino acids during digestion.

32. Discuss two examples of countertransport in mammalian cells.

1. The **sodium-hydrogen exchanger** takes advantage of the electrochemical gradient for Na^+ that is established by the ATP-driven Na^+, K^+ pump to transport H^+ out of the cell by secondary active transport. In this process, the binding of extracellular Na^+ and intracellular H^+ to the opposite faces of the transport protein results in a conformational change in protein structure whereby the sidedness of the protein is reversed in the membrane. The subsequent transport of Na^+ into the cell and extrusion of H^+ act as a buffering mechanism to prevent intracellular acidification.

2. The **sodium-calcium exchanger** also takes advantage of the electrochemical gradient for Na^+ established by the ATP-driven Na^+, K^+ pump. This exchanger transports Ca^{2+} out of the cell by secondary active transport. Although the Na^+, Ca^{2+} exchanger, similar to other transport proteins, can transport substrates in either direction across the cell membrane, Na^+ ions are present in tenfold higher concentration at the outside surface of the cell membrane. Hence extracellular Na^+ ions usually bind to the external face of the transport protein. The cobinding of Ca^{2+} to the cytosolic face of the same transport protein results in a conformational change in protein sidedness within the membrane, resulting in the exchange of extracellular Na^+ for intracellular Ca^{2+} (see figure). The stoi-

chiometry of the Na^+, Ca^{2+} exchanger is unclear in some tissues but may involve the exchange of extracellular Na^+ for intracellular Ca^{2+} on a 2-for-1 basis (electrically neutral) or a 3-to-1 basis (electrogenic). Regardless, the subsequent decrease in the intracellular concentration of Ca^{2+} will inhibit Ca^{2+}-dependent excitation processes, such as neurotransmitter release and muscle contraction.

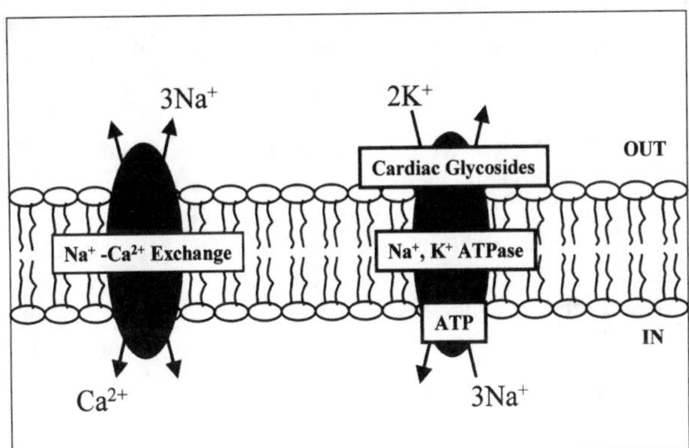

Coexpression of the Na^+, K^+ pump and the Na^+ and Ca^{2+} counter-transporter in the cardiac cell membrane.

33. How do digitalis glycoside drugs take advantage of secondary active transport to increase the force of contraction of the heart?

Digitalis glycosides are therapeutic agents used to increase the force of contraction of the failing heart. These drugs bind to the external face of the α-subunit of the Na^+, K^+ pump to inhibit its activity. As a consequence of blocking active Na^+ extrusion from the cell, the intracellular concentration of Na^+ rises. This build-up of Na^+ at the inside surface of the cell membrane indirectly affects Ca^{2+} transport because it reduces the electrochemical gradient for Na^+ and thereby also reduces the activity of the Na^+, Ca^{2+} countertransporter. The subsequent buildup of Ca^{2+} in the cell cytoplasm provides an increased supply of intracellular Ca^{2+} to activate the contractile proteins in cardiac muscle cells, thereby enhancing the force of contraction of the heart.

THE ELECTRICAL PROPERTIES OF CELLS

34. What is an ion channel?

Ion channels are specialized proteins in the membrane that provide a passageway through which charged ions can cross the cell membrane down their electrochemical gradient. The resulting ionic current, generated by the movement of charged ions through membrane channels, is sometimes regarded as a form of facilitated diffusion because it involves a transport protein (see figure in question 9).

35. What is the general structure of ion channels?

Most ion channels are multiunit protein structures, similar to the carrier proteins in the membrane. The channel pore is composed of amino acid sequences called **α-subunits,** which are arranged around a central shaft that spans the membrane. Other regulatory subunits (β, δ, γ) influence the gating behavior of the pore-forming α-subunits and may regulate their level of expression in the membrane. The pores of most ion channels have a **selectivity filter,** which makes the channel selectively conduct only one type of ion. Hence, sodium channels preferentially conduct Na^+ ions over other ion species, whereas potassium channels primarily conduct K^+ ions and reject other ion species.

36. How does an ion channel differ from a pore?

Membrane pores are openings in the membrane between lipid molecules that permit simple diffusion. **Ion channels** are gated pathways that can exist in open or closed states to regulate the rate of ion flux across the membrane. Ions can traverse channels only when in the open state.

37. What are the three main conformational states of an ion channel?

- The **resting state** of an ion channel refers to a channel that is closed but is available for opening if challenged by a chemical or voltage stimulus.
- The **activated state** of an ion channel refers to a channel that is open and permits the passage of ionic current.
- The **inactivated state** of an ion channel refers to a channel that is closed and is not available for activation. Generally the inactivated state occurs immediately after the successful activation (opening) of the channel by a chemical or voltage stimulus.

38. How is the behavior of single ion channels studied?

The patch-clamp method is commonly used to measure current through single ion channels. The open tip of a glass pipette is placed on the membrane surface of a cell, and a high-resistance seal is made between the pipette wall and the cell membrane. Ionic currents resulting from the opening of single ion channels in the membrane patch formed within the pipette tip are detected and recorded by a high-resolution amplifier (see figure). Using this method, the functional characteristics of ion channels in different types of cells can be studied, and the action of therapeutic drugs on ion channel behavior can be explored.

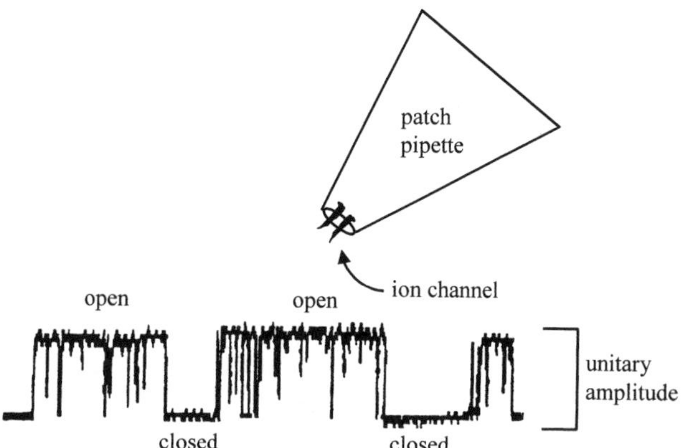

The patch-clamp technique for measuring current through single ion channels.

39. Which factors determine the total amount of ionic current that can be generated across a cell membrane?

The total amount of ionic current (**I**) that crosses a membrane is described by the equation:

$$\mathbf{I = n \times i \times p}$$

where **n** = the number of channels in the membrane, **i** = the amplitude of unitary current through a single channel, and **p** = the probability that a single channel is in the open state.

40. Discuss some types of ion channels and how they participate in cell function.

Ligand-gated ion channels, also called **chemical-gated ion channels,** are channels that are closely associated with a membrane receptor. Binding of a chemical messenger to the receptor causes a conformational change in the channel, which causes it to shift from the resting state to the open state. Ligand-gated channels often are **nonselective** ion channels, which conduct more than one type of similarly charged ion species in the open state. For example, the binding of acetylcholine to its postjunctional receptor on the skeletal muscle membrane activates a ligand-gated ion channel, which permits the passage of Na^+ into and K^+ out of the muscle cell at physiologic levels of membrane potential.

Voltage-gated ion channels are opened by changes in cell membrane potential. Changes in the electrical field surrounding the channel protein trigger the movement of positively charged amino acids in the α-subunits, which form the ion-conducting shaft of the channel. As a result of this conformational change, the channel is converted to its open state. Most ion-selective channels inherently involved in cell excitability, such as Na^+, K^+, and Ca^{2+} channels, represent voltage-gated ion channels.

41. What is resting membrane potential?

The difference in electrical potential (voltage) between the inside and outside membrane surfaces under resting (unstimulated) conditions. At rest, cells have an excess of negative charges at the inside surface of the membrane and show a negative membrane potential.

42. Why does the resting membrane potential show a negative charge?

1. The resting cell membrane is preferentially permeable to K^+ ions. For example, most mammalian cell membranes are 20–100 times more permeable to K^+ than to Na^+, Ca^{2+}, or other ion species. Because the K^+ concentration inside the cell is much higher than the outside concentration, K^+ moves out of the cell through K^+ channels and leaves an excess of negative charges at the cytoplasmic side of the cell membrane.

2. The electrogenic Na^+, K^+ pump is active at resting membrane potentials and acts as a second force to generate negativity at the inner membrane surface. Hence, the resting membrane potential is the sum of the negative electrical potentials generated by both K^+ efflux and the Na^+, K^+ pump.

43. What are the relative contributions of K^+ efflux and the Na^+, K^+ pump to resting membrane potential?

In mammalian cells, K^+ efflux primarily generates the electrical potential generated across the cell membrane. Resting membrane potential varies between –50 mV and –90 mV in different types of mammalian cells, and the contribution of the Na^+, K^+ pump to this potential is estimated at about 5–20% of the total voltage.

44. What is an equilibrium potential?

The equilibrium potential for an ion is the membrane potential that would exist if the cell membrane suddenly became selectively and completely permeable only to that ion species. Under these conditions, the distribution of the ion across the membrane would be at equilibrium (equal rates of influx and efflux).

45. How is equilibrium potential predicted?

$$\textbf{Nernst equation: } \mathbf{V} = \frac{\mathbf{RT}}{\mathbf{FZ}} \ \mathbf{ln} \ \frac{\mathbf{C_o}}{\mathbf{C_i}}$$

where **V** = the equilibrium potential in volts, **R** = the gas constant (2 cal/mol/°K), **T** = the absolute temperature (°K), **F** = Faraday's constant (9.65×10^4 coulombs/mole), **Z** = the valence of the ion, **ln** = logarithm to the base e, $\mathbf{C_o}$ and $\mathbf{C_i}$ = the outside and inside concentrations of a positively charged ion. The numerator and denominator of the $\mathbf{C_o/C_i}$ ratio are reversed to calculate the equilibrium potential for an ion that is negatively charged.

46. What are the predicted values for the K^+ and Na^+ equilibrium potentials for a mammalian cell using the Nernst equation?

By replacing the constants with their numerical values and converting from the natural log to the base 10 log, the following equation predicts the equilibrium potential (in millivolts) for K^+:

$$E_K = -60 \log \frac{[K_i]}{[K_o]} = -60 \log \frac{[140]}{[4]} \approx -90 \text{ mV}$$

By using the same approach, the following equation predicts the equilibrium potential (in millivolts) for Na^+:

$$E_{Na} = -60 \log \frac{[Na_i]}{[Na_o]} = -60 \log \frac{[14]}{[140]} \approx +60 \text{ mV}$$

47. What do the equilibrium potentials for K^+ and Na^+ reveal about the ionic basis of the resting membrane potential in nerve cells?

The resting membrane potential in nerve cells ranges between −80 mV and −90 mV, near the K^+ equilibrium potential. Because the membrane potential of these cells approaches the K^+ equilibrium potential, their plasma membrane must be highly and selectively permeable to K^+ rather than to Na^+ under resting conditions.

48. What is the Goldmann constant-field equation?

The final level of membrane potential depends on the concentrations of K^+, Na^+, Cl^-, and other ions across the membrane and on the relative permeability of the membrane to each of these ions. The Goldmann constant-field equation can be used to predict the contribution of different ion permeabilities to resting membrane potential:

$$V = \frac{RT}{F} \ln \frac{P_{K+} [K_o^+] + P_{Na+} [Na_o^+] + P_{Cl-} [Cl_i^-] + P_x [X]}{P_{K+} [K_i^+] + P_{Na+} [Na_i^+] + P_{Cl-} [Cl_o^-] + P_x [X]}$$

where **V** = membrane potential, **R** = gas constant, **T** = absolute temperature, **F** = Faraday constant, $\mathbf{P_x}$ = permeability of the membrane to x, and **[x]** = concentration of ion x on the inside or the outside of the cell membrane.

49. Which definitions are commonly used to describe changes in membrane potential?

- **Firing threshold:** the level of membrane potential at which sufficient depolarization has occurred to initiate an action potential
- **Depolarization:** the cell membrane potential becomes less polarized (e.g., moves toward 0 mV from a more negative potential level)
- **Repolarization:** the cell membrane potential becomes polarized again (e.g., moves away from 0 mV to a more negative membrane potential)
- **Hyperpolarization:** the cell membrane potential becomes more polarized (negative) than the original resting membrane potential level

50. What is the ionic basis for the action potential in nerve cells?

An **action potential** is the series of membrane potential changes that follow a suprathreshold stimulus and results in cell excitation. The following series of events characterizes the action potential in neurons.

- An excitatory stimulus induces the nerve cell to reach the firing threshold for the initiation of an action potential.
- The initial change in membrane potential causes a conformational change in the Na^+ channel protein, which converts it from its resting to its activated state. As the Na^+ channels open, Na^+ begins to rush into the cell down its electrochemical gradient. This influx of positively charged Na^+ on the inside surface of the cell membrane depolarizes the cell further, and more Na^+ channels open. This chain of events has a snowball effect, and the action potential is now **all or none** and runs its full course regardless of other cell changes. Membrane permeability to Na^+ may increase several thousand-fold during the early stages of the action potential, owing to the almost simultaneous activation of a dense population of Na^+ channels in the plasma membrane of the nerve cell.
- As the cell depolarizes further, voltage-dependent K^+ channels open more and K^+ begins to flow through the cell membrane from inside to outside down its electrochemical gradient. Concurrently the Na^+ channels are inactivated by the sustained depolarization. The slowing of Na^+ influx and the exit of the positively charged K^+ ions begin to repolarize the cell and return it to its original level of resting membrane potential. In many cells, this repolarization process temporarily exceeds the original level of resting membrane potential, resulting in cell hyperpolarization. Increases in membrane K^+ permeability may exceed thirtyfold during the latter stages of the action potential and for a short period thereafter.

- After the cell returns to its original level of resting membrane potential, the Na^+ and K^+ channels return to their resting state.

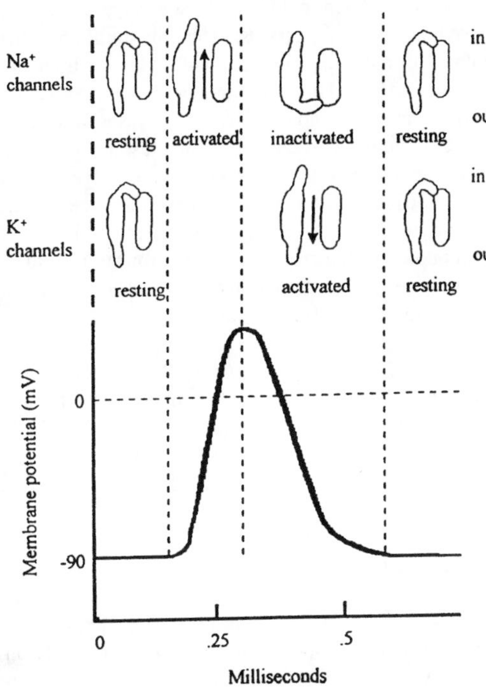

The conformational changes in voltage-gated Na^+ and K^+ channels, which underlie the action potential in nerve cells.

51. Why do voltage-gated Na^+ channels activate before voltage-gated K^+ channels in response to a depolarizing stimulus?

Na^+ channels are more **voltage-sensitive** than K^+ channels (i.e., they are activated at more negative membrane potentials). Just a small depolarization from a resting membrane potential level of −70 or −90 mV is adequate to activate Na^+ channels, which open rapidly to permit Na^+ influx into the cell and induce cell depolarization. Larger changes in membrane potential consistent with further cell excitation are required to activate the less voltage-sensitive K^+ channels, so increases in membrane K^+ permeability are observed later.

52. Why do action potentials of nerve, cardiac, and smooth muscle cells differ?

Different types of ion channels and their relative densities in the membrane vary greatly among nerve, cardiac, and smooth muscle cells. The ion channel profile of each cell membrane probably has evolved over millions of years to reflect the functional requirements of the cell. The complexity of ion channel expression is tremendous because multiple types of α-subunits and regulatory subunits can interact to form many subtypes of a channel. Furthermore, the alternative splicing of mRNA sometimes leads to many isoforms of the same channel. Regardless, it is important to understand the basic interrelationship between ion channel expression, action potential configuration, and cell function for different types of tissues.

Nerve cells must fire rapidly and repetitively to transmit electrical impulses throughout the nervous system. Their action potential reflects this functional requirement, showing rapid changes in potential and a short duration (see figure, *A*). The rapidly activating Na^+ channels provide the upstroke of the action potential. Their almost immediate inactivation coupled to the activation of K^+ channels accounts for the rapid course of repolarization. Voltage-gated, neuronal-type (**N-type**) Ca^{2+} channels also are activated during the action potential, and the resulting Ca^{2+} influx provides the signal for neurotransmitter release. The N-type Ca^{2+} channels show rapid inactivation, which permits the duration of the action potential in neurons to remain short.

Cardiac muscle cells of the ventricular myocardium also show a resting membrane potential between −80 mV and −90 mV. The duration of their action potential is several hundred-fold longer than the length of the action potential in neurons (see figure, *B*). The long duration of the cardiac action potential reflects the functional task of these muscle cells, which is to contract and relax the cardiac ventricles at a relatively slow rate of 60–90 times per minute. Notably, voltage-gated Na^+ and K^+ channels contribute to the depolarization and repolarization phases of the cardiac action potential, similar to their role in excitation of neuronal cells. The plasma membrane of cardiac cells expresses a different type of voltage-gated Ca^{2+} channel than the N-type found in neuronal cells. Depolarization of cardiac cells triggers the activation of voltage-dependent, long-lasting (**L-type**) Ca^{2+} channels, which inactivate slowly and provide a sustained influx of Ca^{2+} into the muscle cell. This Ca^{2+} influx, coupled to the release of Ca^{2+} from intracellular stores, provides the activator Ca^{2+} required for the vigorous contraction of the cardiac ventricles. The sustained influx of Ca^{2+} also acts to maintain depolarization and accounts for the long **plateau phase** of the action potential. Notably, the pacemaker cells in the sinoatrial and atrioventricular node have a different action potential configuration. Resting membrane potential is less negative in these cells, and they show spontaneous depolarization. Also, importantly, the upstroke of the action potential is mediated by Ca^{2+} influx primarily through L-type Ca^{2+} channels rather than by Na^+ influx as occurs in neuronal and cardiac ventricular cells (see figure, *C*).

Smooth muscle cells populate a heterogeneous group of tissues, including blood vessels, bladder, uterus, and gastrointestinal tract. Their electrical properties vary greatly among different tissues. What generally distinguishes the electrical properties of these cells from neuronal or cardiac ventricular cells is (1) the absence of voltage-gated Na^+ channels in their plasma membranes and (2) the setting of their resting potential at less negative potentials between −45 and −60 mV. In this range of potentials, voltage-gated Na^+ channels (if present) are largely inactivated and hence not available to participate in cell excitation. Thus, smooth muscle cells rely primarily on voltage-gated, L-type Ca^{2+} channels for electrical excitation. The influx of Ca^{2+} through voltage-gated Ca^{2+} channels is responsible for the upstroke of action potentials in smooth muscle cells and

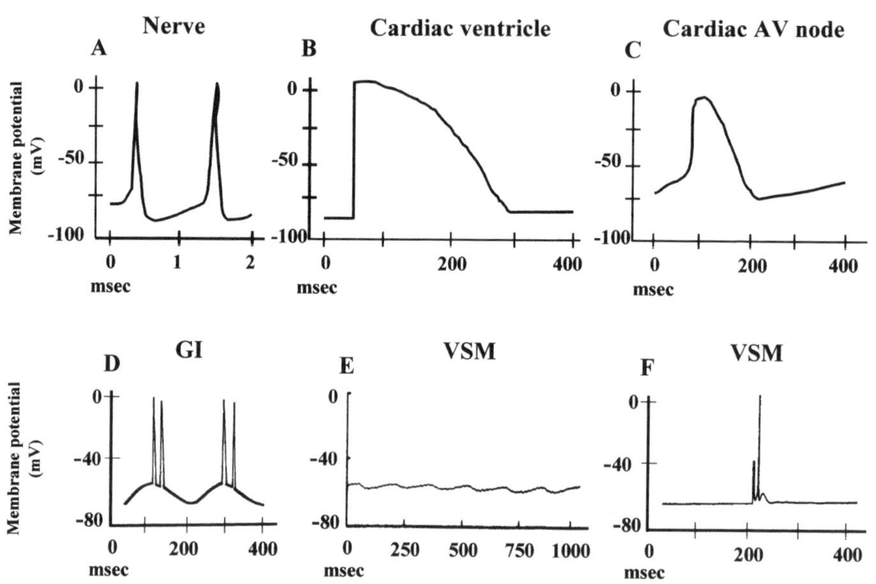

Cells from different types of tissue show different action potential configurations.

provides Ca^{2+} for muscle contraction. These action potentials may be sustained or show a spiking configuration as may occur in gastrointestinal (GI) smooth muscle cells (see figure, *D*). In addition, many smooth muscle cells do not show action potentials but rely on graded changes in membrane potential to provide activator Ca^{2+} (see figure, *E*). The excitability patterns of different kinds of smooth muscle cells reflect their functional role in the body. Some gastrointestinal smooth muscle cells that participate in rhythmic contraction designed to support peristalsis show rhythmic Ca^{2+}-dependent action potentials. Vascular smooth muscle cells, which require a continual influx of Ca^{2+} to maintain arterial tone and prevent rapid changes in blood pressure, generally show a relatively constant level of resting membrane potential coupled to voltage-gated Ca^{2+} influx. However, even under these circumstances, a sudden excitatory stimulus may trigger a Ca^{2+}-dependent action potential (see figure, *F*).

53. What is a refractory period?

The period of time after an action potential during which another action potential **cannot** be initiated is called the **refractory period**. The continued inactivation of the voltage-gated Na^+ channels after the firing of an action potential makes them unavailable for opening and provides the physiologic basis for the refractory period.

54. How does a refractory period protect the cell from overexcitation?

A refractory period is required to allow a recovery period between action potentials in the same cell and thereby protect the cell from extremely rapid, repetitive stimulation, which would compromise its function. For example, in neuronal cells, the refractory period protects the cell from the hyperrepetitive firing of action potentials, which could trigger chaos within the nervous system and result in pathologies such as seizures. In the cardiac ventricular cell, the refractory period also prevents rapid, repetitive action potentials, which could trigger a rapid heart rate (tachycardia) or disorganized cell-to-cell conduction patterns resulting in cardiac arrhythmias and death.

55. What are the two types of refractory periods?

1. The **absolute refractory period** begins when the Na^+ channels are inactivated during the action potential and lasts until the Na^+ channels begin to return to their resting state after restoration of the resting membrane potential. During this period, a second action potential cannot be initiated regardless of the strength of the stimulus.
2. The **relative refractory period** refers to the time period immediately after an action potential, when a second action potential can be triggered if a suprathreshold stimulus is applied. During this period, some of the Na^+ channels have returned to their resting state and are available for activation. The relative refractory period always follows the absolute refractory period in the course of an action potential.

NERVES AND NEUROTRANSMISSION

56. What are the three main anatomic regions of a motor neuron?

1. The **soma** is the main cell body of the neuron, which acts as a processing center for the nerve fiber.
2. The **dendrites** are antenna-like processes that project out from the soma and increase the cell surface area for the reception of signals from other neurons, which they subsequently transmit to the cell body. The plasma membrane of the dendrites is densely populated with ligand-gated receptors to provide high-affinity binding sites for chemical transmitters released by surrounding neurons.
3. The **axon** is a larger projection that transmits action potentials away from the soma. The axon originates at the axon hillock (a bulge in the soma) and ends in a nerve terminal. This terminal contains vesicles filled with chemical neurotransmitters, which can be released when an action potential is propagated down the axon. Hence the axon ultimately provides an electrochemical connection to other neurons.

57. How is an action potential propagated along a nerve axon?

An action potential initiated at one site in the nerve plasma membrane is propagated throughout the rest of the nerve fiber by a self-perpetuating process (see figure). This process involves the local flow of current (positive charge) from depolarized sites on the inside surface of the cell membrane to adjacent, normally polarized membrane sites available for activation. Hence the original action potential does not propagate along the nerve fiber but rather results in the sequential generation of identical action potentials, which propagate unidirectionally away from the site of the original action potential. The refractory period that follows the action potential along the axon prevents the backward flow of current toward the initial excitation site and acts to restrict the frequency of action potential transmission.

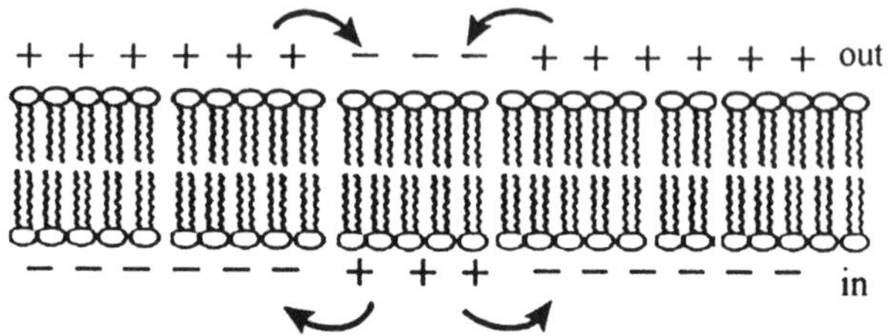

Propagation of an action potential along a membrane by the local flow of current.

58. What is saltatory conduction?

The axons of some nerves are populated by cells called **oligodendrocytes** (in the brain and spinal cord) or **Schwann's cells** (in peripheral nerves). The plasma membrane of oligodendrocytes and Schwann's cells contains a high density of a lipid called **myelin,** and the thick layering of the plasma membranes of these cells at periodic sites along the nerve axon forms myelin blocks, which insulate the underlying nerve cell membrane from excitatory stimuli. Between the myelin blocks are the **nodes of Ranvier,** which are myelin-free sites where the cell membrane remains exposed to the extracellular fluid and is densely populated with voltage-gated Na^+ channels to promote action potential generation. **Saltatory conduction** refers to the unidirectional jumping of depolarization from one node of Ranvier to the neighboring node, which provides a rapid propagation of nerve impulses for long distances.

59. Which two factors are the main determinants of the velocity of action potential propagation?

1. **Myelination** increases the speed of action potential propagation along the axon. The nodes of Ranvier provide a sequence of highly efficient sites to transmit the nerve impulse as it jumps between nodes. Myelination can enhance the velocity of action potential propagation by as much as fiftyfold. The requirement of myelin for normal motor function is revealed by the motor deficits observed in patients with **multiple sclerosis,** a demyelinating disease of the central nervous system of possible autoimmune origin.

2. The **diameter** of nerve fibers also positively influences the velocity of action potential propagation. Large myelinated nerve fibers, such as those innervating skeletal muscle, show the highest conduction velocity. Small, unmyelinated nerve fibers, such as the sympathetic postganglionic fibers, show a low speed of impulse propagation.

60. How are chemical messages transmitted between nerve cells?

Nerve synapses represent the communicating structure between the axon terminal of one nerve (the **presynaptic neuron**) and the dendrites or cell body of a second, target nerve (the **postsynaptic neuron**). The space between the two adjacent nerves that must be spanned to permit the continuation of the nerve signal is called the **synaptic cleft**. When a nerve impulse is propagated to the axon terminal of the transmitting nerve, the influx of Ca^{2+} through voltage-gated Ca^{2+} channels in the plasma membrane of the presynaptic nerve terminal triggers the release of chemical neurotransmitters from vesicles stored in the axon terminal. These neurotransmitters diffuse across the synaptic cleft and bind to specific high-affinity receptors on the plasma membrane of the postsynaptic neuron. If the chemical signal is adequate, the activation of these ligand-operated receptors initiates intracellular signals that alter the electrical and functional properties of the postsynaptic neuron.

61. Which four factors determine the concentration of neurotransmitter in the synaptic cleft?

- The amount of neurotransmitter released by the presynaptic nerve terminal
- The passive diffusion of the transmitter down its concentration gradient from the synaptic cleft to adjacent areas of extracellular fluid
- The active uptake of neurotransmitter by transport proteins in the plasma membrane of the surrounding neurons
- The breakdown of neurotransmitter molecules by enzymes located in the presynaptic cleft or in the plasma membranes of the presynaptic or postsynaptic neurons

62. How do the chemical neurotransmitters from different presynaptic neurons interact to regulate the level of excitability of the postsynaptic neuron?

Presynaptic neurons can release neurotransmitters that either promote or inhibit excitation of the postsynaptic neuron (see figure). Neurotransmitters released from excitatory presynaptic neurons produce a small, local, nonpropagated depolarization of the postsynaptic neuron, which is called an **excitatory postsynaptic potential** (EPSP). Because the amplitude of this depolarization is rarely sufficient to bring the membrane potential to the threshold required for the initiation of an action potential, the additive effect of multiple EPSPs is generally required to initiate an action potential at the postsynaptic membrane. Conversely, neurotransmitters released from inhibitory presynaptic neurons induce a small, local, nonpropagated hyperpolarization when they bind to their receptors on the plasma membrane of the postsynaptic neuron. This local hyperpolarization is called an **inhibitory postsynaptic potential** (IPSP). The algebraic summation of these graded changes in potential determines whether the membrane potential of the postsynaptic nerve cell depolarizes sufficiently to reach its firing threshold and initiate an action potential.

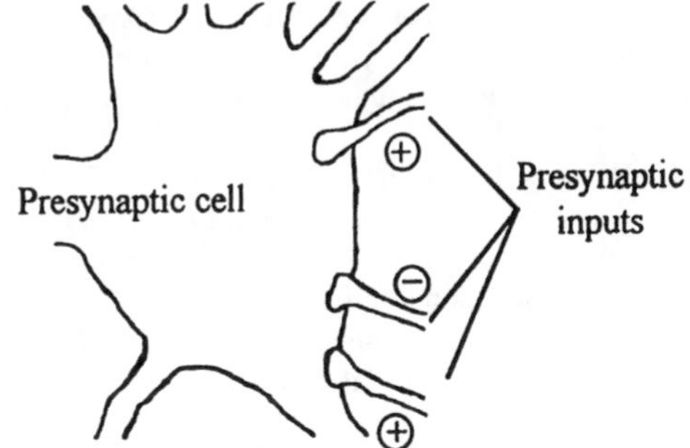

Excitatory and inhibitory presynaptic neurons influence the excitability of the postsynaptic neuron.

63. What is the difference between temporal and spatial summation?

Temporal summation refers to the additive effect of sequential multiple EPSPs or IPSPs **originating from a single presynaptic neuron** on the membrane potential of the postsynaptic neuron. For example, the repetitive firing of a single excitatory presynaptic neuron may result in summated EPSPs, which may depolarize the membrane potential to its firing threshold for action potential generation. Because an EPSP results in only a small increment of membrane depolarization that is not sufficient to inactivate voltage-gated Na^+ channels, a refractory period does not occur. This permits multiple EPSPs to exert a summating, depolarizing effect on the membrane potential of the postsynaptic neuron.

Spatial summation refers to the additive effect of multiple EPSPs or IPSPs simultaneously **originating from different presynaptic neurons** on the membrane potential of the postsynaptic neuron (i.e., the neurotransmitter signals have different geographic origins). Under physiologic conditions, spatial and temporal summation act concurrently to regulate the membrane potential of the postsynaptic neuron.

NEUROMUSCULAR TRANSMISSION

64. How do nerves regulate muscle function?

- In **skeletal muscle,** motor nerves initiate muscle contraction.
- In **cardiac muscle,** sympathetic and parasympathetic nerves modulate the performance of the muscle, even though cardiac muscle contraction is spontaneous and independent of nerve activity.
- In **smooth muscle,** nerves may either initiate contractile activity or modulate the amount of contractile force in the muscle. For example, norepinephrine from adrenergic nerve terminals can increase the level of active tone in a blood vessel above the resting levels of tone that exist as a result of intrinsic excitability of the muscle cells.

65. What is a motor unit?

A motor unit consists of the alpha motor neuron and all the skeletal muscle fibers that it innervates.

66. What is the innervation ratio?

The number of muscle fibers innervated by each alpha motor neuron. If few fibers are innervated by the neuron (low innervation ratio), fine motor control is possible, but the overall strength of contraction is less. If the innervation ratio is high, more powerful contractions are possible, but the movements are less precise. Contraction of motor units with low and high innervation ratios is integrated in the central nervous system.

67. What is the "all or none law" for skeletal muscle?

The all or none law states that when any skeletal muscle fiber is stimulated to threshold, it will contract to the maximum of its ability. If a threshold stimulus is not delivered to the muscle, the muscle will not contract. That is, the force of contraction in an individual skeletal muscle fiber is not graded in intensity. In contrast, contractile force of cardiac muscle fibers can be graded in intensity, depending on the inotropic state (contractility) of the heart.

68. What is the motor end plate?

A specialized region of the muscle fiber membrane with receptors at the top of junctional folds that lie opposite of the terminal region of the presynaptic motor neuron. The skeletal neuromuscular junction (see figure, top of next page) is an excitatory synapse that serves to transfer action potentials from spinal motor neurons to the skeletal muscle fibers. Transmission of the impulse across the synapse is mediated by the chemical transmitter acetylcholine.

69. Describe the process of synaptic transmission at the skeletal muscle neuromuscular junction.

Action potentials in the presynaptic motor neurons release acetylcholine, which is packaged in synaptic vesicles that fuse to the presynaptic membrane and release their contents via exocytosis. The exocytosis of the synaptic vesicles requires Ca^{2+} ions that enter the cell through voltage-gated Ca^{2+} channels that are opened in response to the depolarization of the presynaptic membrane during the action potential. Acetylcholine diffuses across the neuromuscular junction and binds to nicotinic receptors on the plasma membrane of the muscle cell. The binding of the transmitter to the receptor leads to an increase in the permeability of the postsynaptic membrane to both Na^+ and K^+ ions, producing a depolarization that triggers a propagated action potential in the skeletal muscle fiber and a subsequent contraction of the muscle cell.

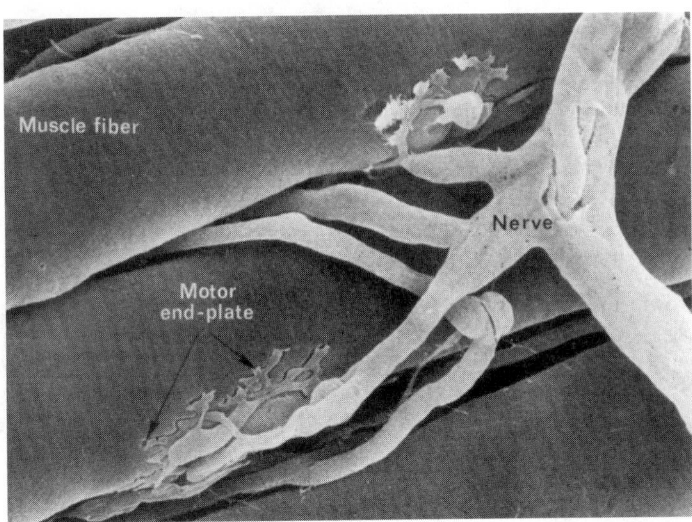

Scanning electron micrograph of skeletal muscle neuromuscular junction. (From Fawcett DW: Bloom and Fawcett's Textbook of Physiology, 12th ed. New York, Chapman & Hall, 1994, with permission.)

70. What is unusual about the nicotinic acetylcholine receptor on the skeletal muscle cell?

The nicotinic acetylcholine receptor in skeletal muscle is an integral part of the ion channel in the postsynaptic membrane that is responsible for the end plate potential. Binding of acetylcholine molecules to the receptor-channel complex leads to opening of the channel, resulting in the motor end plate potential.

71. What is a motor end plate potential and what causes it?

The local depolarization of the end plate region of skeletal muscle fibers that occurs in response to acetylcholine binding to the nicotinic cholinergic receptors located on it. The motor end plate potential is caused by increases in the permeability of the postsynaptic membrane to Na^+ and K^+ ions, causing the postsynaptic membrane to depolarize past the threshold value for an action potential in the skeletal muscle.

72. What is the safety factor for transmitter release at the skeletal muscle neuromuscular junction?

The **safety factor** refers to the fact that acetylcholine is released in quantities many times greater than those required to produce an action potential at the postsynaptic membrane. This ensures that each action potential in the motor nerve triggers a response in the muscle fibers that it innervates. The large safety factor for transmission at the skeletal muscle neuromuscular junction is in contrast to many excitatory interneurons in the central nervous system, where neurotransmitters cause a subthreshold depolarization that needs to be summated (added together) to produce an action potential in the postsynaptic neuron.

73. What is quantal release of neurotransmitter?

The release of neurotransmitter molecules in discrete packages or quanta. An individual quantum corresponds to a synaptic vesicle in the presynaptic neuron.

74. What is a miniature end plate potential?

A small, nonpropagated change in membrane potential that occurs spontaneously on the motor end plates of the skeletal muscle neuromuscular junction. Miniature end plate potentials

(MEPPs) are due to the spontaneous release of individual quanta of the neurotransmitter acetylcholine and the subsequent binding of acetylcholine to receptors on the postsynaptic membrane.

75. How is the action of acetylcholine terminated at the synapse?

The acetylcholine released into the synaptic cleft is rapidly hydrolyzed to acetate and choline by the enzyme **acetylcholinesterase**. This terminates the action of the transmitter on the postsynaptic receptors. Anticholinesterases, such as those found in classic nerve gases, lead to a prolonged action of acetylcholine and subsequently a prolonged contraction of the skeletal muscle cell owing to failure to eliminate the transmitter.

76. What is myasthenia gravis, and how is it related to neuromuscular transmission?

Myasthenia gravis is a neuromuscular disorder that leads to muscle weakness. It is caused by an autoimmune response to the person's own acetylcholine receptors, leading to a reduction in the number of functional receptors in the postsynaptic membrane.

77. How does curare work?

The South American arrow poison curare contains *d*-tubocurarine, a compound that binds to nicotinic receptors at the skeletal muscle neuromuscular junction, inhibiting the binding of the neurotransmitter acetylcholine to the same postsynaptic receptor. Paralysis of the skeletal muscle results from the inhibition of neurotransmission at the junction.

MUSCLE STRUCTURE, CONTRACTILE PROTEINS, AND CROSS-BRIDGE CYCLING

78. Why are skeletal muscle and cardiac muscle called striated muscle? Why is smooth muscle not classified as striated muscle?

Skeletal muscle and cardiac muscle are called striated muscle because of the striations (stripes) in the cells; these striations are absent in smooth muscle cells. The striations in skeletal and cardiac muscle are formed by the orderly arrangement of the thick and thin contractile filaments, which produce alternating areas of light and dark bands, giving the muscle its striated appearance. In contrast, smooth muscle cells do not have a sarcomeric structure, and there is no orderly overlap of thick and thin filaments to cause striations in the muscle cell (see figures).

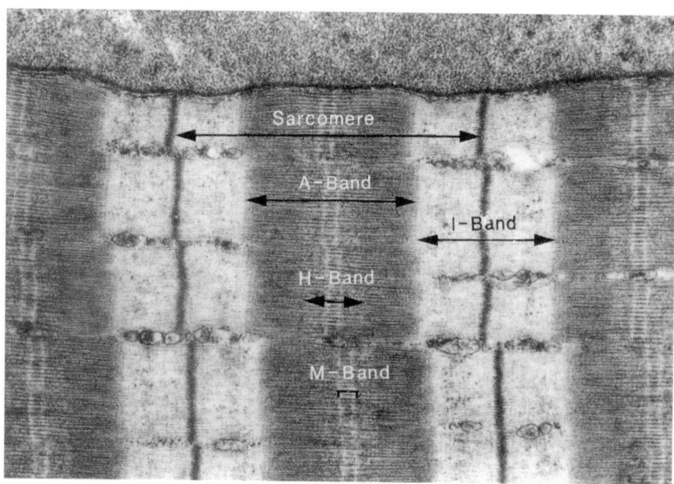

Electron micrograph of an individual sarcomere of skeletal muscle showing the characteristic banding patterns of striated muscle. (From Fawcett DW: Bloom and Fawcett's Textbook of Histology, 12th ed. New York, Chapman & Hall, 1994, with permission.)

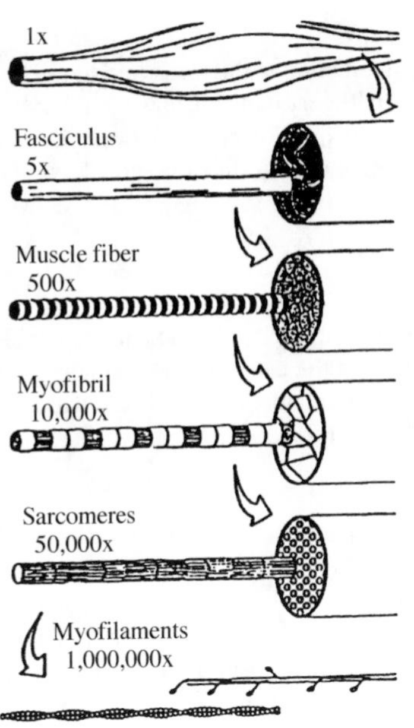

Hierarchical arrangement of structural components of skeletal muscle from the whole muscle through the contractile filament level. (From Rhoades RA, Tanner GA: Medical Physiology. Boston, Little, Brown, 1995, with permission.)

79. What is the hierarchical arrangement of the structural components of skeletal muscle?

The individual skeletal muscle cells are known as **muscle fibers**. Skeletal muscle fibers (and cardiac muscle cells) contain bundles of myofibrils that are composed of many individual **sarcomeres** arranged in series. The sarcomere is the fundamental contractile unit of striated muscle and consists of overlapping thick and thin filaments that produce a characteristic pattern of light and dark bands (see electron micrograph in question 78). The individual fibers are surrounded by a connective tissue layer known as the **endomysium,** which connects the individual fibers to parallel muscle cells. Groups of skeletal muscle fibers make up a **fasciculus,** which is surrounded by a connective tissue layer called the **perimysium**. Bundles of fasciculi make up the muscle itself. The fasciculi, with their associated blood vessels and nerves, are held together by another connective tissue layer, the **epimysium**. The fasciculi, which run the length of the muscle, are surrounded by yet another connective tissue layer, called the **fascia.** The fascia is a strong and dense layer of connective tissue that covers the entire muscle. In addition to separating muscles from each other, the fascia permits frictionless motion and also extends beyond the muscle to become the **tendon**.

80. What are the components of an individual sarcomere?

An individual sarcomere is bordered by two structures known as the **Z-lines** or Z-disks, which serve as the point of attachment for the thin filaments. The thin filaments are attached to the Z-lines by α-actinin, which is a major component of isolated Z-disks. The **I (isotropic) band** is a light band composed of thin filaments only, whereas the **A (anisotropic) band** is a dark band that corresponds to the region of overlap between the thick and thin filaments. As seen in the electron micrograph in question 78, the Z-lines bisect the I band and indicate the borders of the individual sarcomeres. The **H zone** (H-band) corresponds to the center region of the thick filament, which contains the tails but not the heads, of the myosin molecules. Thus, no cross-bridges can be formed in the H zone. A darkly staining **M-line** (M band) in the center of the sarcomere contains proteins that link the thick filaments together to maintain their position. The thick and thin filaments themselves are composed of a collection of individual proteins. Myosin is the primary component of the thick filament, and actin, tropomyosin, and troponin are the major components of the thin filament (see electron micrograph in question 78).

81. What is the sliding filament mechanism of contraction?

This refers to the generation of contractile force by the interaction of thick and thin filaments, causing them to slide between each other. The sliding filament theory explains how the thick and thin filaments move in relation to each other, in order to allow the sarcomeres to shorten. During contraction, the cycling of the cross-bridges causes the thin filaments to slide over the thick filaments; this decreases the distance between adjacent Z lines, allowing the sarcomere to shorten and the muscle to develop force.

82. What is the composition of the thick filament?

The thick filaments are composed of an aggregation of myosin molecules. The myosin molecules are arranged with the tails of the molecules facing toward the center of the filament. This causes the active force to be directionally oriented so that the thin filaments are pulled toward the center of the filament, causing active force generation and shortening of the muscle.

83. What are the biochemical characteristics of myosin?

Myosin is a large protein (470 kD) consisting of six polypeptide chains arranged in pairs. Two of these chains are myosin heavy chains consisting of an α-helical portion and a globular head portion. The globular head portion of the molecule hydrolyzes ATP in the presence of actin and interacts with the thin filaments to generate contractile force. The interactions between the thick and thin filaments are possible because of projections of the myosin molecule known as **cross-bridges,** which extend toward the thin filament. The cross-bridge consists of the globular head of the molecule and part of the α-helical structure. The helical part of the molecule contains two hinges. One of these is located next to the thick filament, and the other is located next to the globular head of the myosin molecule. The hinge near the body of the thick filament allows the cross-bridge to extend toward the active sites on the thin filament, and the hinge near the head of the molecule allows the head to rotate to produce the **power stroke** that generates contractile force. Pairs of cross-bridges are arranged on the opposite sides of the thick filament with a 120° rotation from one set of cross-bridges to another, allowing cross-bridges to reach thin filaments on different sides of the thick filament. Myosin also has two types of polypeptide light chains associated with the globular head of the molecule. These are wrapped around the neck of the molecule, below the myosin head, and appear to stiffen the neck region. One of these chains is called the **essential light chain** and may be important for the ATPase activity of the molecule. The other light chain is known as the **regulatory light chain**. In smooth muscle, phosphorylation of the regulatory light chains allows the myosin molecule to begin ATP hydrolysis, resulting in cross-bridge cycling and the generation of active contractile force.

84. What are the components of the thin filaments?

- **F-actin:** The thin filaments of striated muscle consist of two strands of fibrous actin (F-actin) molecules that are intertwined in a double helical arrangement like two strands of beads. The F-actin is composed of a string of individual globular (G) actin monomers (molecular weight of approximately 42–45 kD) that are arranged in series like a string of beads and contain active sites where the myosin cross-bridges bind and where contractile force is produced by a ratchetlike mechanism involving rotation of the attached myosin head (the **power stroke**).
- **Tropomyosin and troponin: Tropomyosin** is a fibrous protein 38–39 nm in length that has a molecular weight of approximately 50 kD. **Troponin** is a globular protein composed of three different subunits: (1) **troponin C** (18 kD), which binds Ca^{2+} ions; (2) **troponin I** (22 kD), which binds to troponin T and actin; and (3) **troponin T** (22 kD), which binds to the C terminal end of tropomyosin and links troponin I and troponin C to tropomyosin. Troponin molecules are attached to the tropomyosin strands at intervals corresponding to every seven actin monomers. A tropomyosin strand with its associated troponin molecules lies within each of the two grooves of the double helix that is formed by the intertwined F-actin molecules.

85. What is the role of tropomyosin and troponin in muscle contraction?

In striated muscle, the tropomyosin strands mask the active sites on the thin filament. This prevents contraction by blocking the interaction between the myosin cross-bridges and the actin monomers. When cytoplasmic Ca^{2+} levels increase during excitation-contraction coupling, the Ca^{2+} ions bind to troponin C. This changes the force of attraction between the troponin subunits and causes the troponin-tropomyosin complex to move farther down into the groove of the actin filament, exposing the active sites on the thin filament. This allows the myosin cross-bridges to gain access to the active sites, and cross-bridge cycling begins, causing muscle contraction. In smooth muscle (which lacks troponin), the tropomyosin may have a structural function, helping to maintain the integrity of the thin filaments.

86. What are the three major roles of ATP in muscle function?

1. ATP provides energy for the generation of contractile force, when it is hydrolyzed by the globular heads of the myosin molecule. The hydrolysis of ATP provides stored energy that is transformed into contractile force by the conformational change in the myosin head (power stroke) that occurs spontaneously right after the myosin head binds to the active site on the thin filament.

2. ATP binds to the head of the myosin molecule, reducing the affinity of the cross-bridge for the active site. This binding of ATP to the myosin head is essential for muscle relaxation to occur. In the absence of ATP, the myosin cross-bridges cannot release from the thin filament, and rigor complexes are formed. These complexes are responsible for the rigor mortis that occurs when ATP stores are exhausted after death.

3. ATP also provides energy for active transport of ions by various transport proteins that maintain normal ionic gradients across the cell, pump Ca^{2+} back into the sarcoplasmic reticulum, or pump Ca^{2+} out of the cell (in smooth muscle).

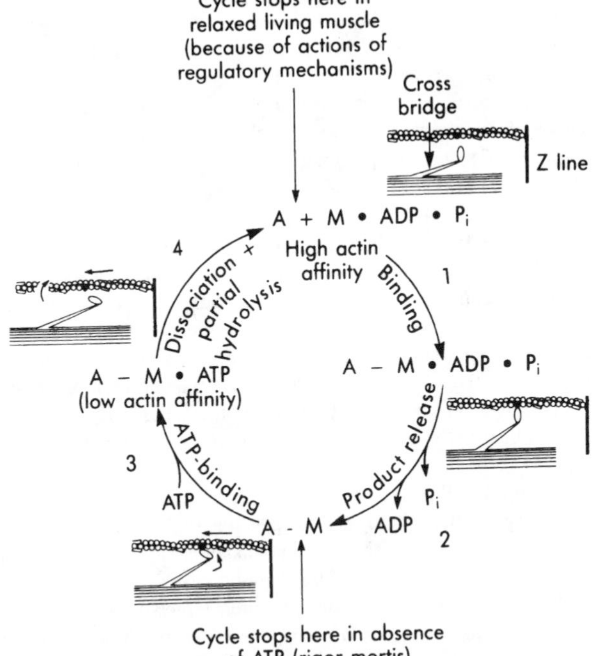

Steps in cross-bridge cycling during the development of contractile force in striated muscle. (From Berne RM, Levy MN: Physiology, 3rd ed. St. Louis, Mosby, 1993, with permission.)

87. What steps are involved in cross-bridge cycling?

The cross-bridge cycling process that generates contractile force in muscle is a ratchet-like mechanism that depends on the cyclic attachment and release of myosin heads at the active sites on the thin filament. The energy for cross-bridge cycling is derived from the hydrolysis of ATP by the myosin head, which acts as an ATPase when it can interact with active sites on the thin filaments. After the ATP is hydrolyzed by the myosin molecule, the ADP and P_i that result from the hydrolysis remain bound to the myosin head. At this point, the myosin head is in its higher energy state, because it has undergone a conformational change in which it stores the energy derived from hydrolysis of the ATP molecule as potential energy that will be released in the next power stroke. This myosin-ADP-P_i conformation of the molecule's head has a high affinity for actin, causing the head to bind to an active site on the thin filament at the first opportunity.

In the presence of elevated Ca^{2+} levels in the cytoplasm, the cross bridges can interact with the active sites on the thin filament. Right after the myosin head on the cross-bridge combines with the active site on the thin filament, the ADP and P_i are released from the myosin head and the power stroke occurs as a result of a spontaneous change in the conformation of the myosin head to the lower energy state. The net result of this conformational change is that the energy that was stored in the myosin head as a result of ATP hydrolysis is converted to mechanical energy that pulls the thin filament toward the center of the sarcomere via the ratchet mechanism.

After the power stroke is completed, myosin has a high affinity for ATP, which binds to the head portion of the molecule. Binding of ATP to the myosin head reduces the affinity of the cross-bridge for actin, causing it to release its attachment to the active site on the thin filament. The ATP is then hydrolyzed by the myosin head, causing the molecular conformation of the globular head to return to the higher energy conformation for the next cycle. The ADP and P_i formed from the hydrolysis of the ATP molecule remain bound to the head, and the cycle repeats as long as the active sites on the thin filament are exposed to allow cross-bridge attachment (see figure in question 86).

EXCITATION-CONTRACTION COUPLING

88. What is excitation-contraction coupling?

The process by which the excitation of a muscle cell (generally involving changes in membrane potential) is coupled to increases in cytoplasmic Ca^{2+} concentration and muscle contraction. The increase in cytoplasmic Ca^{2+} concentration initiates muscle contraction by interacting with regulatory proteins, such as troponin in skeletal and cardiac muscle or calmodulin in smooth muscle. Under some conditions, excitatory or inhibitory agents also can cause changes in cytoplasmic Ca^{2+} concentration and contractile force in smooth muscle without a change in membrane potential (pharmacomechanical coupling).

89. What is the sarcolemma and why is it important?

The sarcolemma is the external cell membrane of the muscle fiber. It is an excitable membrane that generates a membrane potential via mechanisms similar to those giving rise to the membrane potential in neurons. The permeability of the sarcolemma in skeletal muscle is increased by the neurotransmitter acetylcholine acting at the neuromuscular junction. This leads to action potentials that are propagated over the cell membrane and into the center of the fiber via the T-tubules. Propagation of action potentials in skeletal muscle cells occurs via mechanisms that are identical to those operating in nerve cell membranes.

90. What are T-tubules?

Invaginations of the muscle cell plasma membrane (sarcolemma) that occur at regularly spaced intervals on the sarcolemma of skeletal and cardiac muscle. These form a dense interconnecting network that extends throughout the muscle cell cytoplasm (see figure). Smooth muscle cells do not have T-tubules because their large surface area-to-volume ratio allows intracellular Ca^{2+} levels to be increased easily via influx of extracellular Ca^{2+} and by release of Ca^{2+} ions from intracellular stores (sarcoplasmic reticulum).

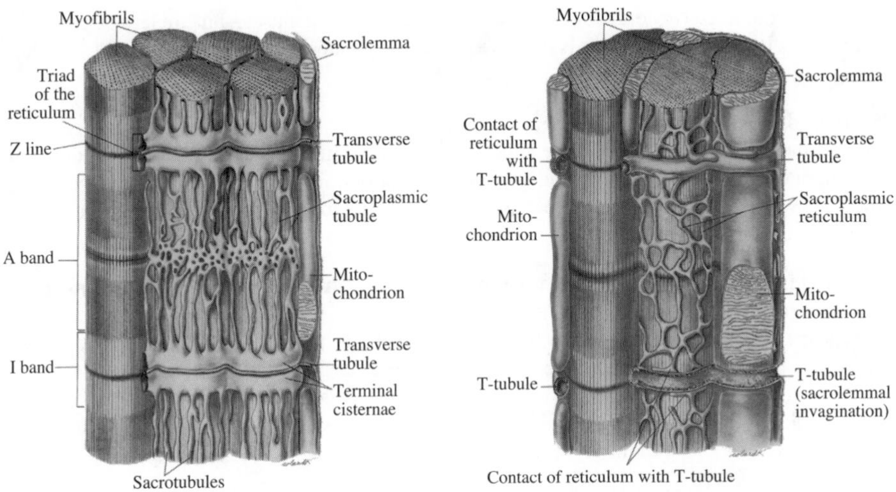

Transverse (T) tubule system from skeletal muscle (left panel) and cardiac muscle (right panel). (From Fawcett DW: Bloom and Fawcett's Textbook of Histology, 9th ed. New York, Chapman & Hall, 1994, with permission.)

91. Why are T-tubules important?

The T-tubule is contiguous with the extracellular fluid and contains voltage-gated Na^+ channels, as indicated by the presence of tetrodotoxin binding sites. The T-tubule system allows action potentials that are conducted over the sarcolemma to be conducted deep into the muscle fiber, providing rapid and coordinated excitation of the muscle cell. Excitation of the T-tubule system by the action potential is coupled to Ca^{2+} release from the terminal cisterna of the sarcoplasmic reticulum to allow a rapid, coordinated mobilization of Ca^{2+} from internal stores. This results in a coordinated contraction of all the myofibrils. This is important because the large volume of the skeletal muscle cell relative to its surface area makes the coordinated activation of the contractile filaments by the influx of extracellular Ca^{2+} ions impossible.

92. What is the sarcoplasmic reticulum?

A highly specialized internal membrane system of the muscle cell, which stores Ca^{2+} ions that are released during excitation contraction coupling. The sarcoplasmic reticulum (SR) is not contiguous with the extracellular fluid. The SR is extremely dense in skeletal muscle, is prominent but less dense in cardiac muscle, and can be either sparse or fairly prominent in smooth muscle.

93. How does the sarcoplasmic reticulum function?

After excitation of the muscle fiber is terminated, Ca^{2+} is actively transported back into the SR by a calcium ATPase. This allows large numbers of Ca^{2+} ions to be stored in the SR. The accumulation of Ca^{2+} in the SR is aided by a protein (**calsequestrin**) that binds Ca^{2+} loosely, thereby reducing the electrochemical gradient opposing the action of the sarcoplasmic reticulum Ca^{2+} ATPase. In striated muscle, Ca^{2+} release from the SR is coupled to depolarization of the T-tubule membrane so that excitation of the T-tubule system leads to Ca^{2+} release from the SR. In skeletal muscle, Ca^{2+} release from the SR depends entirely on depolarization of the T-tubule membrane. In cardiac muscle, increases in cytoplasmic Ca^{2+} ions cause the rapid release of more Ca^{2+} ions from the SR (calcium-induced Ca^{2+} release).

94. What are the terminal cisternae?

The specialized sac-like ends of the sarcoplasmic reticulum in skeletal and cardiac muscle. The terminal cisternae are the storage sites for the Ca^{2+} ions that are released during excitation-contraction coupling. The terminal cisternae are large in skeletal muscle, but are less extensive in cardiac muscle. This arrangement is consistent with the greater role of extracellular Ca^{2+} influx for regulating the contractile force in cardiac muscle.

95. What is a triad?

The structure formed by the close apposition of two terminal cisternae against a T-tubule in skeletal and cardiac muscle. The triad structure is important in the electromechanical coupling process in which the action potential passing through the T-tubule eventually leads to calcium release from the terminal cisternae.

96. What is the relationship among membrane potential, intracellular Ca^{2+} levels, and contractile force in various kinds of muscle?

The membrane potential generally plays an important role in regulating cytoplasmic Ca^{2+} concentration (and therefore contractile force) in muscle cells. Depolarization of the membrane is associated with increased levels of Ca^{2+} in the cytoplasm of skeletal, cardiac, and smooth muscle.

In **skeletal muscle,** action potentials spreading over the sarcolemma in a process similar to action potential propagation in nerve cells eventually cause Ca^{2+} to be released from the terminal cisterna of the SR.

In **cardiac muscle,** depolarization of the membrane not only causes the release of Ca^{2+} from the SR, but also leads to some influx of Ca^{2+} ions from the extracellular fluid. Influx of extracellular Ca^{2+} ions not only contributes to the development of contractile force, but also leads to the release of Ca^{2+} from the SR (calcium-induced Ca^{2+} release).

In **both skeletal and cardiac muscle,** cytoplasmic Ca^{2+} levels reach a peak value rapidly after release from the SR, preceding peak force development. As the Ca^{2+} ions are bound to troponin C, free Ca^{2+} in the cytoplasm falls, while contractile force increases. Peak force develops when all the regulatory sites on troponin are saturated, and the elastic elements in series and in parallel with the contractile filaments are drawn tight by the activity of the contractile filaments. After excitation of the muscle is terminated, Ca^{2+} diffuses off of the regulatory subunit of troponin and is removed from the cytoplasm by active pumping into the SR by the Ca^{2+} ATPase. In cardiac muscle, Ca^{2+} is also extruded from the cell via the Na^{+}, Ca^{2+} exchanger, which is a secondary active transport mechanism.

In **smooth muscle,** depolarization of the membrane opens voltage-gated Ca^{2+} channels, leading to the influx of extracellular Ca^{2+} ions. This triggers contraction by binding to calmodulin, which, in turn, activates myosin light chain kinase. Binding of excitatory substances, such as some neurotransmitters or hormones, to their receptors on the cell membrane also causes Ca^{2+} release from the SR of smooth muscle. This release of Ca^{2+} from the SR is triggered by inositol triphosphate, a second messenger compound that is is formed by the hydrolysis of membrane lipids by phospholipase C. Phospholipase C is an enzyme that is activated by the binding of the excitatory substance to its receptor on the cell membrane. Increases in cytoplasmic Ca^{2+} levels, in turn, lead to activation of myosin light chain kinase, phosphorylation of the regulatory light chains of the myosin molecule, and cross-bridge cycling. Hyperpolarization of the smooth muscle membrane closes voltage-gated Ca^{2+} channels, resulting in smooth muscle relaxation. Many smooth muscle cells exhibit graded changes in membrane potential that are not associated with action potentials. Some types of smooth muscle (e.g., intestinal smooth muscle and portal vein smooth muscle) exhibit spontaneous action potentials, which are usually associated with spontaneous contractions of the muscle. These action potentials are due to Ca^{2+} ions and are eliminated by Ca^{2+} channel blockers or Ca^{2+} free solution. Under some conditions, contractile force in smooth muscle can also change without a change in membrane potential. A change in smooth muscle contractile force without a change in membrane potential is known as **pharmacomechanical coupling**.

97. What conveys the signal between the sarcolemma, T-tubule, and sarcoplasmic reticulum to release Ca^{2+} during excitation contraction coupling in striated muscle?

The release of Ca^{2+} from the SR of striated muscle during excitation-contraction coupling is due to interactions between the T-tubules and the terminal cisternae of the SR. The T-tubule contains dihydropyridine-sensitive voltage sensors that are lined up opposite from the specialized feet on the terminal cisternae of the SR. These SR feet are composed of four identical subunits with a membrane spanning domain and a cytoplasmic domain. The SR feet also are called **ryanodine** receptors because they bind this pharmacologic agent, which causes release of Ca^{2+} from the SR. The ryanodine receptor is part of the Ca^{2+} channel that releases Ca^{2+} from the SR. In skeletal muscle, the opening of Ca^{2+} channels in the SR appears to be controlled by an electrical coupling between the T-tubules and the foot proteins, where the key variable in the signaling process is the electrical potential across the T-tubule membrane. The depolarization that occurs as the action potential passes down the T-tubule is proposed to cause a conformational change in foot proteins of the terminal cisternae. This conformational change is transmitted to the foot proteins via the dihydropyridine receptors and opens the Ca^{2+} channels in the SR. This allows Ca^{2+} ions to enter the cytoplasm down a large electrochemical gradient. In cardiac muscle, the influx of extracellular Ca^{2+} also leads to rapid Ca^{2+} release from the SR (Ca^{2+}-induced Ca^{2+} release).

98. What stops contraction of skeletal muscle?

The signal to stop contraction of skeletal muscle is the cessation of nerve impulses in the motor neuron. When the nerve impulses cease, the signal to release calcium ions from membrane stores is removed, stopping further Ca^{2+} release. The SR re-sequesters any free calcium remaining in the cytoplasm via an active transport mechanism that requires ATP (SR calcium pump). When calcium is removed from the cytoplasm, Ca^{2+} ions bound to troponin diffuse into the cytoplasm and are re-sequestered in the SR. When Ca^{2+} ions are no longer bound to the troponin, the thick and thin filaments can no longer interact, and contraction is terminated.

MECHANICS OF MUSCLE CONTRACTION

99. What is the difference between an isotonic and an isometric contraction?

Isotonic contraction refers to a contraction in which a muscle shortens while it exerts a constant force that matches the load being lifted by the muscle.

Isometric contraction refers to a contraction in which the external length of the muscle does not change because the force being generated by the muscle is insufficient to move the load to which it is attached. In the body, most contractions are a combination of isometric and isotonic components. The isometric phase occurs until the muscle generates enough force to lift the load. At this point, the isotonic phase begins and the muscle shortens at a constant force as it lifts the load. The rate and extent of muscle shortening during an isotonic contraction is less with heavier loads, and the duration of the isometric phase of the contraction is longer with heavier loads.

100. What is the difference between a twitch contraction and a tetanic contraction?

A **twitch contraction** is a single brief contraction of the muscle that occurs in response to a single threshold or suprathreshold stimulus.

A **tetanic contraction,** or tetanus, is a maintained contraction of a skeletal muscle owing to the continuous excitation of the muscle fibers. During a tetanic contraction, the muscle exhibits multiple action potentials, which serve to release Ca^{2+} continually from the SR and to maintain high levels of Ca^{2+} bound to troponin. Cross-bridges cycle continuously, and contractile force is maintained until excitation stops and cytoplasmic Ca^{2+} levels fall below the threshold needed to initiate muscle contraction. Tetanic contractions can arise from rapid stimulation of the muscle at frequencies greater than those at which individual twitch contractions can be resolved. The magnitude of a tetanic contraction is substantially greater than that of a twitch contraction because the elastic elements of the muscle are fully stretched, and the Ca^{2+} regulatory sites are completely saturated.

101. What are temporal and multiple motor unit summation?

Summation refers to the addition of contractile force in skeletal muscle. There are two types of summation. In **temporal summation,** with rapid frequencies of stimulation, the muscle is re-

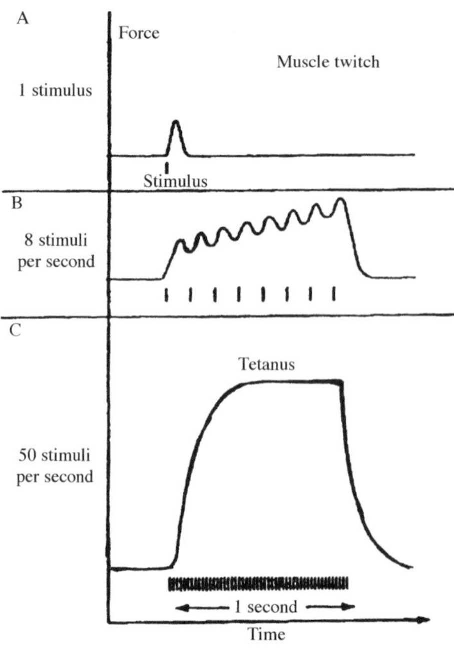

Recordings of contractile force during a twitch contraction (upper panel), temporal summation of contractile force (middle panel), and tetanic contraction of skeletal muscle (lower panel). (From Berne RM, Levy MN: Principles of Physiology, 2nd ed. St. Louis, Mosby, 1996, with permission.)

activated before it is fully relaxed from the previous stimulus. **Multiple motor unit summation** occurs when stronger stimuli cause the activation of additional motor units with lower excitability (i.e., higher thresholds), leading to an increased force of muscle contraction.

102. How can the power output of a muscle be calculated?

The **power output** of a muscle is the mechanical force (work × distance shortened) per unit of time and can be calculated as the **product of load times shortening velocity**.

103. Can twitch contractions be of different magnitudes?

Yes. Single-twitch contractions can be of different magnitudes, depending on the number of motor units that are activated and the position of the muscle on the length-force curve. A motor unit consists of a motor nerve fiber and all of the muscle cells innervated by that nerve fiber. At low stimulus strengths, the more excitable, smaller motor units are activated. With increasing stimulus strength, motor units having higher thresholds (i.e., less excitable, larger motor neurons) are activated, adding to the force of the contraction. A maximal stimulus of the muscle activates all the motor units, and supramaximal stimuli (stimuli that are greater than the maximal stimulus) do not produce any further increase in the magnitude of the twitch contraction. As a muscle is stretched, its position on the length-force curve also changes, and the amplitude of contraction increases with the degree of overlap between thick and thin filaments. At the rest length or optimal length (L_0) of the muscle, the number of myosin heads that can combine with active sites on the thin filament is at its maximum, and twitch contractions have their maximal amplitude for a given set of conditions.

104. What is treppe?

Treppe (or the **staircase effect**) refers either to the progressive increase in the magnitude of twitch contractions of skeletal muscle to a plateau value during repetitive stimulation after a period of rest or to the progressive increase in the magnitude of cardiac muscle contractions to a plateau value that can occur immediately after an increase in heart rate. The phenomenon is due to progressive increases in cytoplasmic Ca^{2+} levels after successive activations of the muscle and reflects the inability of the SR and Ca^{2+} extrusion mechanisms to restore cytoplasmic Ca^{2+} completely to the levels existing before the contraction.

105. What is the difference between preload and afterload?

Preload is the load that a muscle experiences before the onset of contraction. An example of preload is the amount of stretch on a resting muscle during the determination of the length-force relationship or the amount of stretching of cardiac muscle cells as a result of changes in end-diastolic volume.

Afterload is a load that is encountered by the muscle only after it starts to contract. An example is the load being lifted from the floor during a weight-lifting exercise or the arterial pressure that the heart muscle encounters at the onset of systole.

106. What is the length-force (length-tension) relationship?

The **length-force relationship** is the relationship between the length of the muscle and the amount of active and passive force on the muscle, which can be measured by a transducer attached to the muscle. **Active force** refers to the force generated by the contractile machinery when the muscle is activated, and **passive force** refers to the elastic force acting on the muscle because of stretching of the connective tissue and other elastic components of the muscle. **Total force** on the muscle is the sum of the passive and active forces.

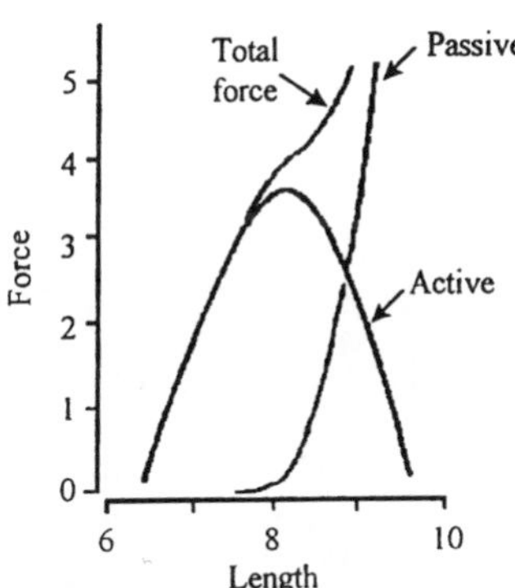

Length-force relationship from skeletal muscle. (From Rhoades RA, Tanner GA: Medical Physiology. Boston, Little, Brown, 1995, with permission.)

107. Describe how the length-force relationship works.

At short muscle lengths, the muscle is slack and the elastic components of the muscle are not stretched. As a result, there is no passive force on the muscle prior to activation, and the active force measured when the muscle contracts is significantly smaller than it is at longer lengths. As the muscle is stretched, the amount of passive force on the muscle increases exponentially because of the stretching of the elastic elements of the muscle. Lengthening the muscle at this point also increases the amount of active force generated by the muscle because the thick and thin filaments are stretched into a more optimal alignment, and more myosin heads on the thick filaments can reach active sites on the thin filament. A muscle generates force that is proportional to the number of cross-bridges that are formed simultaneously. At the rest length (also known as the optimum length [L_o]) of the muscle, all of the myosin heads on the thick filaments can reach active sites on the thin filaments, and the muscle can generate the maximal amount of contractile force. As the muscle is stretched further, the thick and thin filaments are drawn out of optimal overlap, and fewer myosin heads can reach active sites on the thin filaments, leading to a reduction in the active force that can be generated by the muscle. If the muscle is stretched to a sufficient degree, there is no overlap between thick and thin filaments, and the muscle cannot generate any contractile force. At that point, active force is 0, and the passive and total forces are the same. As the muscle is stretched further, passive force increases exponentially until the tissue tears or the muscle becomes dislodged from the force transducer.

108. What is the difference between the rest length (L_0) of a skeletal muscle and the equilibrium length?

The **rest length** of a skeletal muscle is the length at which the contractile force generated by the muscle is maximum. This is also referred to as optimal length of the muscle and is close to the length of a muscle at rest in the body.

The **equilibrium length** of the muscle is the length to which the muscle recoils after the tendon is cut. This is the length at which passive force on the muscle just equals 0. The equilibrium length is shorter than the rest length, and the contractile force exerted by the muscle at the equilibrium length is less than that occurring at rest length, owing to the changes in the length-force relationship.

109. What is the force-velocity relationship?

The hyperbolic relationship between the force generated by a muscle during an isotonic contraction and the velocity of muscle shortening. The velocity of the shortening of an isotonic contraction depends both on the intrinsic properties of the muscle and on the load on the muscle. Although skeletal muscles of different types can vary substantially in their velocity of contraction at a given load, the velocity of shortening decreases as the load is increased, regardless of muscle type.

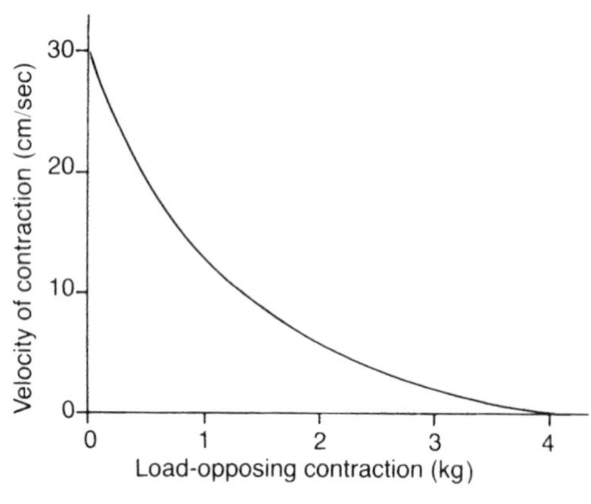

Force-velocity relationship for skeletal muscle contraction. (From Guyton AC, Hall J: Textbook of Medical Physiology, 9th ed. Philadelphia, W.B. Saunders, 1996, with permission.)

110. How does the force-velocity relationship differ among muscle types?

In **skeletal** and **cardiac muscle,** the force-velocity relationships have a similar shape, with an increase in the load on the muscle resulting in a reduced velocity of contraction. As the load on the muscle is increased, the muscle reaches a point where it cannot generate enough force to lift the load, and the contraction becomes isometric. At this load, shortening velocity is 0, and the force-velocity curve intersects the x-axis. As the load on the muscle is reduced, shortening velocity increases. The shortening velocity at 0 load (where the curve intersects the y-axis) is the **maximal velocity of shortening (V_{max})**. In skeletal muscle, V_{max} is constant for a given muscle and is a specific characteristic of the muscle. In cardiac muscle, V_{max} can change as a result of the inotropic state (contractility) of the heart.

Smooth muscle exhibits a similar force-velocity relationship as striated muscle, but the velocity of contraction is much slower than skeletal and cardiac muscle (see figure). The velocity of shortening in smooth muscle can exhibit substantial variation, depending on the level of phosphorylation of the regulatory light chains on the head of the myosin molecule.

111. What determines V_{max} for a specific muscle type?

- V_{max} for specific muscle types is determined by the myosin isoform that exists in the muscle. Different isoforms of myosin have different rates of ATP hydrolysis, and faster rates of ATP hydrolysis correspond to a greater V_{max}.

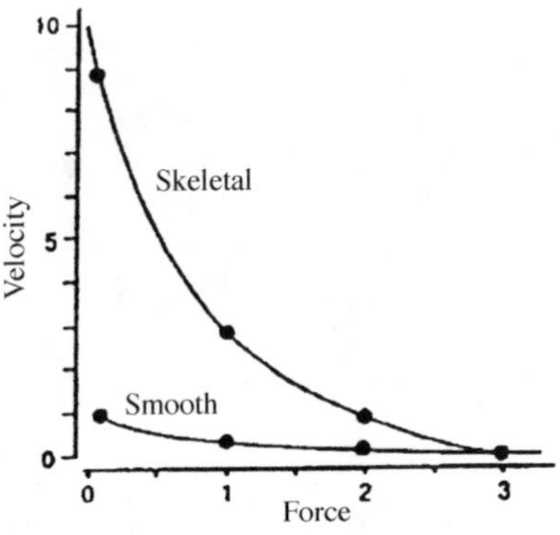

Force-velocity relationship in smooth muscle. Note the much slower velocity of contraction in smooth muscle compared with skeletal muscle. (From Rhoades RA, Tanner GA: Medical Physiology. Boston, Little, Brown, 1995, with permission.)

- In **skeletal muscle,** V_{max} is a constant for a given muscle and is determined by the myosin isoform in that muscle.
- In **cardiac muscle,** V_{max} can change, with increases in V_{max} occurring during positive inotropic states such as sympathetic stimulation and treatment with cardiac glycosides such as digitalis. Decreases in V_{max} occur during negative inotropic states such as vagal stimulation. These changes in V_{max} are generally related to changes in the availability of Ca^{2+} ions in the cytoplasm for excitation-contraction coupling.
- In **smooth muscle,** V_{max} can exhibit substantial variation, depending on the extent of phosphorylation of the regulatory light chains on the myosin cross-bridges (i.e., phosphorylated cross-bridges cycle faster and shortening velocity is greater when more of the cross-bridges are phosphorylated).

COMPARATIVE PHYSIOLOGY OF MUSCLE

112. How does cardiac muscle differ from skeletal muscle?

A major difference between cardiac muscle and skeletal muscle is the property of **automaticity** in the heart, which arises from spontaneous pacemaker potentials that occur as a result of complex changes in ionic conductance in special pacemaker cells. Action potentials in the heart exhibit a substantial regional variation, and cardiac muscle exhibits a number of different ionic currents that are not found in skeletal muscle.

In contrast to skeletal muscle, the heart acts as a **functional syncytium,** with excitation spreading from cell to cell through low-resistance pathways, enabling the contractile activity of the heart to be coordinated to ensure the efficient pumping of blood.

Cardiac muscle also exhibits some differences in **excitation-contraction coupling** (greater reliance on extracellular Ca^{2+} influx) and **mechanical properties** (ability to change V_{max} and a slower contraction velocity) relative to skeletal muscle.

113. What are the two general types of cardiac action potentials?

- **Fast-response action potentials** have a rapid depolarization (phase 0) with a substantial overshoot, a rapid reversal of the overshoot owing to a partial repolarization of the cell (phase 1), a long plateau (phase 2), and a rapid repolarization (phase 3) to return to the resting potential (phase 4).
- **Slow-response action potentials** exhibit a slower initial depolarization, less overshoot, a shorter and less stable plateau, and a repolarization to an unstable resting potential that exhibits a progressive, slow diastolic depolarization that is a major feature of pacemaker activity.

Fast-response and slow-response action potentials both exhibit an effective (absolute) and a relative refractory period.

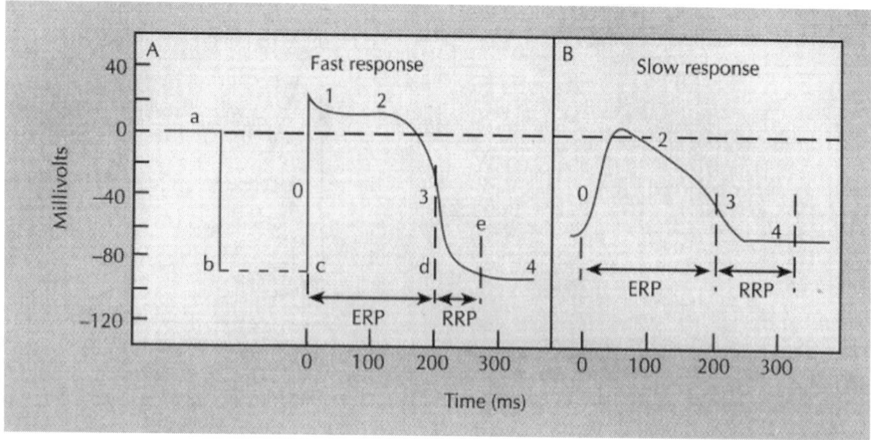

Fast-response and slow-response action potentials from cardiac muscle, showing the different phases of the action potential and the effective (ERP) and relative (RRP) refractory periods. (From Berne RM, Levy MN: Cardiovascular Physiology, 7th ed. St. Louis, Mosby, 1997, with permission.)

114. What is the ionic basis of the fast-response cardiac action potential?

The different phases of the fast-response action potential in cardiac muscle are due to changes in membrane permeability to different ions, which result in complex ionic currents that produce changes in membrane potential (see figure).

- **Phase 0** refers to the initial depolarization phase of the fast cardiac action potential, which is due to the opening of tetrodotoxin-sensitive, voltage-gated Na^+ channels. These channels are rapidly voltage inactivated, stopping the inward Na^+ current.
- **Phase 1** refers to the transient repolarization phase, which is mediated by a transient outward K^+ current that drives the initial repolarization, aided by the inactivation of the fast Na^+ current.

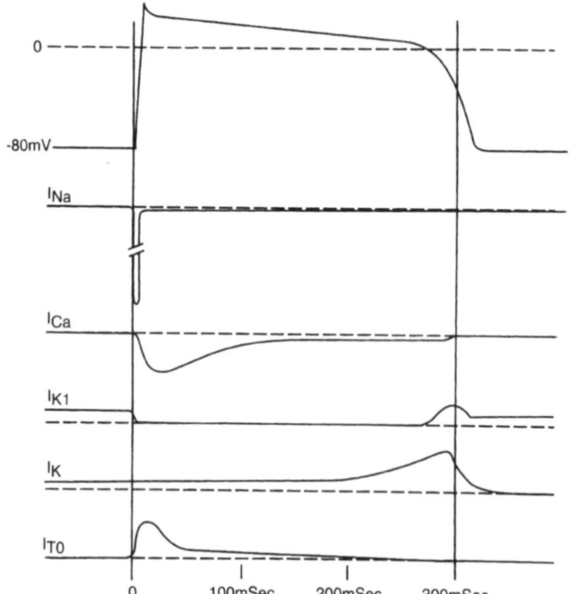

Changes in ionic currents during the action potential of a ventricular muscle cell. I_{Na} indicates inward Na^+ current, I_{Ca} indicates inward Ca^{2+} current, I_{K1} indicates current through inward rectifier K^+ channels, I_K indicates K^+ current through delayed rectifier channels, and I_{TO} indicates transient outward current during partial repolarization phase. (From Sperelakis N, Banks RO (eds): Essentials of Physiology, 2nd ed. Boston, Little Brown, 1996, with permission.)

- **Phase 2** refers to the plateau phase of the action potential, which is mediated by an inward Ca^{2+} current carried by L-type Ca^{2+} channels. The influx of Ca^{2+} ions through these channels contributes to excitation-contraction coupling and to calcium-induced Ca^{2+} release from the SR. The depolarization during the plateau phase of the action potential is also maintained by a low K^+ conductance that allows the inward current to maintain the depolarization. This reduced K^+ conductance is the result of the inward rectifier (K_{IR}) potassium channels, which allow inward K^+ current to be passed much more easily than outward K^+ current. In addition to aiding the depolarization during the plateau phase of the action potential, the decrease in the conductance of the K_{IR} channels at the onset of the action potential is important in preventing excessive K^+ loss from the cell during the action potential.
- **Phase 3** refers to the repolarization of the cell at the end of the plateau, which is mediated by a large, slowly developing K^+ current through delayed rectifier K^+ channels that are activated early in the action potential but exhibit slow activation kinetics. As the membrane potential approaches its normal resting value, the inward rectifying K^+ current, which is a crucial determinant of resting potential, also begins to contribute to the repolarization of the cell.

115. What causes the automaticity of the heart?

The automaticity of the heart is normally mediated via the spontaneous electrical activity of the pacemaker cells in the sinoatrial node. The atrioventricular node and Purkinje fibers can also serve as pacemakers but are normally overridden by the faster rate of the sinoatrial node. The pacemaker cells undergo spontaneous changes in membrane potential because of fluctuations in ionic conductances that allow the membrane potential to reach threshold values and to initiate conducted action potentials throughout the heart (see figure). The pacemaker potential exhibits a slow diastolic depolarization that eventually reaches threshold, resulting in an action potential. The diastolic depolarization is mediated by three different currents. One of these (I_f, or "funny" current) is an inward depolarizing current that is activated by hyperpolarization of the cell and is carried mainly by Na^+ ions through channels that are different from the tetrodotoxin-sensitive, voltage-gated Na^+ channels. The other depolarizing current is an inward Ca^{2+} current, which accelerates the diastolic depolarization, leading to the upstroke of the action potential. These inward currents are opposed by an outward K^+ current that repolarizes the cell after the upstroke of the action potential, then decreases its influence during phase 4 of the action potential, allowing the inward currents to trigger another diastolic depolarization. The heart rate is determined by the

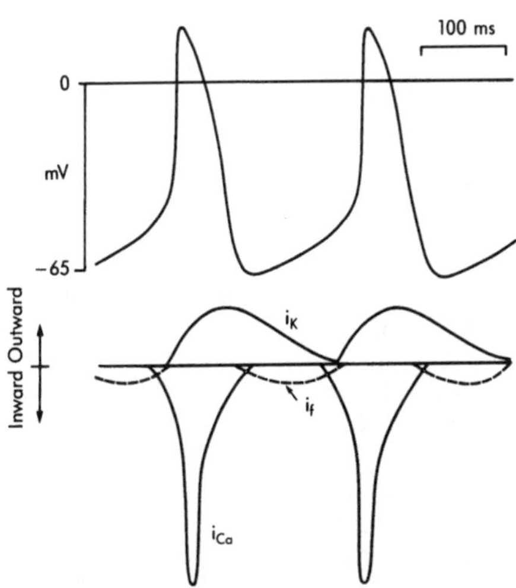

Changes in ionic current during pacemaker potentials in the sinoatrial node of the heart. i_{Ca} indicates inward Ca^{2+} current, i_f indicates inward Na^+ or "funny" current, and i_K indicates outward K^+ current. (From Berne RM, Levy MN: Cardiovascular Physiology, 7th ed. St. Louis, Mosby, 1997, with permission.)

slope of the diastolic depolarization, the absolute value of membrane potential, and the value of the threshold potential, all of which determine how fast the diastolic depolarization reaches the threshold value required to initiate the next action potential.

116. Which two pathways mediate the coordinated spread of excitation and contraction in the heart?

1. The **His-Purkinje system** provides a specialized system for conduction of excitation that consists of modified cardiac muscle fibers that have fewer myofibrils than other cardiac muscle cells.

2. The **intercalated disks** provide low-resistance pathways between individual cardiac muscle cells. The intercalated disks contain gap junctions. The gap junctions are low-resistance pathways composed of connexons, which are hexameric structures consisting of six polypeptides with a central core that serves as a low-resistance pathway for cell-to-cell conduction. The combined function of the His-Purkinje system and the intercalated disks permits the heart to function as a syncytium, enabling cardiac contractile activity to be coordinated to ensure the efficient pumping of blood.

117. Which aspects of excitation-contraction coupling are different in cardiac muscle compared to skeletal muscle?

- The terminal cisternae of cardiac muscle are much less extensive than those of skeletal muscle, and hence excitation-contraction coupling in cardiac muscle is much more dependent on the influx of extracellular Ca^{2+} ions.
- The T-tubules in cardiac muscle are much larger than those of skeletal muscle, allowing easier exchange of ions, nutrients, and waste products between the cardiac myocyte and the extracellular fluid. To aid in their function, the T-tubules also contain negatively charged mucopolysaccharides that bind Ca^{2+} ions, making more Ca^{2+} available for excitation-contraction coupling.
- Changes in the number of Ca^{2+} ions released from the SR can have a much greater effect on cardiac muscle contraction than on skeletal muscle contraction. For example, the increases in cytoplasmic Ca^{2+} that result from sympathetic stimulation of the heart or reduced Ca^{2+} extrusion during treatment with cardiac glycosides result in a greater sequestration of Ca^{2+} by the SR. This ultimately leads to a greater Ca^{2+} release from the SR during the next activation of the cell and to an increased force of contraction.
- Calcium-induced Ca^{2+} release, by which increases in cytosolic Ca^{2+} levels lead to a rapid and massive release of Ca^{2+} from the SR in cardiac muscle cells, does not occur in skeletal muscle.

118. What is the mechanism for changes in the contractility (inotropic state) of the heart?

Changes in the inotropic state of the heart are due mainly to the changes in the concentration of cytoplasmic Ca^{2+} ions available for activation. Any stimulus that can lead to a maintained increase in Ca^{2+} in the cytoplasm (through an increased influx of Ca^{2+} ions, an increased release of Ca^{2+} from the SR, or a reduced extrusion of Ca^{2+} from the cytoplasm) can result in an increase in contractility, or a positive inotropic effect. For example, catecholamines exert a positive inotropic effect on the heart by combining with a β-adrenergic receptor, which activates adenylyl cyclase via a G-protein mechanism. The resulting phosphorylation of the L-type Ca^{2+} channel by a cAMP-dependent kinase leads to an increased influx of Ca^{2+}. Treatment with cardiac glycosides such as digitalis inhibits the Na^+, K^+ pump, resulting in a reduced electrochemical gradient for Na^+ across the cell membrane. The energy for the Na^+, Ca^{2+} exchanger to extrude Ca^{2+} from the cell against its electrochemical gradient is derived from the electrochemical gradient for Na^+, and this results in a reduced Ca^{2+} extrusion via the Na^+, Ca^{2+} exchanger and an increased force of contraction (positive inotropic effect). In contrast, vagal stimulation can lead to a reduced contractility, or negative ionotropic state, owing to reduced Ca^{2+} influx into the cell.

119. What are heterometric and homeometric regulation of contractile force in cardiac muscle?

Heterometric regulation of contractile force in cardiac muscle (see figure, left panel) refers to changes in contractile force occurring as a result of changes in the length of the muscle fiber at a constant inotropic state. These changes can occur during increases or decreases in end-diastolic volume and are due to changes in the position of the muscle fiber on the length-force curve.

Homeometric regulation of contractile force in cardiac muscle (see figure, right panel) refers to changes in the contractile force of cardiac muscle at the same muscle fiber length (or end-diastolic volume). This occurs during changes in the inotropic state of the muscle. For example, sympathetic stimulation or treatment with cardiac glycosides has a positive inotropic effect, resulting in an increase in the force generated by the muscle at a given end-diastolic volume. During heart failure or parasympathetic stimulation, the force of contraction decreases (negative inotropic effect).

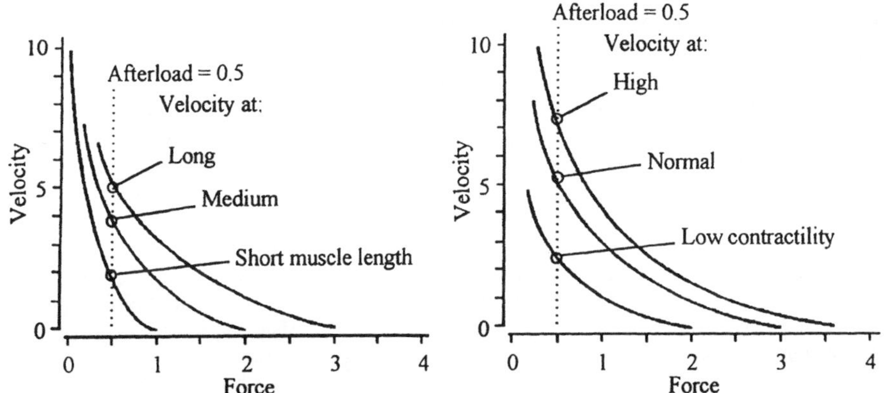

Changes in force-velocity curve of cardiac muscle during changes in fiber length (heterometric regulation of contractile force) in the left panel and during changes in the inotropic state of the heart (homeometric regulation of contractile force) in the right panel. (From Rhoades RA, Tanner GA: Medical Physiology. Boston, Little, Brown, 1995, with permission.)

120. How do the contractile properties of cardiac muscle differ from those of skeletal muscle?

Cardiac muscle has a slower velocity of contraction than skeletal muscle, and cardiac muscle can exhibit changes in the V_{max} during changes in the inotropic state of the heart.

In contrast to skeletal muscle, cardiac muscle normally operates at lengths that are much shorter than the optimal, or rest, length (L_o). This property is important in allowing the heart to increase its force of contraction in response to increases in end-diastolic volume that are associated with increases in venous return (Frank-Starling mechanism or heterometric autoregulation).

121. What are the sources of metabolic energy for cardiac muscle contraction?

Oxidative phosphorylation is the primary source of metabolic energy in the heart. The primary substrates for oxidative metabolism in the heart are either fatty acids or carbohydrates. Lactate is an important substrate, and ketones and amino acids can also serve as substrates during periods of increased activity. Similar to skeletal muscle, cardiac muscle contains creatine phosphate as a buffer system to supply the short-term demands of the contractile system for ATP.

Anaerobic glycolysis can also briefly compensate for a transient lack of aerobic ATP production, but the capacity of anaerobic glycolysis to meet the energy needs of the heart is limited. The formation of ATP depends on a steady supply of oxygen via coronary blood flow. Because of the dependence of the heart on aerobic metabolism, there is a good correlation between the oxygen consumption of the heart and the amount of work performed by the heart. Oxygen consumption is nearly proportional to the product of the tension that occurs in the heart muscle during contraction times the duration of contraction (**tension-time index**).

122. Define single-unit (unitary) and multiunit smooth muscle.

Single-unit or **unitary** applies to a smooth muscle in which the excitation spreads from cell to cell through low-resistance pathways, allowing the muscle to respond as a syncytium, or single unit. Single- unit smooth muscle often exhibits spontaneous activity, as in the intestine.

Multiunit refers to smooth muscle that requires external activation by nerves or hormones to generate contractile force. In multiunit smooth muscle, each individual cell is viewed as an independent unit, and the response of the whole muscle is a result of the response of multiple individual units.

The classification of single versus multiunit smooth muscle, although useful, is far from absolute because many types of smooth muscle exhibit both single-unit and multiunit properties.

123. What are tonic and phasic contractions of smooth muscle?

- **Tonic contractions** are contractions in which muscle contraction is maintained for a prolonged period of time (e.g., the resting tone of arterioles in the microcirculation).
- **Phasic contractions** are relatively rapid contractions followed by complete relaxation (e.g., the spontaneous contractions of smooth muscle in the small intestine).

124. How does excitation spread from cell to cell in smooth muscle?

Through low-resistance pathways termed **gap junctions**. The gap junctions enable membrane potential changes and contractile activity to be coordinated among many cells, leading to coordinated activity of the muscle. In this respect, the smooth muscle represents a functional syncytium, similar to cardiac muscle.

125. Why is coordinated excitation important?

Conducted excitation with coordinated activity of smooth muscle cells is especially important in organs such as the intestine, where extensive areas of the organ work together to mix or propel the luminal contents.

126. How do individual smooth muscle cells serve as integrators of information?

The amount of force that is generated by a smooth muscle at any given time is a function of the overall effect of a variety of excitatory and inhibitory inputs. These can include excitatory and inhibitory neural inputs, circulating hormones, autacoids, or local paracrine factors produced in the tissue. In blood vessels, the endothelium releases a number of contracting and relaxing factors that affect the active tone of the smooth muscle. Many smooth muscles are also sensitive to stretch and to local conditions such as PO_2, PCO_2, and pH. The latter factors are important in regulating physiologic functions, such as the local control of blood flow in the microcirculation. In this way, smooth muscle cells sample excitatory and inhibitory inputs to provide an integrated response that is determined by the combined influence of these inputs.

127. Compare and contrast the contractile proteins of smooth muscle and striated muscle.

Smooth muscle and striated muscle both contain myosin that has cross-bridges, hydrolyzes ATP, and interacts with actin to generate contractile force. In contrast to striated muscle, the thin filaments of smooth muscle contain only actin and tropomyosin, but not troponin. Also in contrast to striated muscle, regulation of contractile activity by Ca^{2+} in smooth muscle is mediated by the binding of Ca^{2+} to calmodulin, which activates myosin light chain kinase and phosphorylates the regulatory light chain of myosin. This results in subsequent ATP hydrolysis and cross-bridge cycling.

128. Compare and contrast the arrangement of the contractile filaments in smooth muscle with that in skeletal muscle.

The arrangement of the contractile filaments in smooth muscle is depicted in the figure. Smooth muscle contains both thick and thin filaments. As in striated muscle, the thick filaments in smooth muscle are composed of myosin. The thin filaments of smooth muscle contain actin and tropomyosin, but no troponin. The contractile filaments in smooth muscle also are not arranged in orderly arrays as in striated muscle, and the actin-to-myosin ratio in smooth muscle (14–16:1) is much greater than that in skeletal muscle (2:1). Thin filaments in smooth muscle are attached to dense bodies rather than Z lines, and myosin cross-bridges from the thick filament can interact with thin filaments along a much greater length of the thin filament, allowing smooth muscle to shorten to a much greater fraction of its length than skeletal muscle.

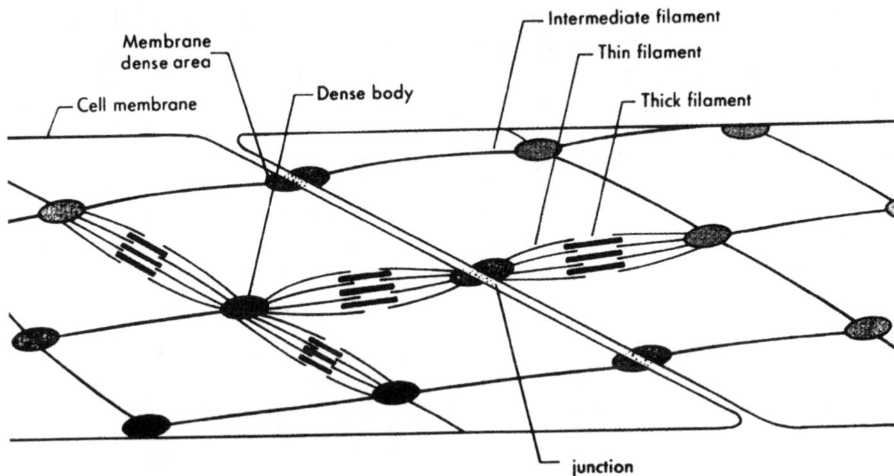

Arrangement of contractile filaments in smooth muscle. (From Berne RM, Levy MN: Principles of Physiology, 2nd ed. St. Louis, Mosby, 1996, with permission.)

129. How do smooth muscle cells shorten if they do not have sarcomeres as in skeletal muscle?

As in the case of skeletal and cardiac muscle, smooth muscle cells shorten as a result of an interaction between thick and thin filaments. In contrast to the regular sarcomeric structure of skeletal and cardiac muscle, thin filaments in smooth muscle are attached to structures in the cytoplasm known as the **dense bodies,** and to dense areas or attachment plaques on the sarcolemma. Dense bodies are connected to each other by **intermediate filaments** generally consisting of the protein desmin, although the intermediate filaments of some smooth muscles contain vimentin. The contractile filaments and dense bodies form an interlacing structure attached to the cytoskeleton. Interaction between the thick and thin filaments with cycling of the myosin cross-bridges results in shortening of the smooth muscle cell.

130. How do the sources of activator Ca^{2+} differ between skeletal, cardiac, and smooth muscle cells?

In both smooth and striated muscle, excitation contraction coupling involves an increase in the cytoplasmic Ca^{2+} levels of the cell. The increase in cytoplasmic Ca^{2+} in skeletal muscle is due entirely to release of Ca^{2+} from the SR stores, whereas in cardiac muscle, both the SR stores and the influx of extracellular Ca^{2+} ions are important in regulating contraction. In smooth muscle, activator Ca^{2+} can either enter the cell from the extracellular fluid or come from the SR. In most cases, smooth muscle depends substantially more on the entry of extracellular Ca^{2+} ions than striated muscle. The contraction of smooth muscles that have a sparse SR is much more sensitive to inhibition by calcium channel blockers and Ca^{2+} free solutions.

131. How do Ca^{2+} ions regulate contractile protein interactions in striated and smooth muscle?

In **striated muscle,** the Ca^{2+} ions bind to troponin C, causing a change in the position of the troponin-tropomyosin complex that unmasks the active sites on the thin filament, allowing the cross-bridge cycling that leads to muscle contraction.

In contrast to striated muscle, **smooth muscle** does not contain troponin, and regulation of contractile force occurs at the level of the thick filament (see figure). Initiation of contraction in response to increases in cytoplasmic Ca^{2+} concentration in smooth muscle cells occurs as a result of the binding of Ca^{2+} ions to calmodulin, a Ca^{2+}-binding regulatory protein that has four high-affinity Ca^{2+} binding sites and is important in activating a number of different enzymes. The calcium/calmodulin complex activates myosin light chain kinase, which phosphorylates the regulatory light chains on the head of the myosin molecule. When the light chains are phosphorylated, the myosin molecule hydrolyzes ATP, and the cross-bridges begin to cycle. The ATPase activity of the actomysin complex under these conditions is proportional to the percentage of phosphorylated cross-bridges. The phosphorylated cross-bridges continue to cycle until they are dephosphorylated by myosin light chain phosphatase. In smooth muscle, Ca^{2+} may also regulate contractile force at the level of the thin filament. This form of regulation involves other proteins (caldesmon and calponin) that are proposed to bind to the thin filament and inhibit myosin ATPase activity in the absence of elevated Ca^{2+} levels in the cytoplasm.

132. Do smooth muscle cells have T-tubules and a sarcoplasmic reticulum?

Smooth muscle cells *do not* have T-tubules. Because of their small size, smooth muscle cells have a large surface area-to-volume ratio that allows the cell to be easily activated by extracellu-

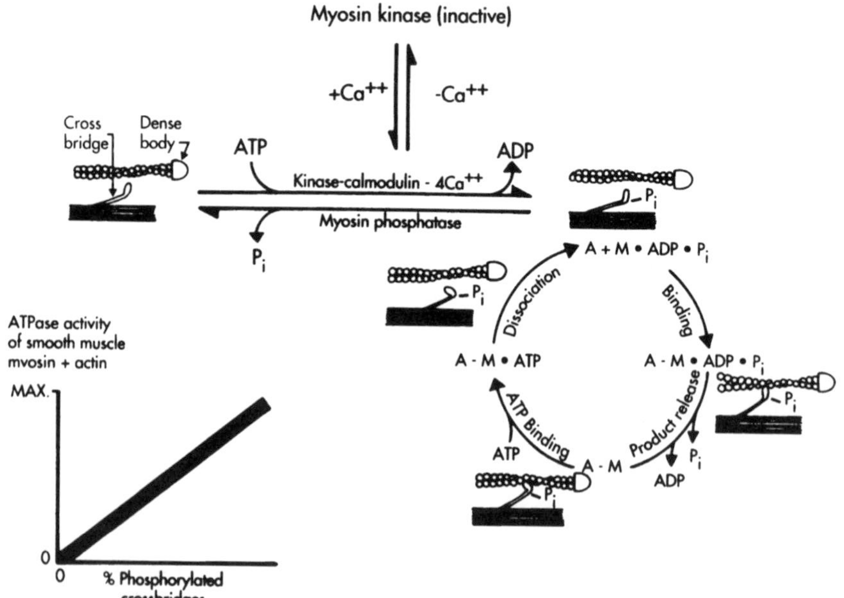

Steps in cross-bridge cycling and effect of cross-bridge phosphorylation on myosin ATPase activity in smooth muscle. (From Berne RM, Levy MN: Principles of Physiology, 2nd ed. St. Louis, Mosby, 1996 with permission.)

lar Ca^{2+} influx without the need for conduction of excitation to the center of the cell by a T-tubule system. Smooth muscle cells *do* have a sarcoplasmic reticulum that can be either fairly extensive or relatively sparse. Smooth muscles with an extensive SR are more resistant to inhibition by reductions in extracellular Ca^{2+} concentration or calcium entry blockers.

133. Which three factors determine the level of cytoplasmic Ca^{2+} in smooth muscle cells?

1. The influx of Ca^{2+} through activation of Ca^{2+} channels in the cell membrane
2. The release of Ca^{2+} ions from the SR
3. The removal of Ca^{2+} from the cytoplasm of the smooth muscle cell by several different mechanisms:
   - The active transport of Ca^{2+} into the SR by the SR-bound Ca^{2+} ATPase
   - The active extrusion of Ca^{2+} from the cell by the sarcolemmal Ca^{2+} ATPase
   - Secondary active transport out of the cell by the Na^+, Ca^{2+} counter-transporter

134. How do ion channels regulate smooth muscle function?

K^+ channels: Several types of K^+ channels are expressed in smooth muscle membranes. These include large Ca^{2+}-activated K^+ channels (K_{Ca}), ATP-sensitive K^+ channels (K_{ATP}), inward rectifier K^+ channels (K_{IR}), and voltage-dependent K^+ channels (K_V). Increases in K^+ conductance lead to the efflux of K^+ from the cell, causing the membrane potential to become more negative. This leads to the inactivation of voltage-gated Ca^{2+} channels, reduced Ca^{2+} influx, and relaxation of the smooth muscle. The role of specific K^+ channel types in regulating membrane potential and contractile force in response to various stimuli can vary among different kinds of smooth muscle.

Ca^{2+} channels: The predominant type of Ca^{2+} channel in smooth muscle membranes is the L-type, voltage-gated Ca^{2+} channel. The L-type Ca^{2+} channels are sensitive to inhibition by dihydropyridine Ca^{2+} entry blockers and control the entry of extracellular Ca^{2+} induced by membrane depolarization. Transient (T-type) Ca^{2+} channels also have been reported and may contribute to pacemaker activity in some smooth muscle cells.

Nonspecific cation channels: These ligand-gated channels are closely linked to membrane receptors and open in response to some contractile agonists. Nonspecific cation channels permit the influx of Na^+ and K^+ as well as Ca^{2+} ions and may provide the initial depolarization that triggers the opening of L-type Ca^{2+} channels.

Chloride channels: These channels may modulate the level of excitability of some smooth muscle cells by regulating electromechanical coupling. Because the Cl^- equilibrium potential is more positive than the membrane potential, opening of Cl^- channels may result in Cl^- efflux and provide a depolarizing influence to promote smooth muscle contraction.

Stretch-activated channels: The properties of these mechanosensitive channels are still being characterized. They appear to be insensitive to pharmacologic block by dihydropyridine drugs and may mediate Ca^{2+} influx during stretch of the smooth muscle cell.

135. How do membrane receptors regulate smooth muscle activity?

Membrane receptors are proteins that serve as targets for binding by specific ligands, such as neurotransmitters, hormones, and other humoral factors. The binding of the ligand to its receptor results in a specific response within the cell. In smooth muscle, excitatory receptors increase cytoplasmic Ca^{2+} and cause contraction by increasing the permeability of the cell membrane to Ca^{2+}, leading to an influx of extracellular Ca^{2+}, or by causing the release of Ca^{2+} from the SR. In other cases, occupancy of receptors by ligands can lead to smooth muscle relaxation. Receptor-mediated relaxation is often associated with hyperpolarization of the membrane mediated by activation of K^+ channels. This hyperpolarization of the cell membrane inhibits Ca^{2+} influx through voltage-gated Ca^{2+} channels. In many cases, the binding of ligands to their receptors causes an elevation in cAMP or cGMP that leads to relaxation of smooth muscle via a variety of mechanisms including activation of K^+ channels, increases in the active transport of Ca^{2+} from the cytoplasm, or alterations in the force-generating capacity of the contractile filaments.

136. How do second messengers regulate smooth muscle function?

Smooth muscle function can be regulated by a number of important second messenger systems, including:

- **Phospholipase C,** which hydrolyzes membrane lipids to produce inositol 1,4,5-trisphosphate (IP_3) and diacylglycerol. IP_3 causes the release of Ca^{2+} ions from the SR, and diacylglycerol can activate protein kinase C (PKC), which leads to activation of membrane ion channels (e.g., a PKC-dependent phosphorylation of the L-type Ca^{2+} channel stimulates Ca^{2+} influx).
- **Phospholipase A_2,** which hydrolyzes membrane lipids to liberate arachidonic acid, whose active metabolites can regulate smooth muscle contractile force.
- **Adenylyl and guanylyl cyclase,** which increase cAMP and cGMP levels.
- **Calcium ions,** which can also be viewed as second messengers because they activate the contractile system via Ca^{2+}-calmodulin–dependent activation of myosin light chain kinase and trigger other responses such as the opening of Ca^{2+}-activated K^+ channels in the cell membrane

137. How do the mechanical properties of smooth muscle differ from those of skeletal muscle and cardiac muscle?

- Skeletal muscle contracts faster than cardiac muscle, which, in turn, contracts much faster than smooth muscle.
- When normalized to cross-sectional area, smooth muscle cells can generate an equal or greater amount of force than cardiac or skeletal muscle cells, can operate over a much wider range of lengths, and can generate contractile force at much shorter lengths than skeletal or cardiac muscle. The ability of smooth muscle to generate contractile force over a wide range of lengths is important in allowing smooth muscle to adapt to large changes in the volume of hollow organs, such as the intestine or urinary bladder.
- The velocity of smooth muscle contraction can change, depending on physiologic conditions. Smooth muscle also exhibits a **latch state,** in which it can generate contractile force for prolonged periods of time with minimal energy consumption.

138. What is the latch state of smooth muscle?

The **latch state** refers to a condition in which the muscle maintains high levels of active force without rapid cross-bridge cycling and with low rates of ATP consumption.

139. What is the mechanism of the latch state?

When smooth muscle is initially activated, the rapidly developing phase of contraction coincides with a transient peak in intracellular Ca^{2+} levels, leading to activation of myosin light chain kinase, phosphorylation of cross-bridges, and cross-bridge cycling with ATP hydrolysis. During the latch state, the initial peak Ca^{2+} concentration falls to a moderately elevated steady-state level while force is sustained. This is accompanied by a reduction in cross-bridge phosphorylation and a reduction in ATP consumption. The existence of high force with moderate levels of cross-bridge phosphorylation means that cross-bridges that are attached but dephosphorylated also contribute to contractile force in the muscle. Therefore, both the number of attached cross-bridges (which determines force) and the cycling rate of the cross-bridges (which determines velocity and ATP consumption) can be regulated.

140. Why is the latch state important?

It enables the muscle to maintain contractile force for prolonged periods of time with minimal energy expenditure in the form of ATP consumption.

141. What is stress relaxation and reverse stress relaxation?

Stress relaxation and **reverse stress relaxation** refer to the ability of smooth muscle to adjust its length after abrupt changes in muscle length or organ volume. When smooth muscle length or organ volume is abruptly increased, the total force on the smooth muscle or the pressure within the organ increases substantially. Over the next minute or so, the force on the muscle or the pressure inside the organ gradually returns to near the control value as the muscle lengthens to accommodate the stretch or the increased volume within the organ. This compensatory response of the smooth muscle to stretch is called **stress relaxation**. When smooth muscle is abruptly shortened or when organ volume is abruptly decreased, the force on the muscle or the pressure inside the organ drops. Muscle force and organ pressure are soon restored to near the control value as the muscle shortens to maintain force at the new length or pressure at the reduced volume (**reverse stress relaxation**). Stress relaxation and reverse stress relaxation result from readjustment of the position of the myosin cross-bridges on the thin filament and are important in allowing smooth muscle to maintain a constant pressure in hollow organs, despite changes in the length of the smooth muscle cells.

BIBLIOGRAPHY

1. Berne RM, Levy MN (eds): Physiology, 4th ed. St Louis, Mosby, 1998.
2. Berne, RM Levy MN: Principles of Physiology, 3rd ed. St. Louis, Mosby, 2000.
3. Berne RM, Levy MN: Cardivascular Physiology, 8th ed. St. Louis, Mosby, 2001.
4. Bloom W, Fawcett DW: A Textbook of Histology, 9th ed. Philadelphia, W.B. Saunders, 1968.
5. Fawcett DW: Bloom and Fawcett's A Textbook of Histology, 12th ed. New York, Chapman & Hall, 1994.
6. Guyton AC, Hall J: Textbook of Medical Physiology, 10th ed. Philadelphia, W.B. Saunders, 2001.
7. Horowitz A, Menice CB, Laporte R, Morgan KG: Mechanisms of smooth muscle contraction. Physiol Rev 76:967–1003, 1996.
8. Johnson LR: Essential Medical Physiology. New York, Raven Press, 1992.
9. Lodish H, Baltimore D, Berk A, et al: Molecular Cell Biology, 3rd ed. New York, Scientific American Books, 1995.
10. Murphy RA: What is special about smooth muscle? The significance of covalent cross bridge regulation. FASEB J 8:311–318, 1994.
11. Nelson MT, Quayle JM: Physiological roles and properties of potassium channels in arterial smooth muscle. Am J Physiol 268(Cell Physiol 37):C799–C822, 1995.
12. Rhoades RA, Tanner GA: Medical Physiology. Boston, Little, Brown, 1995.
13. Sherwood L: Human Physiology, St. Paul, MN, West Publishing Company, 1989.
14. Smith JJ, Kampine JP: Circulatory Physiology: The Essentials. Baltimore, Williams & Wilkins, 1990.
15. Somlyo AP, Somlyo AV: Signal transduction and regulation in smooth muscle. Nature 372:231–236, 1994.
16. Sperelakis N: Cell Physiology Source Book, 2nd ed. San Diego, Academic Press, 1998.
17. Sperelakis N, Banks RO (eds): Essentials of Physiology, 2nd ed. Boston, Little, Brown, 1996.

2. CELL SIGNALING

Meghan M. Taylor, Ph.D., and Willis K. Samson, Ph.D.

CELL SURFACE RECEPTORS

1. Name the three classes of cell surface receptors and give examples of each.
G protein–linked, enzyme-linked, and ion channel-linked.

Examples of Subclasses of Cell Surface Receptors

G PROTEIN-LINKED	ENZYME-LINKED	ION CHANNEL-LINKED
Acetylcholine (M_1, M_2)	Insulin	GABA ($GABA_A$)
Norepinephrine	Growth factors	Glutamate (AMPA, NMDA)
Luteinizing hormone	Interferon	Glycine
Angiotensin	Prolactin/growth hormone	Acetylcholine (N_M, N_N)
Dopamine	Natriuretic peptide	ATP (P_2X)
Thrombin	Interleukins	
Prostaglandins		
ATP (P_2Y)		

ATP = adenosine triphosphate; GABA = gamma aminobutyric acid; AMPA = alpha-amino-3-hydroxy-5-methyl-4-isoxazoleneproprionate; NMDA = N-methyl-D-aspartate.

2. What other classes of receptors are there?
In addition to cell surface receptors, there are cytosolic and nuclear receptors. Most steroid receptors fall into this category.

G-PROTEIN COUPLED RECEPTORS

3. What is a G-protein coupled receptor (GPCR)?
GPCRs form the largest family of cell-surface receptors. They all have similar structure, consisting of a single polypeptide chain that spans the cell membrane seven times. GPCRs interact with heterotrimeric G proteins on the intracellular side of the plasma membrane.

4. What is a heterotrimeric G protein?
A heterotrimeric G protein is composed of three subunits: α, β, and γ. Each subunit has multiple isoforms, which provide specificity to each receptor. The classification of the receptor is based on the α subunit.

Mammalian α Subunits

α SUBUNIT	EXPRESSION	EFFECTOR	RECEPTOR EXAMPLES
α_s	Ubiquitous	↑ Adenylyl cyclase, ↑ Ca^{++} channel	β-Adrenergic, TSH
α_i	Ubiquitous	↓ Adenylyl cyclase, ↑ K^+ channel	α_2-Adrenergic, M_2-muscarinic
α_o	Neural, endocrine	↓ Ca^{++} channel	Somatostatin
α_q	Ubiquitous	↑ Phospholipase C-β_1	α_1-Adrenergic, M_1-muscarinic
α_{11}	Ubiquitous	↑ Phospholipase C-β_1	V_1-vasopressin
α_{13}	Ubiquitous	↑ Na^+/H^+ exchange	Thrombin
α_t	Rod/cone cells	↑ cGMP-phosphodiesterase	Rhodopsin

TSH = thyroid-stimulating hormone; cGMP = cyclic guanosine monophosphate.

5. Describe what happens to the G proteins upon ligand binding to the GPCR.
The receptor protein undergoes a conformational change that alters the intracellular surface of the receptor. This change enables the receptor to interact with a G protein. The α subunit exchanges its guanosine diphosphate (GDP) molecule for guanosine triphosphate (GTP). This

causes the G protein to break up into two separate molecules, the α subunit and the $\beta\gamma$ complex. These molecules can diffuse freely along the plasma membrane and interact directly with target molecules, which can in turn relay the signal to other molecules. The longer these targets have an α or $\beta\gamma$ subunit bound to them, the stronger and more prolonged the relayed signal will be. The intrinsic GTPase eventually converts the GTP to GDP on the α subunit. This results in the α and $\beta\gamma$ subunits reassociating and the signal is shut off (see figure).

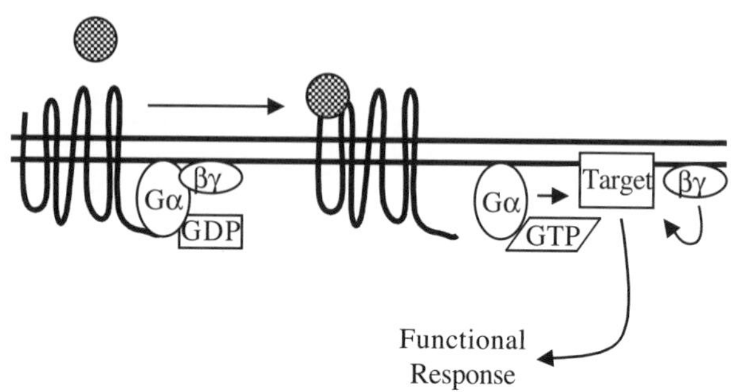

The Gα subunit of a heterotrimeric G protein binds GDP in the inactive state. When a G protein–coupled receptor is bound by its ligand, GDP is exchanged for GTP. The α and $\beta\gamma$ subunits then dissociate. Both the subunits can signal to target molecules resulting in a functional response of the cell. Eventually, the GTP is hydrolyzed to GDP and the G-protein subunits reassociate, terminating the signal.

6. Cyclic adenosine monophosphate (cAMP) is a common second messenger that is produced following GPCR stimulation. Describe the effect of activating the $G\alpha_s$ subunit on cAMP levels.

$G\alpha_s$ stimulates the enzyme adenylyl cyclase. Adenylyl cyclase catalyzes the formation of cAMP from adenosine triphosphate (ATP).

7. How does activation of $G\alpha_i$ alter cAMP levels?

$G\alpha_i$ is an inhibitor of adenylyl cyclase; therefore, levels of cAMP are decreased following activation of $G\alpha_i$.

8. How does *Bordetella pertussis* toxin affect G-protein signaling?

Pertussis toxin transfers an ADP-ribosyl moiety from oxidized nicotinamide adenine dinucleotide (NAD^+) to the α subunit of a G_i protein. This decreases the molecule's affinity for GTP and therefore blocks the ability of G_i to become activated. Furthermore, ADP-ribosylated G_i cannot interact with receptors. This results in elevated levels of cAMP in cells and prevents the actions of ligands that act via G_i signaling. Pertussis toxin does not interfere with the signaling of other G proteins.

9. Explain how cholera toxin alters G-protein signaling.

Cholera toxin transfers an ADP-ribosyl moiety from NAD^+ to the α subunit of G_s. This prevents GTP hydrolysis and therefore results in a persistently activated system. The continued accumulation of cAMP mimics ligand-stimulated activation of adenylyl cyclase. Actions of stimulatory ligands are obscured, because of overactivation of the system. Cholera toxin does not interfere directly with the signaling of other G proteins.

10. How does the increased activity of adenylyl cyclase result in changes in cellular function?

There are several pathways, but one of the most common is the activation of cAMP-dependent protein kinase A (PKA). PKA then can activate (by high-energy phosphate transfer) a number of other key regulatory enzymes within cells. For example, increased cAMP levels can activate hormone-sensitive lipase, resulting in lipolysis and the release of free fatty acids and glycerol into the circulation. Elevated cAMP levels can also result in the phosphorylation of enzymes with the resultant decrease in their activity (e.g., glycogen synthase). This catabolic effect mirrors the lipolytic effect just mentioned. These effects are rapid. (See figure.)

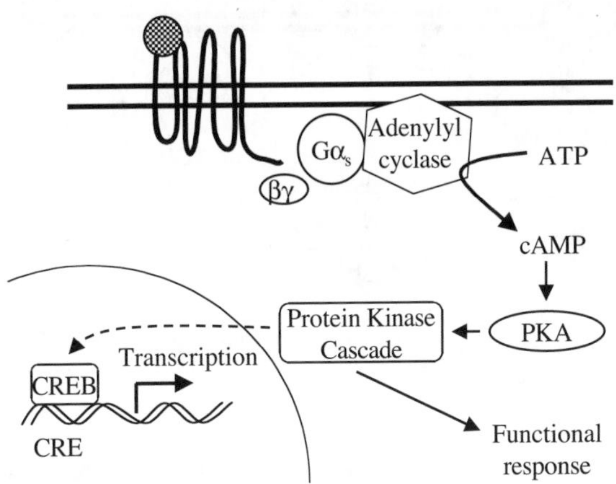

A G protein–coupled receptor that stimulates $G\alpha_s$ leads to the activation of the enzyme adenylyl cyclase. Adenylyl cyclase converts ATP to cyclic AMP, which then activates protein kinase A (PKA). This leads to a protein phosphorylation cascade that will activate or inhibit molecules that regulate transcription of certain genes (e.g., cAMP response element-binding protein [CREB]).

11. Describe how activation of PKA by elevated cellular levels of cAMP also results in more delayed, transcriptional events.

Activated PKA can also phosphorylate a transcription factor (a DNA-binding protein) called **cyclic AMP response element binding protein (CREB).** CREB shuttles to the nucleus where it binds to cyclic AMP response elements (CREs) on the DNA. This binding results in the recruitment of co-activator proteins that facilitate the binding of RNA polymerase II and gene transcription.

12. What is forskolin?

Forskolin is a diterpene that potently stimulates adenylyl cyclase through direct interactions with the catalytic subunit of the enzyme. Forskolin's effects do not depend on the presence of G proteins.

13. What "shuts-off" the cAMP signaling event?

Cyclic nucleotide phosphodiesterases metabolize cAMP to its inactive 5′-adenosine monophosphate configuration. Several hormones, including insulin and α-adrenergic agents, signal by activating cAMP phosphodiesterases, which lower intracellular levels of cAMP.

14. A frequently targeted enzyme for G-proteins is phospholipase C (PLC). For example, vasopressin activates the V_1 receptor in the vasculature via a PLC-dependent pathway. Describe the signaling pathway.

Although vasopressin signals in the kidney via a cAMP-dependent pathway (activation of the V_2 receptor), in vascular smooth muscle the signaling pathway is activation, via G proteins, of membrane-associated phospholipase C (PLC). PLC catalyzes hydrolysis of phosphatidylinositol 4,5-biphosphate (PIP_2) to form diacylglycerol (DAG) and inositol 1,4,5-triphosphate (IP_3). DAG remains in the membrane, where it activates protein kinase C (PKC). When activated, PKC phosphorylates other cellular proteins leading to the biologic response. IP_3 is water soluble, so it diffuses into the cytosol where it associates with a receptor on the endoplasmic reticulum, releasing intracellular stores of free calcium into the cytosol (see figure).

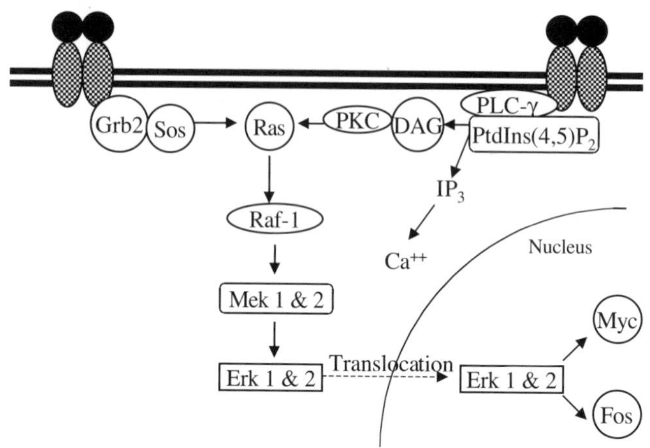

Activation of a receptor tyrosine kinase can activate the MAP kinase cascade through two separate pathways. PLC-γ = phospholipase C-γ; DAG = diacyl glycerol; PtdIns(4,5)P_2 = phosphatidylinositol diphosphate; PKC = protein kinase C; IP_3 = inositol triphosphate; Grb2 = growth factor receptor binding protein; Sos = son of sevenless protein (an adaptor protein).

15. How does activation of PKC by DAG result in biologic responses?

PKC phosphorylates (i.e., activates) serine and threonine residues on a variety of cellular proteins (enzymes). PKC also activates a transcription factor known as **activator protein 1 (AP-1),** which consists of a dimer of two proteins c-*fos* and c-*jun*, both immediate early gene products.

16. A major target of cytosolic free Ca^{++} is the protein calmodulin. Describe calmodulin.

Calmodulin (CAM) is a highly conserved single-chain polypeptide that is found in all eukaryotic cells. The protein contains four Ca^{2+} binding sites. Upon binding of calcium, calmodulin changes conformation and binds to target proteins, which activates them. Calmodulin itself is not an enzyme. A class of molecules that are frequently activated by calmodulin are referred to as CAM kinases, which includes myosin light-chain kinase (MLCK).

17. How do calcium channel blockers cause vasodilation?

Calcium channel blockers decrease the influx of calcium into a cell, reducing the formation of calcium-calmodulin complexes. This reduces the level of activation of MLCK. Activated MLCK phosphorylates myosin light chains, resulting in interaction with actin and contraction. Less calcium entry into the cell means less phosphorylation of the myosin light chains and relaxation.

18. For Ca^{++} to be an effective second messenger, cells must keep their cytoplasmic Ca^{++} levels low. Explain how this is accomplished.

Ca^{++} ATPases on the plasma and endoplasmic reticulum membranes actively pump Ca^{++} out of the cytosol. In addition, the plasma membrane contains Na^+, Ca^{++} pumps. Cytoplasmic Ca^{++} is also actively transported into the mitochondria. Much of the remaining cytoplasmic Ca^{++} is bound by calcium-binding proteins.

19. Adrenergic agonists of the β_2 subclass (e.g., isoproterenol) cause vasodilation by activating adenylyl cyclase. Describe the subsequent step in signaling that causes the vasodilation.

Activation of adenylyl cyclase in vascular smooth muscle results in increased cellular levels of cAMP. This is thought to facilitate phosphorylation of MLCK, converting the enzyme to a less active state.

20. Muscarinic, cholinergic receptors are members of the seven-transmembrane domain receptor family. Once activated, how do they signal?

Muscarinic receptors link via G proteins to signaling cascades that result in activation of phospholipase C (G_q), inhibition of adenylyl cyclase (G_i), or activation of potassium channels (G_i).

21. In addition to activating adenylyl cyclase via a G-protein–linked mechanism, dopamine signals by activating ion channel opening. How does it do this?

Binding of dopamine to the D_2 receptor results in dissociation of the $\beta\gamma$ subunit from the G proteins linked to the dopamine receptor. This $\beta\gamma$ subunit interacts directly with G-protein–linked inward-rectifying potassium channels (GIRKs) resulting in opening of the potassium channels and hyperpolarization, as the ion diffuses out of the cell down its concentration gradient.

22. Describe the mechanisms of prostaglandin signaling.

At least five main types of prostaglandin receptors have been identified, and all signal through G-protein coupled receptors. The signaling mechanisms are cell specific and include stimulation of adenylyl cyclase and PLC activity in platelets and smooth muscle but inhibition of adenylyl cyclase in adipocytes (antagonizes epinephrine's action) and epithelial tissues (blocks the action of vasopressin in renal tubules).

23. Explain how thromboxanes cause platelet aggregation.

Thromboxanes bind to unique receptors on platelets and, through G-protein coupling, subsequently activate PLC. The resultant formation of IP_3 causes calcium release from intracellular stores, promoting aggregation and production of additional thromboxane A_2.

24. What signaling pathway mediates leukotriene-induced bronchoconstriction?

PLC.

25. Describe the two subgroups of purinergic receptors.

The P_1 subgroup is composed of receptors for adenosine (thus adenosine receptors [AR]), whereas the P_2 subgroup is composed of receptors for ATP, ADP, uridine triphosphate (UTP), and uridine diphosphate (UDP).

26. The two subclasses of ARs (P_1 receptors) signal via differing pathways, all utilizing G proteins. What are those pathways?

A_1R in some cells is coupled to the inhibition of adenylyl cyclase via a pertussis toxin–sensitive pathway ($G_{i/o}$). In other tissues, A_1R activation results in increased PLC and PLD activity and in changes in ion channel activity. **A_2R** signals via cholera toxin–sensitive (G_s) adenylyl cyclase and also via PLC (G_q). A_2R activation also results in opening of voltage-gated calcium channels (the P_2X-R subtype) and increases in intracellular calcium via a PLC-dependent mechanism (P_2Y-R subtype).

RECEPTORS AS ENZYMES

27. List the 5 classes of enzyme-linked receptors.

1. Receptor guanylyl cyclases
2. Receptor tyrosine kinases
3. Tyrosine kinase–associated receptors
4. Receptor tyrosine phosphatases
5. Receptor serine threonine kinases

28. What is a receptor tyrosine kinase (RTK)?

RTKs are a large family of receptors that possess a tyrosine kinase domain in their intracellular tail. With the exception of the insulin receptor, all RTKs are composed of a single peptide that spans the plasma membrane once. Most growth factor receptors are RTKs.

29. Describe the events that follow the binding of a growth factor to its receptor.

Most growth factors that bind RTKs are dimers and therefore bind two receptors at the same time. Ligand binding brings two receptors into close enough proximity to allow for autophosphorylation, with each receptor phosphorylating its partner. The insulin receptor is an exception to this general rule. It exists as a preformed dimer. Upon insulin binding, the receptor changes conformation, permitting autophosphorylation. Autophosphorylation of RTKs further activates the tyrosine kinase domain so it is able to phosphorylate other substrates. Furthermore, the phosphorylation of the receptor provides binding sites for signaling molecules, facilitating the initiation of a signaling cascade (see figure).

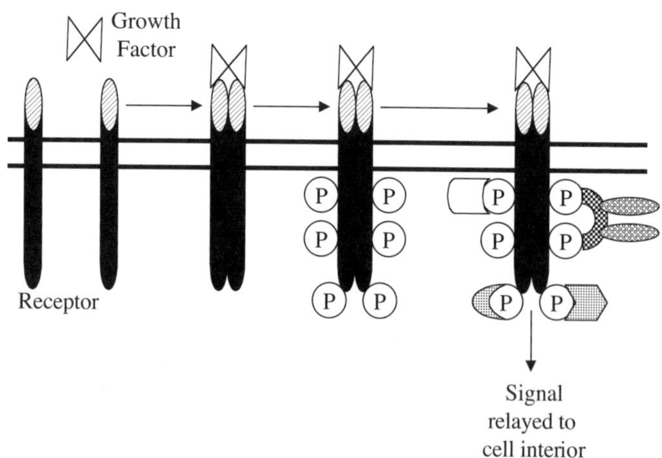

Receptor tyrosine kinases exist as inactive monomers in the plasma membrane. Ligand binding results in dimerization of the receptor and, each receptor transphosphorylating its partner. The phosphorylations provide docking sites for signaling molecules and adaptor proteins (hatched symbol) which relay the signal to the cell interior.

30. Explain the *src* homology 2 (SH2) domain.

SH2 domains bind exclusively to phosphotyrosine residues. SH2 domains are found on many intracellular proteins, including signaling molecules and adaptor proteins. There are often multiple SH2 or other phosphotyrosine-binding domains on each molecule. Each SH2 domain binds to a specific target sequence providing specificity to the down-stream signaling cascade activated by each receptor.

31. What is an adaptor protein?

An adaptor protein, such as Rab2, has no known enzymatic activity but rather contains binding sites for multiple proteins. This allows an adaptor protein to bring several proteins together into a complex that allows interactions among the various components (see figure in question 29).

32. How are RTKs inactivated?

RTKs are inactivated in one of two ways. The cell contains protein tyrosine phosphatases that remove the phosphate moieties from the cytoplasmic tail of the RTK and thus inactivate it. A second method cells use to inactivate RTKs is to dispose of them through endocytosis and then digest the receptor in a lysosome.

33. RTKs activate the GTP-binding protein Ras. Describe Ras and point out the differences between it and the heterotrimeric G proteins.

Ras is a member of a family of small GTP-binding proteins. Ras is monomeric and resembles the α subunit of heterotrimeric G proteins. Similar to the α subunit, Ras cycles between an active state when GTP is bound and an inactive state when GDP is bound. Ras-activating proteins increase the exchange of GDP for GTP thus activating Ras. GTPase-activating proteins (GAPs) increase the hydrolysis of GTP to GDP and switch Ras to an inactive state. Ras promotes the activation of a kinase cascade that ultimately alters the activity of transcription factors resulting in a change in the pattern of gene expression (See figure in question 14.)

34. Ras activates the mitogen-activated protein (MAP) kinase cascade. Detail the members of this cascade.

Ras activates Raf-1 (one of the MAP kinase kinase kinases), which phosphorylates Mek 1 and 2 (two of the MAP kinase kinases), which in turn phosphorylate Erk 1 and 2 (two of the MAP kinases). Phosphorylated Erk is translocated to the nucleus where it activates several transcription factors including c-*fos*, c-*myc*, and C/EBPβ. (See figure in question 14.)

35. Normal cells divide only when stimulated by growth factors. Cancer cells, however, have escaped the control of growth factors and divide autonomously. Describe several mechanisms by which cancer cells escape controlled growth.

Cancer cells often have mutations in genes involved in signaling pathways. In fact, p53, a cell cycle regulatory protein, is one of the most frequently observed mutations in cancer. Other mutation examples include the retinoblastoma protein, Ras, and other G proteins. A second mechanism cancers cells use to escape controlled growth is to mutate an important signaling receptor, leading to a constitutively active pathway.

36. Phospholipase D (PLD) catalyzes the conversion of phospholipids to phosphatidic acid (PA). PA is then converted to diacyl glycerol (DAG), which stimulates PKC activity. What turns on PLD?

Platelet-derived growth factor (PDGF) activates a receptor tyrosine kinase resulting in increased PLC activity and the formation of DAG. DAG activates not only PLC, but also PLD. In addition, PLD activity is directly stimulated by low–molecular-weight G proteins that are activated by yet uncharacterized mechanisms.

37. Drugs in the nitrite/nitrate group, including nitroglycerin and sodium nitroprusside, are remarkable vasodilators. How do they signal?

All agents in this class of drugs cause the formation of nitric oxide (NO) or act as nitric oxide donors. NO activates a soluble guanylyl cyclase resulting in the formation of cGMP. Through still incompletely understood mechanisms, the elevated levels of cGMP cause dephosphorylation of myosin light chains (thus decreasing their interaction with actin) and relaxation (see figure in question 40).

38. Membrane phospholipids serve as substrates for arachidonic acid production. What membrane-bound enzyme catalyzes the conversion of phospholipids to arachidonic acid?

Phospholipase A_2 (PLA_2) (see figure, top of next page).

39. List the potent regulatory molecules derived from arachidonic acid.

Prostaglandins
Prostacyclins
Thromboxanes
Leukotrienes

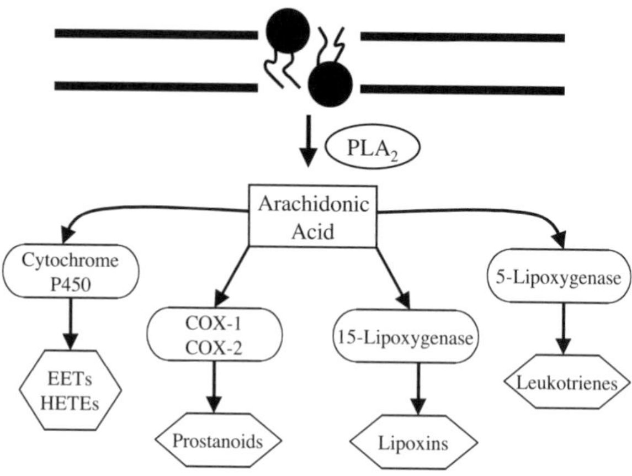

Phospholipase A_2 releases arachidonic acid (AA) from membrane phospholipids. AA itself can act as a messenger molecule or can be metabolized by several enzymes to the eicosanoid messengers. Cytochrome P450 enzymes metabolize AA to the EETs and HETEs family of molecules. Cyclooxygenase 1 and 2 convert AA into the prostanoid family of molecules, which includes the prostaglandins and the thromboxanes. 15-Lipoxygenase converts AA into the lipoxins, lipoprotein A (LPA) and lipoprotein B (LPB). Finally, 5-Lipoxygenase metabolizes AA into leukotrienes.

40. The natriuretic peptides (NPs) are potent vasodilators that act by stimulating the formation of cGMP. How do they do this?

NPs bind to receptors that span the lipid bilayer with a single alpha-helical transmembrane domain. Their cytosolic arm is the catalytic portion of the molecule, including protein kinase and guanylyl cyclase domains. Binding of the ligand (e.g., atrial natriuretic peptide) to the receptor results in activation of its guanylyl cyclase and cGMP formation (see figure).

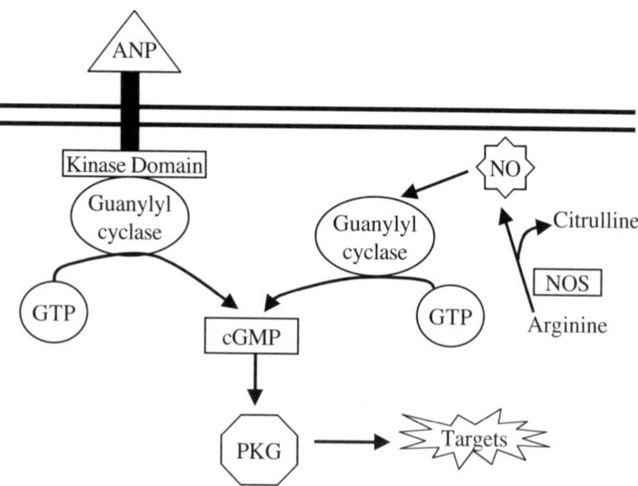

The formation of the second messenger cGMP can be induced through two separate pathways. The natriuretic peptide receptors contain a guanylyl cyclase in their cytoplasmic domain. Additionally, nitric oxide (NO) can stimulate a soluble guanylyl cyclase to produce cGMP. Cyclic GMP then activates protein kinase G (PKG), which begins a protein kinase cascade. ANP = atrial natriuretic peptide; NOS = nitric oxide synthase.

41. What activates PLA_2?

Cardiac PLA_2 is thought to be involved in the actions of lipopolysaccharide, tumor necrosis factor, and mitogenic growth factors. The activity of the enzyme is thought to be secondary to PLC activation, calcium entry, and phosphorylation of MAP-kinase (see figure, top of page 48).

42. Arachidonic acid can be converted to prostaglandins (PGs) and thromboxanes by what enzyme family?

Arachidonic acid is converted first to PGG_2 and then PGH_2 by PGH synthase I (cyclooxygenase 1 [COX-1]) and PGH synthase II (cyclooxygenase 2, [COX-2]). The arachidonic acid cascade is outlined in the top figure on page 48.

43. How do COX-1 and COX-2 differ?

COX-1 is a constitutively expressed enzyme, whereas COX-2 expression is inducible. COX-2 expression is rapidly "turned-on" by lipopolysaccharide (endotoxin) and therefore is an early response gene product of inflammation.

44. How does aspirin influence the inflammatory response?

Aspirin acetylates and inhibits COX-1 and COX-2, blocking the production of prostaglandins and thromboxanes.

45. How do nonsteroidal anti-inflammatory drugs (NSAIDs) work?

They block COX-1 and COX-2 activity. Importantly, selective COX-2 inhibitors are available so that the gastric cytoprotective action of COX-1 can be left unabated, and yet the anti-inflammatory effect of COX-2 inhibition is expressed.

46. Arachidonic acid can also be enzymatically processed to bioactive compounds called the leukotrienes. What enzyme is responsible for the initiation of this pathway?

Lipoxygenase converts arachidonic acid to hydroperoxy-eicosatotranoic acids (HPETEs) and then the hydroxy derivatives, hydroxy-eicosatetraenoic acids (HETEs), and leukotrienes. Leukotrienes are potent bronchoconstrictors, and common asthma therapies target their production or receptor binding. These therapies include lipoxygense inhibitors, phospholipase A_2 inhibitors, and leukotriene receptor antagonists.

47. The transforming growth factor β (TGFβ) superfamily of receptors are serine–threonine kinase receptors. Describe the differences between TGFβ receptors and RTKs.

TGFβ receptors are single transmembrane proteins that exist as disulfide bonded dimers. RTKs also span the plasma membrane once; however, they usually exist as monomers. After ligand binding, the TGFβ receptors form heteromeric complexes, whereas RTKs form homodimers. The type 2 TGFβ receptor is constitutively active. When in close proximity to a type 1 receptor it phosphorylates the receptor on specific serine and threonine residues (as opposed to tyrosine

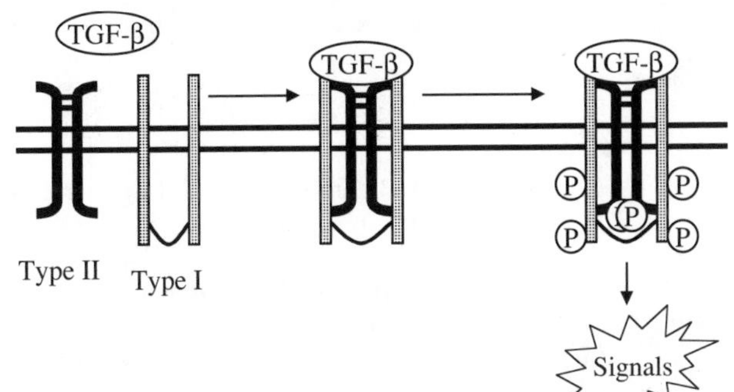

Transforming growth factor β (TGFβ) is an example of a ligand that binds to a serine threonine kinase receptor. Two types of TGFβ receptors exist as homodimers. TGFβ causes the heteromultimerization of the type 1 and type 2 receptor complexes. The two receptor types transphosphorylate each other, activating the receptor complex to relay signals to the interior of the cell.

residues on RTKs) and activates it. The TGFβ type 2 receptor then transphosphorylates its partner initiating a signaling cascade (see figure).

48. List the major classes of ligands for the cytokine class I receptor.

1. Receptors sharing gp130 signal transduction components: interleukin 6 (IL-6), IL-11, leukemia inhibitory factor (LIF), ciliary neurotrophic factor (CNTF), and cardiotropin 1
2. Receptors with a ligand-specific subunit and an associated βc subunit: IL-3, IL-5, and granulocyte-macrophage colony stimulating factor (GM-CSF)
3. Receptors with a ligand-specific subunit and an associated γc subunit: IL-2, IL-4, IL-7, and IL-9
4. Receptors with a ligand-specific subunit and no additional, required subunit: IL-12, erythropoietin (EPO), granulocyte colony stimulating factor (G-CSF), thromopoietin (TPO), prolactin (PRL), and growth hormone (GH)

49. Cytokines that bind to the hematopoietin and interferon receptors (cytokine class I receptors) activate a family of tyrosine kinases called Janus kinases. How do those Janus kinases transduce the signal of cytokines such as IL-2 and IL-3?

These cytokines signal through a heterodimeric family of tyrosine kinase receptors (Janus kinases) that phosphorylate cytoplasmic proteins called **signal transduction activators of transcriptions** (STATs). This leads to dimerization of these proteins and translocation to the nucleus where they activate specific genes. Many of those genes are necessary for growth and differentiation (see figure).

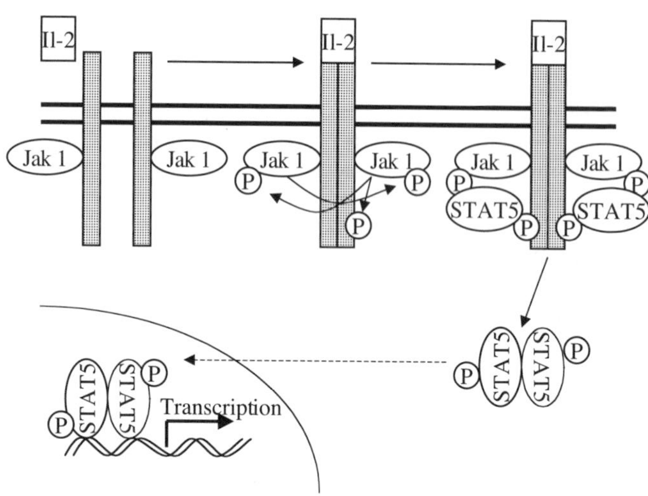

Interleukin 2 (Il-2) binds to its receptor causing dimerization and activation of Janus kinases (Jak). These kinases then phosphorylate STAT proteins which translocate to the nucleus where they activate gene transcription.

50. Name the two classes of ligands that class II cytokine receptors recognize.

Class II cytokine receptors bind **interferons** and **IL-10.**

51. Signaling through the cytokine II receptors leads to transcriptional activation via activation of what promoter elements in the DNA of inducible genes?

Type I interferons signal via IFN-stimulatable response elements (ISREs) and gamma activation sites (GAS). IL-10 also activates GAS.

52. Lipopolysaccharide (LPS) and other microbial products can activate lymphocyte production of the transcription factor nuclear factor (NFκB), as can the cytokine IL-1. What do these two signaling pathways have in common?

LPS signals through the Toll receptor, which has a unique sequence in its cytoplasmic tail. This sequence, known as the TIR domain (Toll/IL-1R), is shared by the IL-1 receptor. Binding of either LPS or IL-1 results in activation of the TIR, which then recruits and activates a cytoplasmic adapter protein called myeloid differentiation factor 88 (MyD88). MyD88 also possesses a domain important for protein–protein interactions known as the death domain. Through a series of intermediary steps, this leads to the dimerization and activation of two kinases that phosphorylate another protein called IκB. IκB is a cytosolic protein that binds to and inhibits the activity of another cytosolic protein NFκB. Phosphorylation of IκB releases it from NFκB. NFκB then enters the nucleus and acts as a transcription factor, activating genes responsible for adaptive immunity and the production of cytokines (see figure).

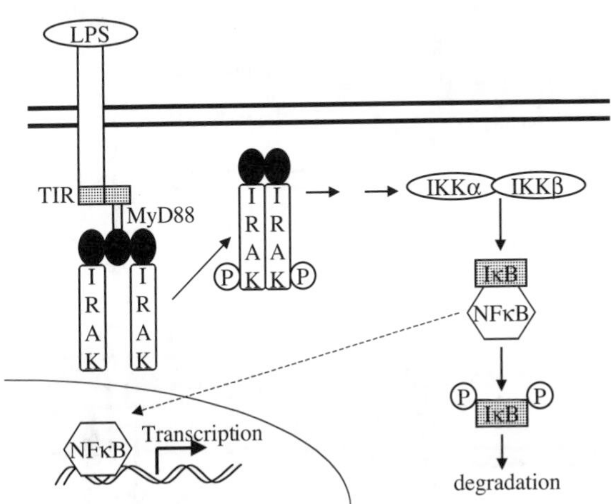

The endotoxin lipopolysaccharide (LPS) binds to a Toll receptor. The receptor contains a TIR domain that recruits myeloid differentiation factor 88 (MyD88), an adaptor protein, which also contains a TIR. The tail of MyD88 contains a death domain that binds to the death domain of an Il-1 receptor–associated kinase (IRAK), facilitating its activation. IRAK then initiates a cascade that results in activation of the Iκ kinases (IKKα and β), which phosphorylate IκB (inhibitor of NFκB). IκB is degraded, allowing NFκB to translocate to the nucleus and induce transcription of the gene associated with apoptosis.

ION CHANNEL–LINKED RECEPTORS

53. Glycine and gamma aminobutyric acid (GABA) are inhibitory neurotransmitters in the brain and spinal cord. How do they signal?

GABA and glycine receptors belong, along with nicotinic cholinergic receptors, to a class of neurotransmitter receptors called **ligand-gated ion channels.** Whereas acetylcholine-activated channels conduct sodium and potassium (with sodium predominating, thus the acetylcholine receptors are excitatory ligand-gated channels), both the glycine and the GABA channels conduct chloride. When chloride diffuses down its concentration gradient into a cell, it carries with it a negative charge, further hyperpolarizing the cell.

54. Glutamate is the major excitatory neurotransmitter in brain. How does glutamate signal?

Glutamate binds to excitatory amino acid (EAA) receptors. Of the five classes of EAA receptors, four are ligand-gated channels (called **ionotropic EAA receptors**). The fifth is known as the **metabotropic EAA** receptor.

55. The two major classes of ionotropic EAA receptors can be distinguished by their ligand specificity and their ion selectivity. One binds N-methyl-D-aspartate (NMDA) and the other does not. Explain how they differ in terms of their gating properties.

Non-NMDA EAA receptors open in the presence of glutamate, allowing entry of sodium and the exit of intracellular potassium. Because the sodium flux is greater than that of potassium, the effect is to depolarize the cell. NMDA receptors have a high permeability for calcium in addition to sodium and potassium. The NMDA receptor is blocked by physiologic levels of magnesium, and that block is released upon depolarization. Thus, glutamate acts first via the non-NMDA receptors (also called AMPA and kainate receptors because of their selectivity for the synthetic ligands alpha-amino-3-hydroxy-5-methyl-4-isoxazole propionic acid [AMPA] and kainate, respectively), causing rapid phase depolarizations called **excitatory postsynaptic potentials (EPSPs).** Then the NMDA receptor is activated (when the inhibition by magnesium is released) and calcium flows into the cell, further depolarizing the membrane. The presence of glycine enhances the activity of glutamate on the NMDA receptor (see figure).

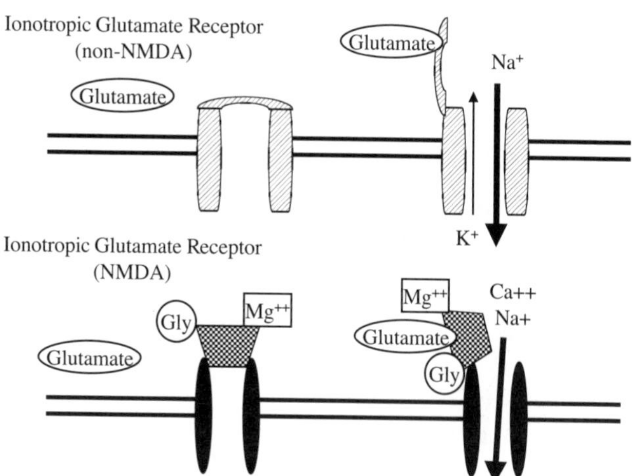

Glutamate causes rapid sodium entry into cells by binding to ionotropic, non-NMDA receptors. These localized membrane depolarizations facilitate opening of a second class of ionotropic glutamate receptors, NMDA receptors, by releasing the inhibitory action of magnesium. Once this blockade is released, the NMDA receptor opens, facilitated by an associated glycine molecule. Both calcium and sodium enter the cell, causing a more sustained depolarization to threshold and, therefore, increased action potential frequency.

56. How do metabotropic EAA receptors signal?

Metabotropic EAA receptors signal via G-protein linked pathways. Excitatory metabotropic EAA receptor activation can activate PLC with the formation of IP_3 and closure of potassium channels due to increasing cytosolic calcium levels. Closure of the potassium leak channels results in local depolarization of the membrane. A similar mechanism is thought to underlie the activation of adenylyl cyclase by the metabotropic EAA receptor. Inhibitory metabotropic EAA receptor activation hyperpolarizes the membrane due to closure of calcium channels, decreasing calcium conductance.

57. How do nicotinic cholinergic receptors signal?

Nicotinic cholinergic receptors, present in neuromuscular junctions, are composed of five subunits derived from four unique genes. These subunits surround a channel through which ions can cross the lipid bilayer. When activated, the channel permits primarily the diffusion of sodium into the cell (i.e., down its concentration gradient), resulting in depolarization.

STEROID RECEPTORS

58. How do steroid hormones exert long-term actions on cells?

Steroids enter the cell and bind to receptors present in the cytosol or nucleus. Once the ligand-receptor complexes have formed, they act as transcription factors, altering the expression of genes related to cell growth and differentiation.

59. What steroid hormone receptors are present in the cytosol and how are they maintained in that compartment?

Receptors for glucocorticoids, progesterone, estrogen, androgens, and mineralocorticoids are present in the cytosol as monomers, associated with chaperone proteins (heat shock proteins [HSPs]). Once the steroid binds, the HSPs are released and the receptors dimerize. After translocation to the nucleus, these receptor-hormone complexes bind to hormone response elements (HREs) in the DNA, recruit co-activators, and initiate transcription (see figure).

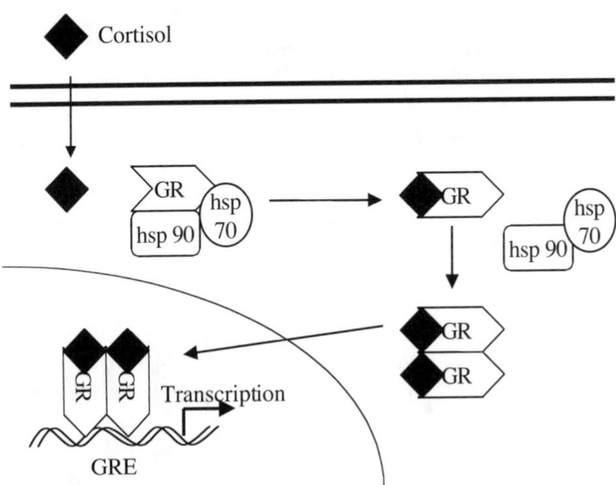

Cortisol enters a cell where it associates with its cytosolic receptor. This releases the receptor from inhibitory chaperone molecules allowing receptor dimerization. The complex then enters the nucleus and associates with other transcription factors, leading to gene activation.

60. What steroid hormone receptors are present in the nucleus and where are they?

Receptors for thyroid hormones, retinoic acid, and 1,25-dihydroxyvitamin D are not complexed with HSPs but instead are associated, as dimers, with the HREs in the DNA. Binding of the hormone activates these HREs.

61. The activated estrogen receptor binds to a unique HRE; however, a single HRE is shared by the activated gluco- and mineralocorticoid receptors and the progesterone and the androgen receptors. What then determine specificity of cellular response to these four hormones?

Because these four hormone-receptor complexes recognize the same HRE, specificity is dictated by the unique cellular expression of one or more of these receptors.

62. In the absence of ligand, the thyroid hormone receptor binds to its HRE in the DNA in association with the retinoid-X receptor (RXR). This receptor recruits co-repressors of transcription. Describe how this occurs.

The "free" thyroid hormone receptor–RXR associates with complexes containing histone deacetylases that maintain the heterochromatin in the closed state. Upon binding of thyroid hormone to its receptor, the co-repressors are replaced by co-activators containing histone acetylases. The heterochromatin then is in the open configuration and transcription initiates.

63. Are all steroid receptors intracellular?

Evidence has accumulated that steroids also bind to cell surface receptors, stimulating rapid cellular responses through nongenomic signaling pathways. For example, estrogen can alter the membrane polarization state in hypothalamic neurons and cultured vascular smooth muscle cells by a combination of effects on neurotransmitter receptors and ion channels. Estrogens have also been demonstrated to signal through phospholipase C and adenylyl cyclase.

64. What anti-inflammatory drugs are thought to act at least in part by inhibiting PLA_2 activity?

Glucorticoids (e.g., prednisone).

65. In addition to inhibiting PLA_2 activity, where do glucocorticoids act in the arachidonic acid metabolism pathway to express their anti-inflammatory actions?

Glucocorticoids inhibit cyclooxygenase (decrease prostaglandin and thromboxane production) and block the action of leukotrienes. Glucocorticoids also act directly to suppress immune cell function.

66. What is the cause of hyperthyroidism with diffuse goiter (Graves' disease)?

Graves' disease is caused by autoantibodies that recognize the thyroid-stimulating hormone (TSH) receptor on the thyroid follicular cells. Binding of the antibodies to the TSH receptor activates the receptor cascade, resulting in increased production and release of thyroid hormones. Normally, TSH secretion is suppressed by increasing levels of thyroid hormones, but in this disease the autoantibodies are not affected by circulating hormone levels so the stimulation of the follicular cell goes unabated, accounting for the high circulating levels of T_3 and T_4 and the enlargement of the gland.

67. Autoantibodies can also result in inflammatory destruction of a particular cell type and organ. What are two examples of this receptor-mediated phenomenon?

Autoantibodies are the basis of tissue destruction in Hashimoto's disease (autoimmune thyroiditis) and primary adrenal insufficiency (Addison's disease).

RECEPTOR KINETICS

68. What defines the specificity of a receptor?

The specificity of a receptor is defined by its affinity for the primary ligand relative to its ability to bind related molecules.

69. How does the binding of a few ligands to their receptors lead to a large cellular response?

The signal is amplified at each step. For example, the activation of one receptor may activate 10 heterotrimeric G proteins. Each α and $\beta\gamma$ subunit activates 10 target molecules (so a total of 100 of each target molecule is activated). The amplification continues through all the signaling steps so that numerous molecules of the final target are activated.

70. How is the affinity of a receptor for a given ligand defined?

The **equilibrium dissociation constant (K_d)** defines the affinity of a receptor for its ligand. If there is only a single class of binding sites, the K_d is the concentration of ligand needed to bind half of the receptors at equilibrium.

71. Describe the difference between K_d and median effective concentration (EC_{50}).

K_d is the amount of ligand required to occupy 50% of its receptors. EC_{50} is the amount of ligand required to obtain 50% of the maximum response.

72. What is a competitive antagonist?

A **competitive antagonist** is a ligand that binds to a receptor but does not activate the normal biologic response. Competitive agonists are said to *compete* with the primary ligand for sites on the receptor (see figure).

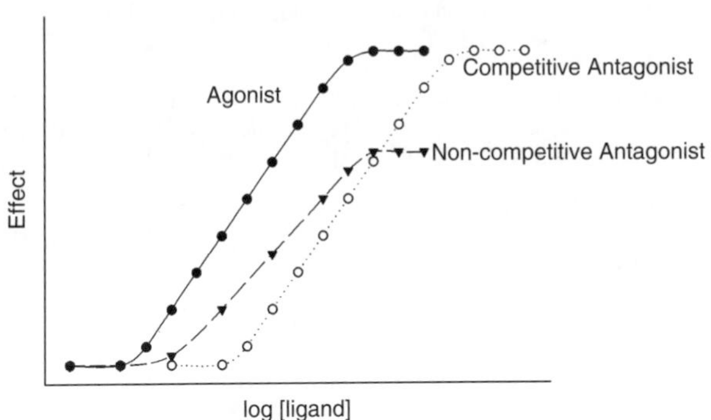

An agonist is a compound that binds to a receptor, eliciting a dose-related, characteristic biologic response. A competitive antagonist binds to the same receptor as the agonist, blocking its binding. This results in higher concentrations of agonist required to elicit full biologic activity. Importantly, this right-dose shift does not alter the maximum response that can be generated. A noncompetitive antagonist binds to the same receptor but cannot be displaced by high concentrations of agonist. This shifts the response curve to the right and lowers the maximum attainable biologic response.

73. What is a noncompetitive antagonist?

A **noncompetitive antagonist,** also called an **irreversible antagonist,** is a ligand that binds the receptor with such high affinity (and does not elicit a biologic response) that the receptor is unavailable for binding to the primary ligand. The maximum effect elicited by the primary ligand even if higher doses are present is, therefore, reduced. (The figure question 72 compares a competitive antagonist to a noncompetitive antagonist.)

74. How does receptor desensitization differ from receptor downregulation?

Receptor downregulation occurs when the number of receptors on the cell surface declines. This is often a result of binding of ligand and subsequent internalization of the ligand-receptor complex. If the rate of replacement of new receptors into the cell membrane does not keep pace, fewer receptors are available for binding to the ligands appearing at the cell surface. Desensitization does not involve a decrease in receptor number but instead involves an "exhaustion" of the signaling cascade downstream from the receptor. In the case of the β-adrenergic receptor, binding of ligand results in phosphorylation of serine moieties in the receptor's cytoplasmic tail by the enzyme β-adrenoreceptor kinase. The phosphorylated serines increase the binding of the cytoplasmic tail to beta-arrestin, a molecule that, once bound, hinders the interaction of the receptor with its G protein (G_s), resulting in less agonist response.

75. The amount of any protein, including receptors and members of the signaling cascades, can be regulated in three different manners. Describe them.

1. **Transcriptional regulation.** The amount of RNA produced can be altered.
2. **Translational regulation.** The amount of protein produced can be altered, usually by changing the stability of the RNA.

3. **Protein modification.** This includes the phosphorylation state, glycosylation, ubiquitination (degradation), and other posttranslational modifications that alter the proteins function or location in the cell.

BIBLIOGRAPHY

1. Alberts B, Bray D, Lewis J, et al: Molecular Biology of the Cell, 4th ed. New York, Garland Publishing, 1998.
2. Gomperts BD, Kramer IM, Tathom PER: Signal Transduction. San Diego, Academic Press, 2002.
3. Griffin JE, Ojeda SR (eds): Textbook of Endocrine Physiology, 4th ed. New York, Oxford Press, 2000.
4. Hardman JG, Limbird LE (eds): Goodman & Gilman's The Pharmacologic Basis of Therapeutics, 9th ed. New York, McGraw-Hill, 1996.
5. Heldin CH, Purton M (eds): Signal Transduction. Cheltenham, UK, Stanley Thornes Ltd, 1998.
6. Johnson LR (ed): Essential Medical Physiology, 2nd ed. Philadelphia, Lippincott-Raven, 1998.
7. Katzung BG (ed): Basic and Clinical Pharmacology, 7th ed. Stamford, CT, Appleton & Lange, 1998.

3. PHYSIOLOGIC GENOMICS: ATTACHING BIOLOGY TO THE GENOME

Anne E. *Kwitek, Ph*.D.

1. What is a genome?

The **genome** is, collectively, all of the DNA on all chromosomes in the nucleus of a cell, including genes and regulatory sequences.

2. Define genomics.

Genomics is the study of the structure and function of very large numbers of genes undertaken in a simultaneous fashion.

3. What is physiologic genomics?

Physiologic genomics, or functional genomics, is the merging of physiology and genomics to determine disease mechanism, essentially attaching biology and pathobiology to the genome.

4. What are the differences among monogenic, polygenic, and multifactorial diseases?

A **monogenic** disease is one that is caused by dysfunction of a single gene. An example of this type of disease is cystic fibrosis, which is caused by a mutation in *CFTR*. These types of diseases have a very clear pattern of inheritance and are relatively rare.

A **polygenic** disease is one that is caused by the action of multiple genes. These genes may act in an additive or interactive manner to cause a particular phenotype.

A **multifactorial** disease is one that is caused by both genetic and environmental factors. Multifactorial diseases are by far the most common form of human disease. Essential hypertension, autoimmune disease, obesity, heart disease, and behavioral and psychiatric disorders are just a few examples of this type of human disease involving genetic components. In the case of hypertension, for example, an estimated 30–50% of the variation in blood pressure is due to the genetic contribution, with the remainder due to environment. Studies indicate not only that environmental stressors and genetic factors independently affect blood pressure, but also that gene–environment interactions play an important role in hypertension. Individuals having the same genetic predisposition to hypertension may or may not be hypertensive, depending on their environment, and individuals in the same environment may or may not develop hypertension, depending on their genetic makeup.

5. What is the difference between a qualitative and a quantitative trait?

A **qualitative** trait is one that is either present or absent, such as sickle cell anemia or cystic fibrosis. A **quantitative** trait is one with a continuous distribution of measurement, such as height, weight, and blood pressure.

6. Why are inbred strains used to study the genetic contribution to quantitative traits?

All members of an inbred strain are essentially biologic twins, generated by consecutive breeding of brother–sister pairs for at least 20 generations. Inbred strains for a particular trait are generated by selecting offspring at one extreme of a phenotypic distribution for the next generation of breeding. More than 200 inbred strains of rats are currently available, primarily polygenic models of human disease with unique biology. Using inbred strains for genetic mapping of quantitative traits is advantageous because they provide natural variants but with reduced heterogeneity (both genetic and etiologic). Crosses between disease and control strains of inbred animals can be used to link traits to the genome.

7. Describe how genetics can be used to generate a linkage map.

Mammals are diploid organisms, meaning they contain two copies of their genetic information, one maternally inherited and one paternally inherited. Thus, each gene is present in two copies; these copies may have slightly different variants, or alleles.

During meiosis, when germ cells are being generated, homologous chromosomes sometimes recombine, exchanging homologous genetic material. Two genes that segregate independently (i.e., on different chromosomes) show up in the progeny in parental combinations 50% of the time and in a new, recombinant combination 50% of the time. However, genes on the same chromosome will remain in parental configuration unless there is a crossover between them; the farther apart two genes are, the more likely that there will be a crossover between them. The percentage of recombinant offspring can be used as a measure of physical distance, making a genetic **linkage map**.

Linkage maps are based on probability, so there is always some uncertainty in marker location. Linkage is defined as $< 50\%$ recombination, but 47% recombination is not a reassuring or reliable distance. Therefore, a genetic map needs many **genetic markers**.

8. What is a genetic marker?

A **genetic marker** is a chromosomal locus with allelic variation that can be directly assayed by methods such as the polymerase chain reaction (PCR). The outcome of these assays provides **genotypes,** or a score of the two alleles of that genetic marker. Commonly used genetic markers include:

- **Simple sequence-length polymorphisms (SSLPs)**. SSLPs are short tandem stretches of repetitive nucleotide sequence (e.g., $(CA)_n$) that vary in length. These markers occur approximately every 30 kilobase pairs of DNA and generally have multiple alleles (variation in length).
- **Single nucleotide polymorphisms (SNPs)**. SNPs are single nucleotide variants that arise as random mutations and are quite common; two unrelated individuals differ by about 1 SNP every 1000 base pairs (bp). To be useful, an SNP must occur at a frequency greater than 1% in the general population.

9. What is quantitative trait locus mapping?

Quantitative trait loci (QTL) are regions of the genome containing a gene that plays a role in a quantitative trait. These regions of the genome are determined by identifying a genetic link between a particular trait and a specific genetic marker that tags the genome region.

10. How are genetic crosses used to find QTL?

A cross between two inbred strains can be used to link a phenotype to the genome, if the alleles differ between the two strains (see figure). Two inbred strains (P_0), one selected for a high

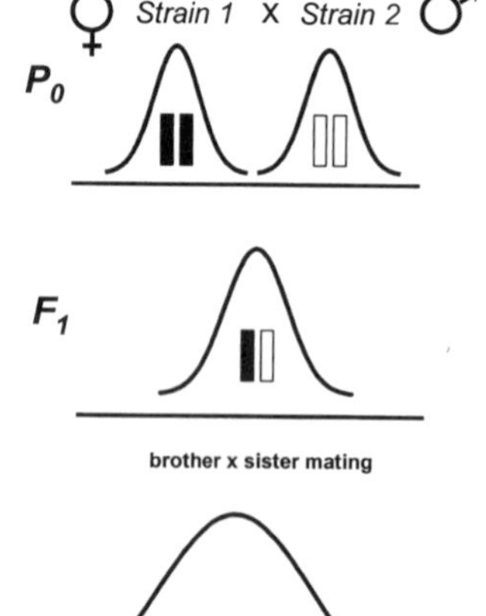

A cross between two inbred strains (P_0) with differing alleles, generating offspring called the first filial (F_1) generation. Brother-sister mating within the F_1 generation produces the second filial (F_2) generation. These offspring can be used to map quantitative trait loci (QTL).

distribution of a quantitative trait (e.g., high blood pressure) and one with a low distribution of a quantitative trait (e.g., low blood pressure) can be crossed to generate offspring, called the first filial (F_1) generation. The variance of the phenotype in both the P_0 and the F_1 populations is due to the environment, because, in each population, all of the animals are genetically identical. Intercrossing the F_1 offspring produces F_2 offspring that can be used for genetic analysis. These animals have various combinations of alleles from the grandparental strains, due to recombination, and have a wider distribution of the phenotype, because of genetic and environmental contribution. However, the environmental contribution can be estimated from the variation due to environment in the parental (F_1) and grandparental populations. Generally, genotypes are determined for markers distributed across the entire genome to determine the cosegregation of the phenotype with a particular genetic marker, thus linking it to a specific region of the genome (a genome scan).

11. What are intermediate phenotypes?

Almost by definition, complex, multifactorial traits are quite far removed from the direct effects of causative genes, because the final phenotype is determined by the interaction of multiple genetic and environmental factors. Consequently, a QTL is not very precise, genetically speaking, which presents a major limitation with respect to identifying the responsible gene. An **intermediate phenotype** is a more precise measurement, directly resulting from the effect of a single allele. If intermediate phenotypes were known, they would be measured and studied rather than, or in addition to, the multifactorial trait. Intermediate phenotypes need to be identified before invoking their use to find genes responsible for QTL. To be more precise, the definition of intermediate phenotype should include genetic evidence that a phenotype maps to a single QTL, rather than simply picking a phenotype that, based on physiologic or other biologic data, could potentially contribute to the phenotype.

12. What are likely determinant phenotypes?

In the absence of actual knowledge, phenotypes that *may* contribute to a trait can be defined as **likely determinant phenotypes**. If a likely determinate phenotype maps to a QTL, it does not immediately qualify as an intermediate phenotype, because it may itself be a complex trait still too far removed from the gene to be useful for positional cloning. For example, QTLs for blood pressure and peripheral vascular resistance map to the same region. There are many ways to modify peripheral vascular resistance, so, although it is perhaps closer to an intermediate phenotype, it does not meet the definition of being caused by a single gene. In fact, it could be argued that in advance of identifying the gene within the QTL, the intermediate phenotype is unknown. Likely determinant phenotypes are currently underutilized but should become more common, because some of these will lead to intermediate phenotypes that can be used for studies in human and other mammals.

13. Once a QTL has been identified, what steps can be taken to determine the genes contributing to the QTL?

To effectively reduce the complexity of a multigenic disease, one can design animals with only a region of interest (ROI) containing a QTL from one strain introgressed onto the background of another. One such type of "designer" strain is the **congenic rat,** which is produced by performing a series of backcrosses and using genetic markers to select for the region of interest, followed by an intercross to fix the selected region (see figure). Each backcross fixes 50% of the genome for the recipient strain while retaining the ROI from the donor strain. By generating reciprocal congenics (i.e., the ROI from the disease strain introgressed onto the background of the control strain, and the ROI from the control strain introgressed onto the background of the disease strain), a classic two-by-two design can be generated for functional studies. One would expect the first congenic to have a phenotype more similar to that of the disease strain, even though the majority of the genome comes from the control strain and vice versa for the second congenic. It is also possible to combine congenic regions in a single animal by simply crossing the two different congenics, allowing reconstruction of the disease pathway in a controlled fashion. Furthermore, positional cloning efforts can be aided with congenic strains. Because of recombina-

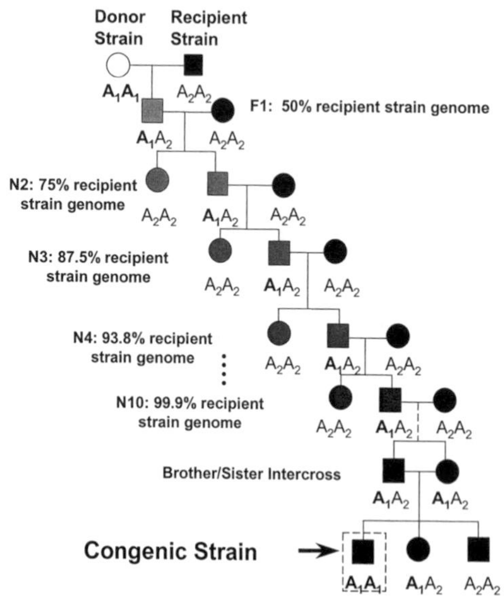

A congenic strain is produced by backcrossing and using genetic markers to select for the region of interest (ROI). Each backcross fixes 50% of the genome for the recipient strain while retaining the ROI from the donor strain.

tion, backcrossing the congenic to the parental strain, intercrossing the offspring and comparing the phenotypes of the F_2 can narrow the interval containing the QTL.

Another powerful method of transferring a region containing a gene of interest in the rat is the **consomic,** or chromosome transfer, approach. By breeding techniques similar to that of congenics, an entire chromosome, rather than only a region of interest, is transferred from one strain to another. Consomics are useful for many reasons. By comparing a trait between a panel of consomics and their respective control animal, one essentially can map a trait to a chromosome without performing a total genome scan. Consomic animals also can be used to produce congenics by a backcross to the background strain followed by an F_1 intercross. Furthermore, modifier loci can be detected by crossing a consomic to the strain for which the consomic chromosome is fixed and then performing an F_1 intercross. This cross results in animals fixed for the consomic chromosome, with the rest of the genome a mixture between the test and the control strains. A total genome scan can then be performed to map modifier loci.

14. How is positional cloning used to identify a gene causing a trait?

Positional cloning involves using linkage mapping to determine the location of a disease gene. Using additional genetic markers in the mapped region, the critical region of interest is pinpointed by relating genotype with phenotype at high resolution. Then, available genomic resources are used to isolate the DNA from the region, to identify and sequence the disease gene, and to identify mutations.

15. What are the downfalls of QTL mapping for complex disease studies?

Although QTL mapping has become easier with the availability of larger numbers of genetic markers, identifying the genes that underlie QTL associated with common phenotypes has proven to be a challenge. Too many genetic variants in humans, too few alleles in inbred animal models, and the potential involvement of many genes within a single QTL have hindered our ability to prove unequivocally the causal role of a gene in a QTL

16. What are other means of linking biology to the genome?

1. A direct way to identify genes affecting a particular trait is to alter genes (**mutagenesis**) and determine if the trait is affected.

- A very powerful and much used mutagenesis approach is **targeted mutagenesis,** generating a loss-of-function mutation of a specific gene of interest by knockouts, or conditional and inducible knockouts, and determining if the trait is affected.

- Another, more comprehensive approach is **gene-trap mutagenesis,** whereby genes expressed under a specified set of conditions are disrupted and screened for interesting phenotypes.
- The most global mutagenesis approach is **ENU (N-ethyl-nitrosurea) mutagenesis**. In this approach, genes are randomly mutated by chemical mutagenesis. A series of phenotypes can be evaluated to determine traits that are affected by the mutations. Traditional mapping and positional cloning approaches can then be used to identify the disrupted gene.

The disadvantage of mutagenesis is that knocking out one gene that affects a complex trait may not result in a phenotypic outcome, because of interacting or modifying genes or homeostasis. Furthermore, gene knockout technology is not available in rats because there are no viable embryonic stem cell lines

2. **Microarray analysis** can be used to evaluate global gene expression in altered disease states and potentially lead to the discovery of new disease genes and pathways. This approach involves spotting minute amounts of cDNA (DNA corresponding to gene sequences) onto a glass slide and hybridizing a pooled sample of mRNA from tissue from "disease" and "nondisease" individuals or animals, each labeled with a different fluorescent dye (see figure). The relative

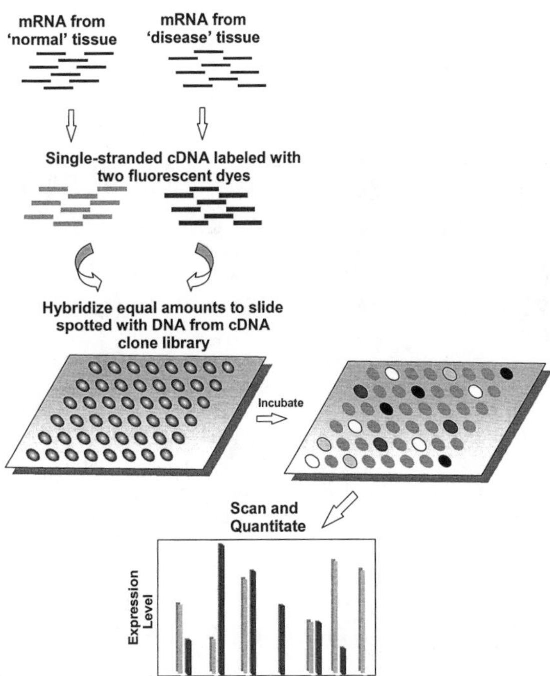

Microarray analysis.

amount of each mRNA is calculated based on the fluorescence intensity corresponding to the relative level of gene expression in the two tissues. Comparing the expression levels in the disease and nondisease tissue can determine which genes are upregulated or downregulated with respect to disease state. Because the identities of the genes spotted on the slide are known (i.e., their sequence has been determined), candidate genes for the trait, either causal or within the disease pathway, can be found and subjected to further analysis.

17. What is comparative mapping and how can it be used to study complex traits?

The primary selection criteria for the animal models have been disease-based phenotypic characteristics similar to human. Indeed, many rat and mouse models share pathobiologic characteristics similar to a human condition. However, in order to determine that genes contributing to a disease in a model organism also contribute to the clinical outcome, model organisms should match human at both the phenotypic and genotypic level.

Comparative mapping identifies regions of a genome that are evolutionarily conserved with that of another species, a phenomenon seen in mammalian species. Evolutionarily, mouse and rat are separated by approximately 10–15 million years, and human and murine (including rat and mouse) are separated by about 80 million years. Consequently, fewer evolutionary genome rearrangements exist between the rat and mouse as compared to rat and human. As genetic and physical maps of human and model organisms developed with the advent of the Human Genome Project in the 1990s, and as the number of identified genes increased, the number of possible integration points dramatically enhanced the potential quality and density of comparative maps. Sequence comparisons have helped to identify orthologous genes (homologous genes in different species evolving from the same common ancestral gene). When mapped in both species, these orthologs serve as anchors useful in identifying conserved segments between species (see figure).

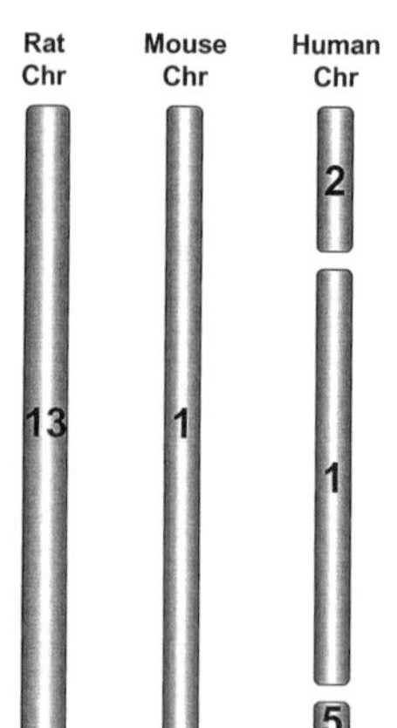

Comparative mapping of rat, mouse, and human genomes. Rat chromosome 13 (*left*) is evolutionarily conserved with a portion of mouse chromosome 1 (*middle*) and portions of human chromosomes 2, 1, and 5 (*right*).

The wealth of genomic resources available in the rat facilitates the generation of a mammalian genome platform among rat, mouse, and human. This platform, which merges the genomes of these three species by comparative mapping, allows transfer of data between the rat (with the bulk of the physiologic and pharmacologic data), the mouse (with the bulk of the gene discovery tools), and the human (with complete genome sequence and clinical data).

BIBLIOGRAPHY

1. Jacob HJ, Kwitek AE: Rat genetics: Attaching physiology and pharmacology to the genome. Nature Rev Genetics 3:33–42, 2002.
2. Rapp JP: Genetic analysis of inherited hypertension in the rat. Physiol Rev 80:135–172, 2000.
3. Schork NJ, Chakravarti A: A nonmathematical overview of modern gene mapping techniques applied to human diseases. In Mockrin S (ed): Molecular Genetics and Gene Therapy of Cardiovascular Diseases. New York, Marcel Dekker, 1996, pp 79–109.

II. Organ System Physiology

4. CARDIOVASCULAR PHYSIOLOGY

Jeanne L. Seagard, Ph.D.

BLOOD

1. What are the components that make up blood?

Blood is a two-phased fluid consisting of formed cellular elements suspended in a liquid medium, the **plasma**. The formed elements are **red cells (erythrocytes), white cells (leukocytes)**, and **platelets**.

2. What are the parts of the plasma?

The plasma, or fluid fraction of the blood, normally occupies about 55% of the blood volume. The normal concentrations of some of the constituents of plasma are as follows:

	PLASMA (mOsm/L OF H_2O)
Na^+	142
K^+	4.2
Ca^{++}	1.3
Mg^+	0.8
Cl^-	108
HCO_3^-	24
HPO_4^-, $H_2PO_4^-$	2
SO_4^-	0.5
Amino acids	2
Creatine	0.2
Lactate	1.2
Glucose	5.6
Protein	1.2
Urea	4
Others	4.8
Total mOsm/L	301.8
Corrected osmolar activity (mOsm/L)	282.0
Total osmotic pressure 37°C (mmHg)	5443

3. What is the hematocrit?

If a blood sample from an adult is centrifuged in a graduated test tube, the relative volume of the packed red cells is termed the *hematocrit*. For a normal adult, this volume is about 40–45% of the total. That is, the red cells occupy about 40–45% of the total volume of the blood in the body. The white blood cells, which are less dense than the red cells, form a thin layer (the so-called buffy coat.) The remaining 55–60% of the volume is the plasma. An increase in hematocrit occurs in people acclimatized to high altitude, where there is an associated decrease in oxygen level. The hematocrit in this case can be 60–65% of the total blood volume.

4. How many red blood cells are there?

In a normal adult, there are between 4.5 million and 6 million red blood cells per milliliter of peripheral blood. More than the normal red cell volume or a greater hematocrit is known as **polycythemia**. A decreased hematocrit is known as **anemia**.

5. How many white blood cells are there?

The number of white cells in the circulation can be quite variable. In a normal individual, there are between 5000 and 10,000 white blood cells per milliliter of normal peripheral blood. The white cells are mainly involved in the immune process. Thus, an infection normally results in an increase in white cells known as **leukocytosis**. A reduction in white cells below the normal level is known as **leukopenia**.

6. How many platelets are there in the circulation?

There are about 150,000–300,000 platelets per milliliter in normal peripheral blood. Because of their small size (2–3 μ), they make up only a small fraction of the blood volume. Platelets are involved in blood coagulation.

7. What is the blood volume of a normal person?

The normal blood volume of an adult remains constant over time, but there is considerable variation from one person to another. The values in a normal adult generally range from 70 to 75 mL per kilogram of body weight. Thus, a 70-kg adult might have a total blood volume of about 5000 mL. About 55%, or 2750 mL, of this blood volume is plasma, and about 45%, or 2250 mL, is total red cell mass. One situation in which blood volume is dramatically increased is in pregnancy. Blood volume can increase to nearly 50% above baseline by about 32 weeks, whereas the erythrocyte mass increases to about 30% above baseline.

8. How does the blood carry oxygen?

The vast majority of oxygen carried in the blood is bound to **hemoglobin,** a protein consisting of globin, four polypeptide chains attached to four iron-containing **heme** groups, which are the binding sites for oxygen. Hemoglobin is the primary constituent of the erythrocyte and combines reversibly with oxygen to form **oxyhemoglobin**. In normal whole blood, the concentration of hemoglobin is about 15 g/dL. When blood is exposed to high oxygen pressure, all the hemoglobin combines with oxygen to form oxyhemoglobin. Under these conditions, the hemoglobin is said to be **fully saturated**. Fully saturated hemoglobin can accommodate about 1.39 mL of oxygen per gram of hemoglobin. Thus, blood with a hemoglobin concentration of 15 g/dL has an oxygen capacity of about 20.8 mL/dL of blood, or 20.8 volume percent. The amount of oxygen that is carried by hemoglobin depends on the partial pressure of oxygen (PO_2) to which the hemoglobin is exposed. This relationship is defined by the **oxygen dissociation curve.** Under normal conditions, the PO_2 level found in the lungs results in blood being about 97% saturated. In this case, when arterial blood has a hemoglobin concentration of 15 g/dL, the oxygen content is about 20 mL/dL.

9. What is the venous oxygen content after the blood has given up oxygen to the tissues?

When the blood has reached the large veins, a lot of the oxygen has been given up to the tissues. Blood in the large veins is referred to as **mixed venous blood,** and its PO_2 value falls to about 40 mmHg. This mixed venous blood has an oxygen saturation of about 75% and therefore a blood oxygen content of about 16 mL/dL. Under this condition, blood releases about 4 mL of oxygen for each 100 mL of blood flow to the tissues.

10. What other factors determine the oxygen content of the blood?

pH, PCO_2, temperature, and the concentration of 2,3-diphosphoglycerate (2,3-DPG) may cause a shift in the **oxygen hemoglobin dissociation curve** and cause the additional unloading of oxygen from hemoglobin. Decreased pH, increased P_{CO_2}, increased temperature, and increased 2,3-DPG all cause a rightward shift of the oxyhemoglobin dissociation curve, which allows more oxygen to be unloaded at the level of the tissues. Conversely, the presence of fetal hemoglobin shifts the curve to the left, which aids in oxygen delivery to fetal tissues.

11. How do white blood cells contribute to the properties of blood?

Although white blood cells represent only a small portion of the cells in the blood, they may have a great effect on the ability of the blood to flow through the vessels. Because white cells are rather large and stiff, and because under some conditions they may stick to the venular endothelial cells, white blood cells can contribute dramatically to the resistance of blood flow. Although under normal conditions the contribution of white cells to the viscosity of the blood is small, under conditions when white cell counts become high, this effect may be dramatic and may cause large increases in vascular resistance.

12. How much do the red blood cells affect the viscosity of the blood?

Under normal conditions in which the hematocrit is about 40%, the contribution of red blood cells to the viscosity of blood is relatively small. A rise in the hematocrit ratio from 40% to 70%, which may occur in polycythemia, can increase the viscosity more than twofold, with direct effect on the resistance to blood flow. This increase in resistance is quite large and may cause a substantial effect on the arterial blood pressure.

13. What is the difference between viscosity and shear stress?

Viscosity may be thought of as the thickness of the blood or the difficulty in forcing it to flow through a tube. Because blood is composed of a suspension of formed elements and plasma, the viscosity of the blood varies as a function of the hematocrit. Increasing hematocrit causes an increase in viscosity. Normal blood has a viscosity that is about 2.5 times that of water. That means that about a 2.5 times greater pressure drop is required to drive the same amount of blood through a given tube as it would for water.

Shear stress is the force that the blood exerts on the vessel wall as it flows. The greater the rate of blood flow in a vessel, the greater the force on the vessel wall, or the shear force. This shear force is important because it is the force sensed by endothelial cells that line the blood vessel. It has been suggested that shear sensitivity is a major mechanism by which endothelial cells sense their environment and alter such functions as permeability of the vascular wall and biosynthetic activity of endothelial cells.

14. What is a blood type?

Blood type refers to the presence of antigens on the surface of red blood cells. Hundreds of such antigens have been found in human blood cells, but most of them are weak. Two antigens—**type A** and **type B**—occur on the surfaces of red blood cells and are those commonly measured in blood typing. Another antigen, the **type D Rh antigen,** is the basis for most Rh typing. A person who has the D antigen is said to be **Rh positive,** whereas a person who does not have the D antigen is said to be **Rh negative**. There are antibodies in the plasma that can interact with the antigens on the red cells to cause agglutination. Because of this, the antigens are referred to as **agglutinogens,** and the antibodies are referred to as **agglutinins**. In general, transfusions are made with the same type of donor blood as that of the recipient. However, **type O** blood has no agglutinogens to be agglutinated, and therefore type O blood can be given to any recipient. Type O is called the **universal donor blood**. Conversely, **type AB** individuals have no agglutinins in their plasma; therefore type AB plasma is referred to as **universal plasma,** and type AB subjects are called **universal recipients**. The agglutinogens, agglutinins, and percent of the population that have each blood type are shown below:

BLOOD TYPE	AGGLUTINOGEN	AGGLUTININ	RH ANTIGEN	PERCENT IN POPULATION
A positive	A	anti B	present	36.0
A negative	A	anti B	absent	6.0
B positive	B	anti A	present	8.5
B negative	B	anti A	absent	1.5
O positive	none	anti A and B	present	37.0
O negative	none	anti A and B	absent	7.0
AB positive	A and B	none	present	3.4
AB negative	A and B	none	absent	1.0

15. How does blood clot?

An injury to a vessel disrupts the endothelium and results in exposure of connective tissue, including collagen. **Platelets** are attracted to the collagen, where they adhere and are triggered to release adenosine diphosphate (ADP) and a prostaglandin, **thromboxane A_2**. These substances attract more platelets and cause the adhered platelets to become "sticky," so new platelets adhere to the old ones and a platelet plug is formed. If the injury is small, this plug may be sufficient to stop bleeding. However, with a larger injury, a clot may be needed. A clot results from a cascade of activation of thirteen factors that circulate in inactive form in the plasma. The final steps of the cascade are conversion of **prothrombin** (plasma protein) to **thrombin** by activation of **factor X** in the presence of calcium. Thrombin converts **fibrinogen** (soluble plasma protein) to **fibrin** (insoluble strands). Strands of fibrin combine to form a network that traps red blood cells and platelets, producing a clot. Activation of factor X can result from activation of either an intrinsic or extrinsic clotting pathway. The intrinsic pathway consists of factors that are all present in blood, whereas the extrinsic pathway includes release of **tissue thromboplastin** from damaged tissues. For the intrinsic pathway, exposure of plasma to collagen activates a plasma protein called factor XII, which triggers a cascading activation of other factors leading to activation of factor X. For the extrinsic pathway, tissue thromboplastin serves as the initiating factor for the cascade of activation. Vitamin K is a necessary contributor to clotting, because it is required for production of many clotting factors by the liver.

16. What is hemophilia?

Hemophilia is an inherited genetic disorder that is linked to the X chromosome. Blood from hemophiliacs is slow to clot, due to delayed formation of fibrin. Hemophilia A results from a defective factor VIII, whereas hemophilia B results from a defective factor IX (Christmas factor).

17. How do anticoagulants work?

Common anticoagulants are **heparin** and the **coumarin** derivatives **warfarin** (Coumadin) and **dicumarol**. Heparin prevents clotting by activating a plasma protein called antithrombin III, a serum protease inhibitor that prevents activation of needed serum proteases at several steps in the clotting cascade process. Coumarin derivatives are competitive inhibitors of vitamin K that prevent the vitamin-induced production of clotting factors by the liver. Dicumarol was the first anticoagulant that could be administered to humans orally. The successor to dicumarol was warfarin, which first became known after it was introduced as a rodenticide. Warfarin's effectiveness led to its widespread success, and it has become the most widely prescribed anticoagulant drug in the nation. Anticoagulants do not break up clots that already have formed in the vessels.

18. How does aspirin "thin" the blood?

Aspirin does not actually thin the blood, but it does interfere with the production of thromboxane A_2, a platelet aggregator. Therefore, aspirin will decrease the ability of platelets to adhere to each other and form a platelet plug.

HEART

19. What is the basic anatomy of the heart?

The heart comprises two separate pumps: **a right heart** and **a left heart**. The right heart pumps the blood through the lungs, and the left heart pumps the blood through the peripheral organs. Each side of the heart, the right and the left, is composed of two pumps in series: one is the **atrium** and the other is the **ventricle**. The role of the atrium is primarily to move the returning blood rapidly into the ventricle to propel the blood through either the pulmonary or the systemic circulation. Intrinsic mechanisms within the heart provide the rhythmicity of the cardiac muscle to cause the heart's constant beating.

20. What are the major types of cardiac muscle?

- Atrial muscle
- Ventricular muscle
- Purkinje fibers, a specialized type of conductive fiber found in the walls of the ventricles

21. How do cardiac muscles contract?

Contraction of atrial and ventricular cardiac muscle is similar to that of skeletal muscle, except that the duration of the contraction is much longer and that some of the calcium that participates in contraction enters as a current-carrying ion during depolarization. The conductive fibers of the heart do not contract significantly; however, they provide pathways for the electrical activation to spread throughout the heart.

22. What is responsible for the spontaneous rhythmic excitation of the heart?

Virtually all of the contractile and electrical generating cells in the heart are capable of spontaneous excitation. Specialized cells within the **sinoatrial (SA) node,** which is located in the superior lateral wall of the right atrium, have the highest rate of spontaneous activation. These cells determine the intrinsic heart rate.

23. What is the mechanism of the sinus node rhythmicity?

Pacemaker activity of cells of the SA node is due to a slowly increasing inward current of calcium, which slowly depolarizes the cells. This slow depolarization takes the cells from a resting membrane potential of only about –55 mV to a threshold potential of –40 mV, at which point other channels become activated. This leads to a rapid entry of both calcium and sodium ions, causing an action potential. Repolarization occurs when the sodium channels become inactivated and potassium channels open.

24. How is the cardiac action potential transmitted throughout the heart?

The electrical discharge from the SA node travels outward from the node and across the atrial muscle mass at a velocity of about 0.3 m/s. Because the ventricles are electrically isolated from the atria, the depolarization from atrium to ventricle must travel through a specialized conductive route. This pathway is known as the **atrioventricular (AV) node** and is located in the posterior septal wall immediately behind the tricuspid valve. Transmission of the electrical impulse through the AV node occurs only in one direction from the atrium to the ventricle and introduces a delay of approximately 100 ms, which allows time for the ventricles to fill after atrial contraction. Once the depolarization passes through the AV node and into the ventricles, it is carried by a specialized conductive system known as the **Purkinje fibers**. These fibers carry the depolarization rapidly throughout the ventricle, resulting in a uniform contraction of ventricular muscle.

25. How is the rhythmicity of the heart controlled?

The heart is supplied with both **sympathetic** and **parasympathetic** nerves. The parasympathetic nerves, which run in the vagus, are distributed mainly to the SA node and the AV node. The sympathetic nerves are distributed throughout the heart.

Stimulation of parasympathetic nerves to the heart decreases the rate of depolarization of the SA node and slows the rate of conduction across the AV node. Parasympathetic nerve stimulation causes an increase in potassium conductance, which slows the rate of depolarization and lowers the resting membrane potential of the nodal cells. These changes result in generation of a slower heart rate.

Sympathetic stimulation causes the opposite effects on heart rate by increasing the spontaneous rate of firing of the SA node, reducing the delay across the AV node and increasing the force of contraction of cardiac muscle. Sympathetic stimulation produces an increase in calcium conductance, which increases the rate of depolarization and raises the resting membrane potential of nodal cells. These changes result in generation of a faster heart rate.

26. What is an electrocardiogram (ECG)?

The ECG is a record of the electrical activation of the heart. It represents a summation of the action potentials of the individual cardiac cells. As this wave of excitation progresses though the heart, the area that is depolarized is electrically negative relative to the resting muscle in areas not yet depolarized. This makes the heart a dipole, or an electrical source consisting of asymmetrically distributed electrical charge. Due to the ions present in body fluids and structures, the body acts as a volume conductor, which allows the electrical activity generated by the heart to be conducted to the surface of the body. This permits the electrical currents generated by the heart to be recorded on surface electrodes, resulting in recording of the ECG. The ECG represents a well-characterized pattern of activity produced by the sequence of depolarization–repolarization of the cardiac muscle. The normal ECG is composed of the following:

- **P-wave,** which represents atrial depolarization (80–100 ms)
- **QRS complex,** which represents ventricular depolarization (60–100 ms)
- **T-wave,** which represents ventricular repolarization (100–250 ms)

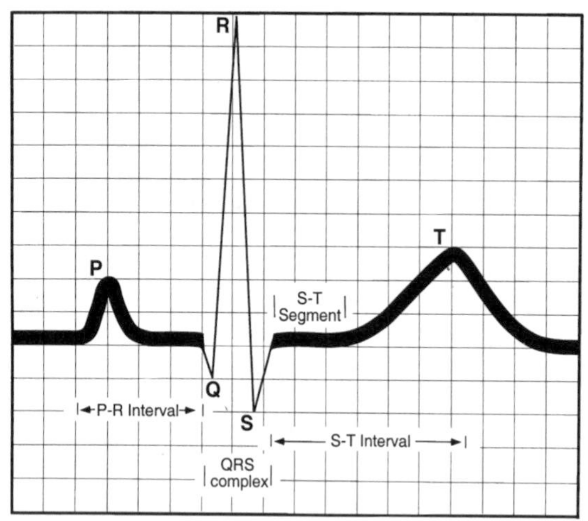

A typical electrocardiogram (ECG) showing the prominent waves and intervals. Scale for the tracing is that adopted for conventional clinical recordings, with vertical lines spaced at 0.4-sec intervals and horizontal lines representing 0.1 mV increments.

Heart rate is often estimated by the **R–R interval,** or the time that occurs between the R-waves of sequential beats in the ECG. The R-wave is selected because it is one of the most striking features of the ECG. The appearance of the ECG is greatly influenced by the positions of the leads on the surface of the body, and thus twelve conventional arrangements have been adopted to standardize the lead arrangements.

- Three **standard limb leads,** which are bipolar recordings because they display the difference in electrical activity between two different points on the body:

  Lead I—Electrodes on the right arm and left arm
  Lead II—Electrodes on the right arm and left leg
  Lead III—Electrodes on the left arm and left leg

- Three **augmented limb leads,** which are unipolar recordings because they record voltages at only one point on the body relative to an indifferent reference point:
  AVR—Electrode on right arm
  AVL—Electrode on left arm
  AVF—Electrode on left leg
- **Six precordial leads,** which are unipolar recordings in which the active electrode is placed at one of six positions in an arc pattern on the chest around the heart, starting at $\mathbf{V_1}$, located in the fourth intercostal space just to the right of the sternum, and ending at $\mathbf{V_6}$, located in the fifth intercostal space at the left midaxillary line

27. What is the structure of cardiac muscle?

Cardiac muscle differs from skeletal muscle in that the cardiac muscle fibers are arranged like latticework. The fibers divide then recombine to form what is known as a **syncytium**. Similar to skeletal muscle, cardiac muscle is striated and contains typical myofibrils made up of actin and myosin filaments.

28. What is the significance of the syncytial nature of cardiac muscle?

From a functional point of view, the syncytial nature of cardiac muscle provides easy movement of cardiac action potentials so that when one cardiac cell becomes excited, the action potential spreads to all the adjoining cells, moving from one cell to another throughout the entire heart chamber. The atrial syncytium and the ventricular syncytium are actually separated from one by a ring of fibrous tissue around the valvular openings. Normally, action potentials are not conducted from the atrium into the ventricle except through the Purkinje system.

29. What is the nature of the cardiac action potential?

Similar to skeletal muscle, the cardiac action potential represents a depolarization from the resting membrane potential. The magnitude of this action potential in cardiac muscle is approximately 105 mV. The most important feature of the cardiac action potential is a long plateau phase of up to 300 ms, which provides time for cardiac filling.

30. What is the refractory period of cardiac muscle?

The interval of time during which normal cardiac impulses cannot reexcite an area of cardiac muscle. The normal refractory period of the left ventricle is about 250 ms. This period is important because it ensures that the wave of electrical activation passes in an organized fashion to cardiac muscle, allowing the individual muscle cells of each chamber to contract almost as a single muscle, or a "functional syncytium." This produces an efficient contraction to eject blood. If damage occurs to parts of the conducting pathway (myocardial infarction) or the heart becomes enlarged (heart failure), conduction may follow an abnormal pathway, and the refractory periods of the muscle cells may no longer line up with respect to time. The wave of depolarization may then affect areas of the heart out of synchrony, leading to inefficient contractions or even arrhythmias.

31. What are the phases of the cardiac contraction?

- Systole—the period during which cardiac contraction occurs
- Diastole—the period during which relaxation and filling occur

32. During what phase of cardiac contraction is the volume in the heart the greatest?

The cardiac chambers fill during diastole; therefore, volume of the heart is at a peak at the end of diastole.

33. Why is the left ventricular wall so much thicker than the right ventricular wall?

The thickness of the walls of the cardiac chambers is indicative of the work that they must do to pump the blood into their respective circulations. The pressure in the systemic circulation is significantly higher than that of the pulmonary circulation, although the blood flow through both circulations is equal. Thus, the left ventricle needs a larger muscle mass to overcome the higher pressures in the systemic circulation.

34. What are the pressures in all of the chambers of the heart?

The **right atrium** is a highly compliant chamber that serves to absorb the blood as it moves from the systemic circulation to return to the heart. Because of its high degree of compliance and the weakness of its contraction, the pressure within the right atrium does not change much. As the chamber fills, pressure rises from approximately 0 to about 6 mmHg with a mean of approximately 4 mmHg.

The **right ventricle,** which pumps the blood into the pulmonary artery, has higher pressures, ranging from 0 mmHg diastolic to 25 mmHg systolic pressure. Pressures in the **pulmonary artery** range from approximately 4 mmHg during diastole to approximately 28 mmHg at the peak of systole.

Blood returning from the pulmonary circulation enters the **left atrium**. Similar to the right atrium, the left atrial pulse pressure is small with a mean pressure of approximately 8 mmHg.

Blood leaves the left atrium and enters the **left ventricle**. The left ventricle pumps the blood into the aorta and the rest of the systemic circulation; therefore, pressures in the left ventricle range from approximately 125 mmHg during the peak of systole to approximately 8 mmHg during diastole. Aortic pressure normally ranges from approximately 120 mmHg systolic to 80 mmHg diastolic pressure.

35. What are the functions of the valves of the heart?

The valves in the heart separate the atria from the ventricles (**AV valves**) and the ventricular chambers from the circulations (**semilunar valves**) into which they pump. The valves on the right side are the **tricuspid valve** and **the pulmonary semilunar valve**. Those on the left side are the **mitral (bicuspid) valve** and **aortic semilunar value**. Because the valves open only in one direction, they force the blood to be propelled out of the heart during contraction. Valve defects or damage to the valves may cause reflux of blood from the circulation back into the heart or from one chamber to another, resulting in inefficient delivery of blood from the heart to the circulation. Backward reflux from the leaking valve may be heard as a **heart murmur**.

36. What are the functions of the papillary muscles?

The **papillary muscles,** which arise from the inner wall of the ventricle, are connected to the valve leaflets via tendinous structures known as the **chordae tendinae**. During cardiac contraction, as the ventricle decreases in size, contraction of the papillary muscles helps to maintain the proper positions of the valve leaflets and prevent the valves from inverting at higher pressures.

37. What are the key features of the cardiac cycle?

The events of the cardiac cycle are summarized in the accompanying figure for the left side of the heart (see figure, next page). Similar events occur for the right side of the heart, but the pressures are all reduced accordingly. **One cardiac cycle** refers to the period comprising the beginning of one heart beat through the beginning of the next heart beat. The cardiac cycle is initiated by the spontaneous generation of an action potential in the SA node. This action potential spreads across both atria resulting in atrial contraction and a rise in atrial pressure (atrial systole). This increase in atrial pressure ejects blood into the left ventricle. As the depolarization spreads through the AV bundle into the ventricles, the ventricles contract with a delay of approximately 100 ms after the atrial contraction. Ventricular pressure increases, resulting in closure of the mitral valve and a period of isovolumetric contraction, when the ventricular muscle begins to contract but both valves are closed. Ventricular contraction results in a rise in pressure within the ventricular chamber and when ventricular pressure exceeds aortic pressure, the aortic valve opens and ejection of the blood into the aorta occurs (rapid followed by slower ejection). After ejection, the cardiac muscle begins to relax and pressure drops, allowing the aortic valve to close (isovolumetric relaxation). When pressure within the ventricle falls below that of atrial pressure, the mitral valve opens and ventricular filling begins (rapid followed by slower ventricular filling), preparing the heart for the next beat.

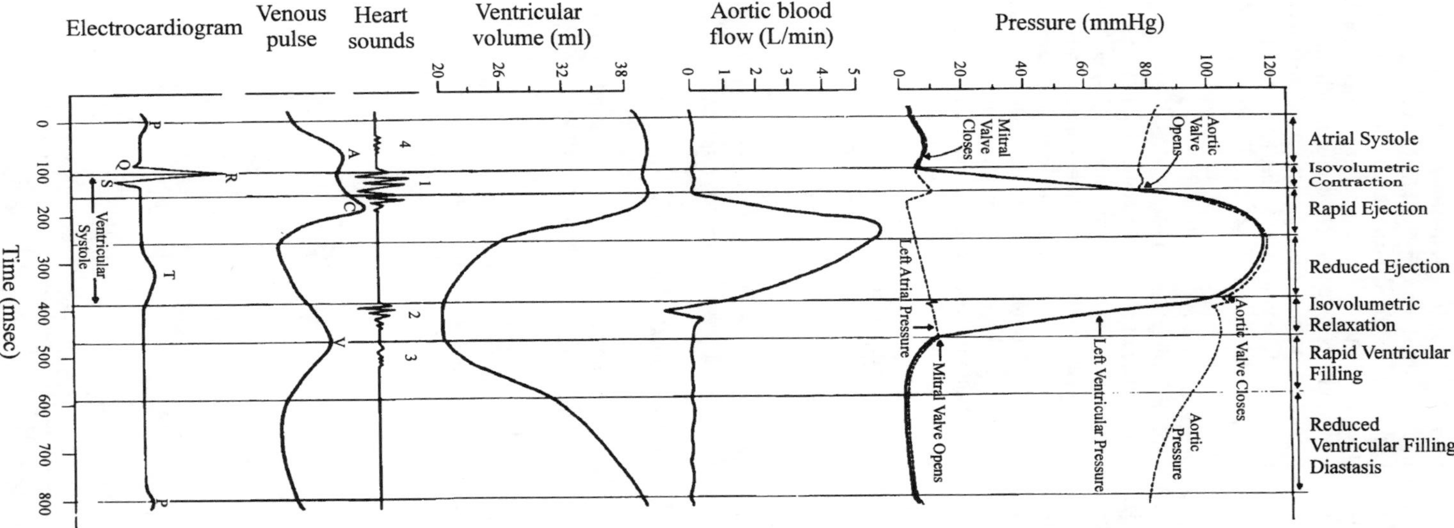

Depiction of the events of the cardiac cycle demonstrating the relationships between the electrical and mechanical events. The upper panel shows the left atrial, left ventricular, and aortic pressures. Note that left ventricular and aortic pressure are equal to each other only during the ejection phase when the aortic valve is open. The aortic blood flow tracing in the second panel illustrates the pulsatile nature of cardiac output and shows that, for the majority of the cardiac cycle, blood flow leaving the heart is zero. Finally, as can be seen by comparing the electrocardiogram in the lower panel with the volume tracing above, changes in electrical activity precede mechanical changes in the heart that lead to contraction.

38. How much of the oxygen required for cardiac contraction comes directly through the ventricular wall as opposed to from the coronary circulation?

Although the left atrium and left ventricle are carrying highly oxygenated blood in large amounts, virtually none of the oxygen required for the cardiac contraction diffuses through the wall of the ventricle. Similar to other tissues, the heart has a complete circulation known as the **coronary circulation**. As in other vascular beds, coronary vessels branch, ultimately forming capillaries where oxygen exchange occurs. Complete blockage of coronary vessels causes regions of the heart to receive no oxygen and therefore ultimately to die, leading to a **myocardial infarction**.

39. Explain Starling's law of the heart.

The **Frank-Starling mechanism,** or Starling's law of the heart, describes the intrinsic ability of the heart to adapt to changes in the amount of blood returned to it by the systemic circulation. The Starling mechanism operates on the principle that as cardiac muscle is stretched, its ability to contract is augmented. Thus, when an extra amount of blood returns into the ventricles, the cardiac chambers are stretched, resulting in a more vigorous contraction that propels the extra blood out of the heart. This relationship between the filling of the heart and the cardiac output is often quantified by graphing filling pressure or preload against cardiac output in a graph referred to as the **cardiac function curve**. The mechanism ensures that both ventricles pump the same volume of blood within one beat, preventing any overfilling of the pulmonary or systemic circulations.

40. Clarify the distinction between preload and afterload.

Preload refers to the pressure or stretch of the cardiac chambers during diastole. Therefore, preload is the load on the heart prior to contraction. Increases in preload cause more vigorous cardiac contractions by the Frank-Starling mechanism.

Afterload is the pressure or resistance into which the heart pumps. Thus, afterload is the magnitude of the load the heart must overcome to eject blood. We often refer to the arterial or pulmonary pressure as the afterload for the left and right ventricles, respectively.

41. Is the preload for the right ventricle equal to the preload for the left ventricle?

Cardiac output from both the left and the right heart is matched; that is, it is equal. The left heart operates at a significantly elevated filling pressure because left ventricular afterload (systemic arterial pressure) is greater than right ventricular afterload (pulmonary arterial pressure).

42. What is a pressure volume loop?

The pressure volume loop charts the changes in ventricular pressure and volume throughout one beat of the cardiac cycle. The element of time is not considered in a pressure volume loop. As shown in the accompanying figure of the left ventricle, one loop represents one beat.

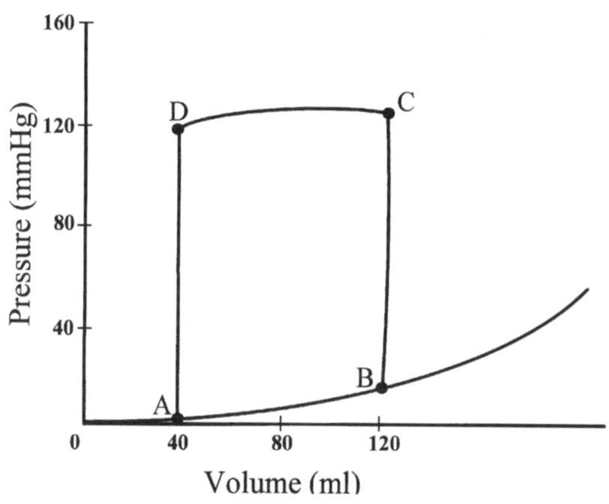

- Beginning at point A and proceeding in a counterclockwise direction around the loop, we move first through the phase in which the left ventricle is filling without a large rise in pressure. This is the **filling phase**.
- At point B, the left ventricle begins to contract, which leads to mitral valve closure; however, the aortic valve has not yet opened, so the period between B and C is the **isovolumetric contraction phase**.
- At point C, the aortic valve opens when sufficient pressure has been generated to overcome aortic pressure, and blood is pumped from the ventricle into the aorta. The period of time from point C to point D is the **ejection phase**.
- At point D, the ventricle has begun to relax, and the pressure rapidly falls, resulting in the closure of the aortic valve. The mitral valve remains closed until point A, at which point left atrial pressure exceeds ventricular pressure and the valve opens to permit filling. Thus, the phase between D and A is the **isovolumetric relaxation phase**.

The segments B-C and C-D represent systole, whereas the segments D-A and A-B represent diastole.

43. Put the work of the heart in perspective.

The heart pumps out about 2.5 ounces of blood on every beat. Each day it pumps at least 2500 gallons, which is nearly 10,000 L of blood. This amount of blood weighs 20 tons. The average adult heart beats 70–75 times a minute. Generally, the smaller the size of the heart, the faster the heart beat; thus women's hearts in general beat six to eight times per minute more than men's hearts do.

44. What is the medical term for a heart attack?

Myocardial infarction.

45. What is a heart attack?

Some of the heart muscle cells die as a result of reduced blood flow through one of the main arteries (often because of arteriosclerosis). The outlook for a patient depends on the size and location of the blockage and the extent of the damage. In the United States, 33% of patients who have a heart attack die within 20 days. It is the leading cause of death in the United States.

46. What is cardiac contractility?

Cardiac contractility is a measure of the performance of the heart at a given preload and afterload. It may be defined precisely as the change in peak isometric force at a given initial fiber length. Contractility is an index that measures the ability of the heart to pump blood. It should not be confused with a direct measurement of the force of cardiac contraction because that depends strongly on the preload (Frank-Starling mechanism). There are several possible operational definitions of contractility:

1. The slope of the cardiac function curve
2. The plateau level of the cardiac function curve
3. The maximal rate of change of left ventricular pressure during systole (dp/dt_{max})

Clinically the ejection fraction is often used as a measure of contractility; however, no index is entirely satisfactory under all conditions.

47. What is ejection fraction?

The percentage of blood pumped by the heart on each beat. It is defined as the volume of blood ejected by one ventricle in one beat (**stroke volume**) divided by the total amount of blood within the ventricle prior to contraction (**end-diastolic volume**). A normal ejection fraction is about 60%.

48. What is the relationship among cardiac output, heart rate, and stroke volume?

$$\text{Cardiac output} = \text{stroke volume} \times \text{heart rate}$$

The **stroke volume** is determined primarily by the preload as defined by Starling's law of the heart. That is, as preload increases, stroke volume also increases until the stroke volume reaches a plateau. Stroke volume also can be increased by sympathetic stimulation of the heart. **Heart rate** changes primarily in response to parasympathetic and sympathetic influences on the heart through the vagus and cardiac sympathetic nerves. Increases in both heart rate and stroke volume can cause increases in **cardiac output,** the amount of blood ejected by one ventricle per minute.

49. What is the relationship between heart rate and cardiac output?

In general, as heart rate increases, cardiac output increases. When heart rate begins to get high (> 150 beats/min), stroke volume begins to decrease significantly with increasing heart rate. This decrease in stroke volume with increasing heart rate causes cardiac output to begin to fall at high heart rates. The reduction in stroke volume at high heart rates is due to a decrease in the length of time the heart spends in diastole and thus a reduction in the time available to the heart for filling.

50. What is the use of the cardiac function curve?

Because cardiac output is proportional to stroke volume and end diastolic pressure is proportional to right atrial pressure, we can create a graph that tells us the pumping ability of the heart is a function of its filling pressure. This cardiac function curve is a useful tool that demonstrates the preload sensitivity of the heart in determining cardiac output.

51. How does the cardiac function change as contractility changes?

Under normal conditions, the cardiac function curve may change both slope and plateau level; an increase in slope or an increase in plateau level corresponds to an increase in contractility of the heart, whereas a decrease of slope or a decrease in the plateau level corresponds to a decrease in contractility. This contractility also is a measure of the pumping efficiency of the heart.

52. What is stroke work?

Stroke work is the amount of work done by the heart on each beat, proportional to the area of the pressure volume loop. An approximation for stroke work is obtained by multiplying stroke volume times arterial pressure. The higher the pressure or the higher the stroke volume, the larger the work done by the heart. Stroke work is also a function of preload because the stroke volume increases as preload increases. In fact, the amount of work done by the right and left ventricles differs not because the stroke volume differs, but because the load into which each ventricle pumps is different. The right ventricle pumps into a low pressure in the pulmonary artery, resulting in a small amount of work, approximately 9 g-m. The left heart pumps into a significantly higher load in the aorta; therefore, for the same stroke volume, its work is much greater, approximately 30 g-m. Thus, even though the output of a left heart and right heart is equal, stroke work is much greater for the left heart because of the greater afterload.

53. If increases in preload increase cardiac output, what do increases in afterload do to cardiac output?

Both the left ventricle and the right ventricle are sensitive to changes in afterload. Increasing afterload decreases stroke volume and therefore decreases cardiac output. Under conditions in which cardiac output is compromised, either by high afterload or by reductions in cardiac function, one of the most effective means for increasing cardiac output is by using afterload reduction. One interesting feature of the heart is that despite the fact that the right and left ventricles are independently afterload-sensitive, the entire heart-lung compartment is remarkably resistant to reductions in stroke volume caused by increases in arterial pressure. It is resistant because, as arterial pressure afterload is increased for the left ventricle, the right ventricle continues to pump blood through the pulmonary circulation, causing an increase in left ventricular preload and thus a compensation for the increase in left ventricular afterload. This compensation results in a normalization of the blood flow through the heart.

54. How do the mechanical properties of the heart change as it goes from diastole to systole?

During diastole, when the heart is in a relaxed state, its compliance is large, making it easy for the heart to fill with blood. As systole begins, the cardiac muscle shortens, but it also stiffens, causing a reduction in compliance and a stiffening of the heart. This change in the mechanical properties of the heart is important because diastolic filling is maximized when the compliance is high and it is easy for the heart to fill with blood. Ejection of the blood, which occurs in systole, is maximized as the heart shortens and stiffens.

55. Are there conditions when the properties of the heart do not change from diastole to systole?

Yes. Immediately after periods of ischemia in the heart, when significant damage occurs to the cardiac muscle, the ischemic region may not change its mechanical properties. Under this condition, as the heart moves into systole, the region that is ischemic remains highly compliant and may bulge out, forming an aneurysm as the pressure in the ventricle increases. Instead of moving out of the aortic outflow tract, blood moves into the aneurysm. During diastole, the blood cycles back into the heart. This bulging of the cardiac muscle can result in a reduced cardiac output as well as potential damage to the wall of the heart. After some time goes by, that region of the wall may form a scar, which has a much decreased compliance (i.e., an increased stiffness), and even though that part of the wall may not contract, it no longer bulges.

56. What is heart failure?

A reduction in cardiac function that can be caused by a metabolic impairment in the heart, an anatomic malformation, elevated arterial or pulmonary pressure, or cardiac ischemia. Heart failure results in a reduction in cardiac output, which sometimes may be compensated for by an increase in preload. Heart failure is often treated by using drugs that increase contractility, decrease preload, and decrease afterload.

57. Why does exercise training cause a reduction in resting heart rate?

Exercise training results in an increase in the size of the heart, which is known as **hypertrophy**. In dynamic exercise training, the hypertrophy occurs in such a way as to increase the size of the cardiac chamber. Because the metabolic needs of the body at rest have not changed dramatically, the resting cardiac output remains constant; therefore, the product of stroke volume and heart rate is constant. Because the heart is larger, stroke volume is increased. If stroke volume is larger, heart rate is lower.

58. Why is a reduction in resting heart rate beneficial?

During exercise performance, cardiac output must increase from approximately 5 L/min to nearly 35 L/min, an increase of nearly sevenfold. An increase in heart rate from a low level of 50 beats/min to a high level of 200 beats/min produces a fourfold increase in cardiac output. Under these conditions, stroke volume needs only to double to get an additional factor of two. If the resting heart rate were not reduced, the individual would quickly reach the point at which increases in heart rate would cause reductions in stroke volume, and it would be difficult to increase cardiac output to the required level.

59. What else does an exercise training program do to the cardiovascular system?

Exercise training also affects the vasculature. Increased use of skeletal muscle results in a growth of capillaries in the skeletal muscle, known as **angiogenesis**. This increase in capillary density increases the availability of oxygen to the skeletal muscle, thus reducing the rate at which skeletal muscle fatigues during exercise performance. In addition, the larger vessels improve in their ability to dilate, thus also facilitating the delivery of blood to working muscle during exercise.

60. What commonly used diagnostic tests are available for evaluating cardiac function?

Echocardiography, gamma scanning, and cardiac catheterization.

61. What is cardiac catheterization?

Cardiac catheterization is the introduction of a catheter directly into the heart to assess the pressures and flows in the cardiac chambers. The catheters may be introduced either from the venous side of the circulation through the femoral vein and into the right atrium, the right ventricle, and the pulmonary artery or from the femoral artery advanced into the aorta and the left ventricle. The results of cardiac catheterization can be used to evaluate the contractile force of the left and right ventricles as well as the competence of the valves in the heart. In addition, catheters can be introduced in the coronary arteries and dye injected to visualize the perfusion of the coronary vasculature and to identify regions of the myocardium that may be underperfused.

62. What is echocardiography?

Echocardiography is a noninvasive imaging modality based on the echo of sound waves from the walls and valves of the heart. It is useful for detecting wall motion and assessing the competency of the cardiac valves.

63. What is a gamma scan or a thallium scan?

Gamma scanning is an imaging technique that relies on the injection of radionuclides that are taken up specifically by the heart. Once the radioactive material is injected and is taken up by the heart, a special camera known as a **gamma camera** is used to record the emissions of the radionuclides. A computer generates an image of the heart that may be interpreted to determine regions that are poorly perfused, shown by an area that has a lack of emission by the radionucleotide. A thallium scan is often combined with an exercise test to evaluate changes in perfusion in going from rest to exercise. This combination helps to determine whether a region of ischemia is due to a structural abnormality or to a metabolic abnormality in the heart.

64. What does an ECG measure?

An ECG shows the pattern of electrical activation of cardiac muscle. Changes in the ECG from normal indicate problems in conduction of depolarizing activity in the heart, the type of which may be assessed by interpreting the ECG. Although the mechanical function of the heart is not assessed by the ECG, experience allows inferences to be made about mechanical abnormalities that are affected by conduction abnormalities.

65. How is the ECG used to show cardiac problems?

Changes in the time needed for cardiac muscle activation or the pathway used for cardiac depolarization, caused by local ischemia or damage to the heart muscle, are reflected by changes in the ECG. For example, **atrial tachycardia** would be characterized by a decreased R-R interval and increased P, QRS, and T waves. The rate may be high enough to cause coincidence of the T and P waves. A **ventricular premature beat** would produce a widened QRS complex with an unusual configuration. It would not necessarily interfere with other normal ECG patterns. Decreases in conduction through areas of the heart are shown by prolonged intervals. For example, a conduction slowing at the AV node (**first-degree heart block**) would result in a prolongation of the P-R interval. Total conduction block (**third-degree heart block**) at the AV node would result in complete dissociation of P waves and QRS complexes so that there would not be any consistent timing relationship between the two wave forms. A slowing of conduction in the bundle branches of the ventricular depolarization pathway would result in a notched QRS complex, because the synchrony of ventricular depolarization would be lost. Cardiac ischemia often produces an elevation or depression of the S-T segment. Carefully reading the ECG can give insights into cardiac functional problems.

66. Is cardiac output determined solely by the heart?

The assumption that if the body needs more blood (e.g., exercise), the heart needs only to pump harder is not true. Because of the high compliance of blood vessels on the venous side of the circulation and a small pressure gradient from the capillaries to the right atrium, as the heart attempts to increase blood flow by increasing stroke volume, the venous vessels collapse. Thus, the amount of blood returning to the heart is actually diminished, which ultimately leads to a reduction in stroke volume. For this reason, cardiac output is largely determined by the venous return or the amount of blood that returns to the heart.

SYSTEMIC CIRCULATION

67. What is vascular resistance?

Vascular resistance is the force that impedes blood flow through the circulation. The resistance (R) of an individual vessel depends directly on its length (l) and the viscosity (η) of the blood flowing through it and inversely on the radius to the fourth power (r^4). Thus, changes in the radius of a blood vessel are the primary means by which resistance is regulated. This relationship is stated in **Poiseuille's law:**

$$R = \frac{\pi\ r4}{8\ \eta l}$$

68. Clarify the distinction between total peripheral resistance, venous resistance, and resistance to venous return.

Total peripheral resistance is the complete resistance that blood encounters as it flows from the arterial (left ventricle) to the venous (right atrium) side of the circulation. **Venous resistance** is generally defined as the resistance that blood encounters as it flows from the capillaries back to the right atrium. The **resistance to venous return** is a concept that incorporates the importance of resistance, compliance, and blood volume and thus describes the dependence of blood flow in the peripheral circulation on these parameters.

69. How long are all the blood vessels in the body?

If all the blood vessels in the human body could be laid end-to-end, they would extend about 60,000 miles, or nearly 100,000 kilometers.

70. Define compliance.

Compliance is a term that describes the ease of stretching a vessel wall. The greater the compliance, the greater the "stretchability" of the blood vessel. Compliance is defined as a change in volume divided by a change in pressure (mL per mmHg). Thus, a highly compliant vessel will have a large change in volume for a small change in pressure. Conversely, a low compliant vessel will have a small change in volume for a large change in pressure. A highly compliant vessel is like a balloon, whereas a noncompliant or stiff vessel is like a steel tube.

71. How is distensibility different from compliance?

Distensibility and compliance are similar, but they differ in one regard. Distensibility is the compliance divided by the resting volume, so it is a normalized measure of compliance. Compliance reflects the total amount of blood stored in a given part of the circulation and is more commonly used than distensibility.

72. Can the compliance of blood vessels change?

Yes. The compliance, or stiffness, of blood vessels is under the control of a number of factors:

- Sympathetic nervous input
- Hormones
- Changing components of the vessel wall, such as occurs in aging

73. List factors that cause compliance to decrease.

- Increased sympathetic outflow
- Increased concentrations of vasoconstrictor hormones such as epinephrine and norepinephrine
- Increasing age

74. What is the relationship between the compliance of arteries and the compliance of veins?

In general, veins of the systemic circulation are 20 times more compliant than arteries. Although there is some difference in the compliance of arteries and veins as you move along the circulation, at almost every level, the veins are larger and more compliant than their companion arteries.

75. List the functions of circulation.

- Delivering nutrients, vitamins, oxygen, water, and electrolytes to the tissues
- Removing products of metabolism
- Conducting hormones from one part of the body to another

76. What are the components of the systemic circulation?

Arteries	Venules
Arterioles	Veins
Capillaries	

The vessels in the circulation that transport blood at high pressure to the tissues are the **arteries**. Arteries have thick walls to withstand the high pressures within them. After several stages of branching and reductions in diameter, the vessels that enter into the tissues are known as **arterioles**. Arteriolar walls have a thick component of smooth muscle that responds to sympathetic stimulation. They therefore can act as the control valves and are the site of much of the control of blood flow in the circulation. The smallest vessels are known as **capillaries,** which have very thin walls. They are responsible for exchanges of fluids, nutrients, electrolytes, hormones, and other substances between the blood and the interstitial fluid. Capillaries are highly permeable to water, oxygen, and other substances, which can move through spaces or "pores" between adjacent capillary endothelial cells or through molecular pores in the cell membrane. After the blood has moved through the capillaries, it is collected into small vessels known as **venules**. Venules have some smooth muscle in their walls that can contract to increase venous resistance and decrease venous compliance, but venules are also highly compliant. Venules coalesce into progressively larger vessels known as **veins,** which are important for the transport of the blood back to the heart. Because so much of the blood volume resides in the veins, they are important areas for storage of blood.

77. What determines the rate of blood flow through a blood vessel?

- The pressure gradient between the two ends of the vessel
- The difficulty of the blood moving through the vessel, known as **resistance**

The blood flow through a vessel can be calculated based on the following equation:

$$\text{Flow} = \text{pressure gradient} \div \text{resistance}$$

For the entire circulation, the flow is equal to the cardiac output, and the pressure gradient is the arterial pressure minus the venous pressure. Resistance to blood flow is often calculated in units called **peripheral resistance units (PRU)**. For the entire circulatory system, the resistance is 100 mmHg divided by a flow of approximately 100 mL/s or 1 PRU.

78. What is delayed compliance?

Delayed compliance is the response of the blood vessel to a sudden change in pressure. When a vessel experiences a sudden change in pressure or volume, the vascular wall slowly stretches to accommodate that increase in volume. As the vessel wall stretches, the pressure within that vessel falls, resulting in the appearance of an increase in compliance. This change in compliance over time is referred to as **delayed compliance,** or **stress-relaxation**.

79. What are the normal levels of arterial and venous pressure in the body?

The pressure in the arteries is highly pulsatile. The peak pressure, known as **systolic pressure,** is approximately 120 mmHg. The trough pressure, known as **diastolic pressure,** is approximately 80 mmHg. The difference between the systolic and diastolic pressure is known as the

pulse pressure. The pulse pressure depends on the amount of blood pumped by the heart on each beat, or the stroke volume, and the compliance of the arteriole tree. As the compliance of the arteries decreases, such as occurs during aging, the pulse pressure will increase.

Venous pressures are much lower than arterial pressure, ranging from about 15 mmHg systolic pressure in the venules just after the capillaries to approximately 0 mmHg as the veins drain into the right atrium.

80. How is the blood volume distributed throughout the circulation?

The vast majority of the blood is in the compliant venous circulation, with nearly 1000 mL or 1 L in the largest veins (the vena cava), and approximately the same amount in the venous branches, including the venules and the terminal veins. Although the number of capillaries is high, their individual volumes are small, so the total blood volume in the capillaries is approximately 200 mL. Similarly, the small size and low compliance of the arteries results in only about 1 L of volume being on the arterial side of the circulation.

81. Graph the relative pressure, velocity, and cross-sectional area of the circulation.

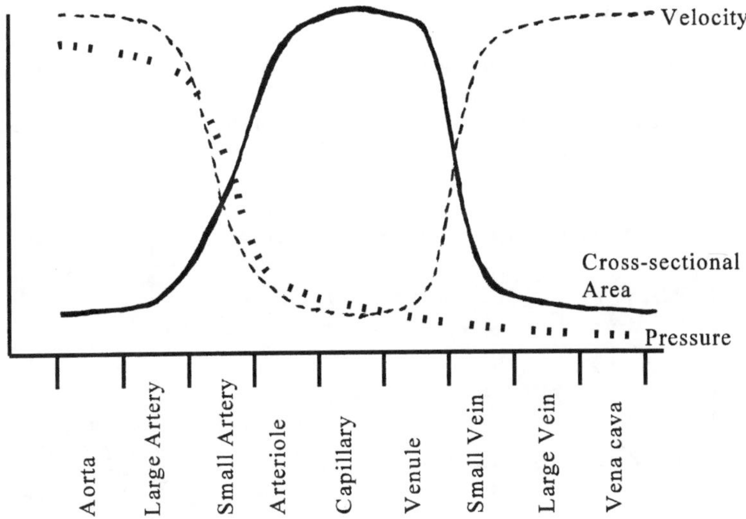

Relative pressure, velocity, and cross-sectional area of the circulation demonstrating the largest fall in pressure in the small arteries and arterioles, as well as the large area and low velocity in the microcirculation.

82. How does gravity influence the blood volume distribution in an upright person?

Because of the weight of the column of blood in an upright human and the high compliance of the veins, blood tends to accumulate in the lower extremities. Several mechanisms facilitate the return of blood from the extremities to the heart:

Venous valves
Contraction of skeletal muscle
Autonomic reflexes, which influence venous tone

Valves, which are found in the larger veins, allow blood to move only toward the heart. The presence of these valves, combined with the squeezing of blood vessels by contracting skeletal muscle, create what is known as the **skeletal muscle blood pump**. This combination of a vascular and an extravascular system results in active pumping of blood from the periphery back to the heart.

83. The words *venodilation, vasodilation, arterial dilation,* and *venous dilation* are often used interchangeably. What does each mean?

- **Venodilation** and **venous dilation**—an increase in the size of veins
- **Vasodilation**—an increase in the size of either arterioles or veins
- **Arterial dilation**—an increase in the diameter of arterioles

For constriction, we refer to arterial constrictions for arteries, venoconstriction for veins, and vasoconstriction for both.

REGULATION OF CARDIAC OUTPUT AND VENOUS RETURN

84. What is the normal value for cardiac output in a human?

Cardiac output is highly variable, depending on the metabolic demands of the organs and tissues of the body. At rest, cardiac output is approximately 5 L/min in a 70-kg person.

85. What happens to cardiac output when the body's need for oxygen increases?

As the needs of the body increase, for example, during exercise, the amount of blood pumped by the heart increases. This increase in blood flow is exactly proportional to the increased demand for oxygen by the tissues.

86. How do the systemic circulation and the heart receive signals to circulate more blood when needed?

There are several mechanisms by which cardiac output can be increased as metabolism is increased. **Sympathetic outflow** to the heart can increase both heart rate and contractility, leading to an increase in cardiac output (see figure). However, this alone does not increase cardiac output effectively. Dilation of the systemic circulation as a result of functional hyperemia or autoregulation increases venous return and thus increases cardiac output.

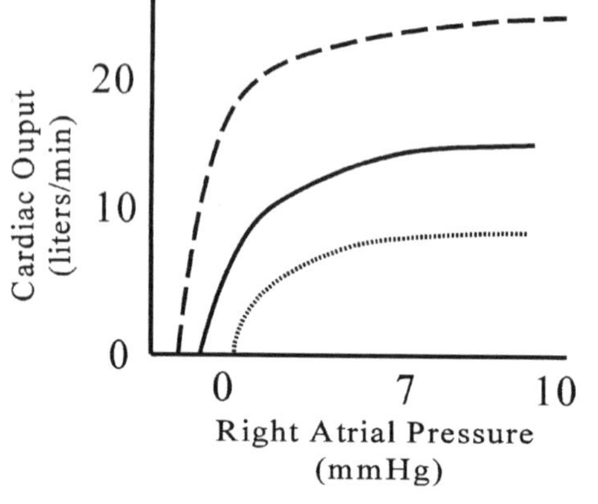

Family of cardiac function curves showing normal (*solid*), increased (*dashed*), and decreased (*dotted*) levels of sympathetic outflow to the heart. Contractility of the heart is proportional to the slope of the cardiac function curve.

87. What is functional hyperemia (active hyperemia)?

Active hyperemia is the increase in blood flow due to an increase in the rate of metabolism of the tissue fed by a given blood supply. As the metabolism of tissue increases, the requirements for oxygen and other substrates are increased. These requirements are met by increases in blood flow that are precisely matched to the increased metabolic demand of the tissue.

88. Contrast active hyperemia and reactive hyperemia.

Although active hyperemia and reactive hyperemia are similar in some respects, reactive hyperemia is the excess blood flow that occurs after a period in which the tissues are not supplied with the appropriate blood flow to meet metabolic needs. After a period in which blood flow has been occluded, for example, by a tourniquet, release of the occlusion results in a blood flow that is greater than that which occurred before the occlusion. The magnitude of the increase in blood flow after the occlusion is proportional to the duration of the period in which the flow was inadequate. This increase in flow above control is sometimes said to be "paying back the oxygen debt" acquired during the period of occlusion.

89. What is blood flow autoregulation?

Autoregulation is the mechanisms by which tissue regulates its own blood supply. For example, when blood pressure is reduced, blood flow tends to fall. This decrease in blood flow is resisted by dilation of arterioles throughout the body. This dilation reduces the resistance to blood flow, thus restoring the delivery of blood to the tissues. Autoregulation is generally divided into the **metabolic response** and the **myogenic response**.

90. Compare the metabolic and myogenic responses in the local control of the circulation.

The myogenic response is a property of a blood vessel resulting in active constriction as pressure rises and in dilation as pressure falls in an effort to maintain a given flow rate. This property originates within the vessel wall and thus does not require interaction with the tissue that the vessel feeds. The metabolic response, which causes constriction as flow increases and dilation as flow falls, arises from the production and washout of dilator metabolites by the tissue. When flow is too low, products of tissue metabolism that are normally washed away build up in the tissue and cause vessels to dilate. When flow is too high, the dilator metabolite concentrations are reduced, resulting in vessel constriction. Under normal conditions, the metabolic and myogenic responses work together to maintain tissue blood flow constant.

91. How do extrinsic control mechanisms of vascular resistance and intrinsic controllers, such as functional hyperemia and the myogenic response, relate to one another?

Extrinsic control of vascular resistance (such as the sympathetic nerves and vasoactive hormones) is superimposed on intrinsic autoregulation. This becomes important in many situations when cardiac output must be **shunted** toward one region or another for the preservation of the organism. An example of this is one that occurs with exercise. At the onset of exercise, there is an increase in sympathetic activity that causes a peripheral arterial vasoconstriction, leading to an increase in peripheral resistance that increases blood pressure. However, because of accumulation of metabolites in exercising muscle, blood flow to these sites is increased due to the local metabolic vasodilatory response.

92. How much do tissues (organs) rely on autoregulation versus extrinsic control mechanisms?

Some organs depend primarily on autoregulation to control blood flow, whereas other tissues are primarily regulated by extrinsic (neural) mechanisms. In general, organs that are thought to be immediately critical to sustain life utilize autoregulation to a greater degree. These include the brain, kidney, and heart. Conversely, the cutaneous circulation is regulated primary by the level of sympathetic vasoconstrictor tone to its vessels. Many tissues utilize both autoregulation and sympathetic neural control, depending on circumstances. For example, skeletal muscle circulation is generally under sympathetic neural control, but this control can be overridden during times of increased metabolic demand by the tissues, such as exercise. Increased sympathetic stimulation of the splanchnic circulation can greatly reduce blood flow through this tissue and release stored blood volume, but over a period of time, the accumulation of metabolites will override the extrinsic neural regulation, and flow will be restored to meet the demands of the tissue.

93. If the amount of blood that flows through the body is regulated by the venous return, then what is it that controls the venous return?

The venous return, or the amount of blood that comes back to the heart, is determined by the following:

- Blood volume
- Compliance of the arteries and veins
- Resistance of the arteries and veins

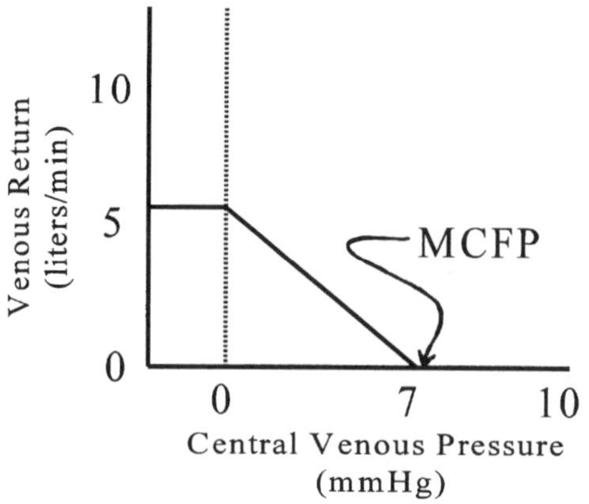

The venous return curve describes the relationship between central venous pressure and venous return. The inverse slope of the curve is the resistance to venous return.

Because vessels are distensible and the heart is preload-sensitive, we can define a relationship that includes Poiseuille's law but also extends it. This relationship is known as the **venous return relationship** (see figure).

To understand the venous return relationship, we must first understand a concept called the **mean circulatory filling pressure (MCFP),** which is defined as the sum of the volume in the arteries + the volume in the veins ÷ the total compliance of the circulation. The MCFP is indicative of the fullness of the circulation. MCFP also represents the pressure that drives blood back to the heart. Therefore, the pressure gradient for venous return is MCFP — right atrial pressure. Because flow = the pressure gradient ÷ the resistance across that gradient, the resistance to venous return (RVR) is defined as the pressure gradient (MCFP — right atrial pressure) ÷ the venous return. This resistance to venous return is not the same as total peripheral resistance because it takes into account the venous resistance (R_V), the arterial resistance (R_A), and the compliance of the circulation:

$$RVR = \frac{R_V + R_A}{20}$$

Clearly the venous return is equal to MCFP — the right atrial pressure ÷ the resistance to venous return. Thus, venous return is regulated by regulation of the MCFP (the fullness of the circulation) and the resistance to venous return (arterial resistance, venous resistance, and compliance).

94. What are the factors that alter the MCFP?

- Changes in blood volume
- Changes in arterial compliance
- Changes in venous compliance

Changes in vascular resistance do not affect the mean circulatory filling pressure.

95. What factors change the resistance to venous return?

The resistance to venous return is determined primarily by constriction or dilation of arteries and veins. Increasing the resistance of the arteries or the resistance of the veins increases the resistance to venous return and therefore decreases the amount of blood returning to the heart. Because resistance of the arterioles can be controlled by local factors, changing the resistance to venous return provides a mechanism by which the needs of the tissues may be met with an increased blood flow.

96. How do vasoconstrictor hormones affect venous return?

Hormones such as norepinephrine, epinephrine, angiotensin, and vasopressin increase both the MCFP and the resistance to venous return. Conversely, hormones such as acetylcholine and drugs such as sodium nitroprusside decrease the MCFP and the resistance to venous return.

97. What do increases in sympathetic nerve activity do to MCFP and resistance to venous return?

- Increase MCFP
- Increase resistance to venous return

98. What is the normal level of MCFP?

MCFP, or the pressure that occurs in the circulation when the flow is equal to 0, is approximately 7 mmHg under normal conditions.

99. What factors can cause increases in the level of MCFP?

- Increases in blood volume
- Increases in sympathetic tone
- Increases in levels of circulating constrictor hormones

100. What is the maximal increase in the level of MCFP?

20 mmHg.

101. What factors may cause decreases in the level of MCFP?

Hemorrhage
Reductions of sympathetic outflow
Vasodilators

102. What is the minimal level of MCFP?

4mmHg.

REGULATION OF BLOOD PRESSURE

103. What is the normal value of blood pressure?

Approximately 120 mmHg for systolic and 80 mmHg for diastolic. This may be quite variable, however. Normal blood pressures in infants may be as low as 90 over 40, and blood pressure tends to increase throughout life. In addition, over a 24-hour period, blood pressure may be somewhat variable, with lower values occurring during sleep and higher values occurring during waking cycles. In most people, the daily average of the mean arterial pressure is normally regulated at about 100 mmHg, with fluctuations of approximately ± 20 mmHg. Despite these fluctuations, blood pressure is fairly stable over life and is well regulated on a moment-to-moment basis, a daily basis, and over the entire life span.

104. Why is regulation of mean arterial pressure needed?

- To provide the organs with blood flow at a constant perfusion pressure so that each organ system can alter its resistance to achieve the desired flow during altered metabolic needs, hydrostatic destabilization, and alter blood volume states
- To optimize the cardiovascular work and minimize cardiac, vascular, and renal damage

105. How is mean arterial pressure regulated?

The basic scheme by which blood pressure is regulated is through a feedback control system consisting of pressure sensors and effector mechanisms that can alter the blood pressure. If pressure becomes altered, such as might occur during hemorrhage, a sensor, or **baroreceptor,** senses the reduction in pressure and activates an effector mechanism to return blood pressure toward its **set point**. This response is termed **negative feedback control**. The degree of effectiveness with which a control system maintains constant conditions (homeostasis) is determined by the gain of the negative feedback. Nearly all body control systems are operated by negative feedback. The primary reflex that helps to control blood pressure on a beat-to-beat basis is the **baroreceptor reflex**.

106. What types of effector mechanisms are important for the regulation of blood pressure?

Extrinsic mechanisms:
Sympathetic nervous system
Parasympathetic nervous system
Hormonal controllers
Intrinsic mechanisms:
Myogenic response
Metabolic response

Hormonal controllers:
Renin-angiotensin system
Vasopressin
Atrial natriuretic peptide
Kallikrein-kinin system
Kallikrein-kinin system

107. How does the sympathetic nervous system act as an effector in blood pressure control?

Sympathetic neurons from the **rostral ventrolateral medulla (RVLM)** descend through the spinal cord in the bulbospinal pathway and synapse on preganglionic neuronal cell bodies in the intermediolateral cell column. Preganglionic sympathetic fibers exit the thoracic and lumbar spinal cord and activate postganglionic nerve cells in ganglia located throughout the body. The postganglionic sympathetic fibers terminate as sympathetic fibers on arterioles, venules, and the heart. These fibers, through release of the neurotransmitter norepinephrine, cause a tonic sympathetic vasoconstriction of arteries and veins and can accelerate heart rate. The tonic constriction of blood vessels is sometimes referred to as **vasomotor** or **vascular tone**. Vasomotor tone keeps vessels partly constricted so that they can both dilate and constrict around this level of **resting tone**.

108. How does the baroreceptor reflex control blood pressure?

Two sites in the cardiovascular system contain baroreceptors, fine nerve endings that are activated by stretch of the vessel walls in which they lie: the carotid sinus and the aortic arch. These pressure-sensitive receptors send afferent nerve activity through the ninth and tenth cranial nerves, respectively, to the **nucleus of the tractus solitarius (NTS),** which activates neurons that serve as the first relay site of the baroreflex. These NTS neurons then activate neurons in the **caudal ventrolateral medulla (CVLM),** which in turn inhibit the neurons in the rostral ventrolateral medulla, which normally excite sympathetic preganglionic neurons in the spinal cord. Thus, activation of the baroreceptors by increases in pressure, or increased stretch of the vessel walls, results in a decrease in sympathetic activity. This decrease in sympathetic activity reduces the vasomotor tone, causing dilation of the blood vessels, and slows heart rate, both of which help to lower blood pressure back to normal. In addition to decreasing sympathetic activity, activation of the baroreceptors increases parasympathetic nerve activity. Neurons in the NTS that are activated by baroreceptor afferent activity also innervate neurons in the **nucleus ambiguus (NA)** in the medulla, which are the preganglionic parasympathetic nerve cell bodies that have fibers in the vagus nerve. These neurons innervate postganglionic neurons contained in ganglia near the heart. Thus, when the baroreceptors are activated, there is an increase in parasympathetic nerve activ-

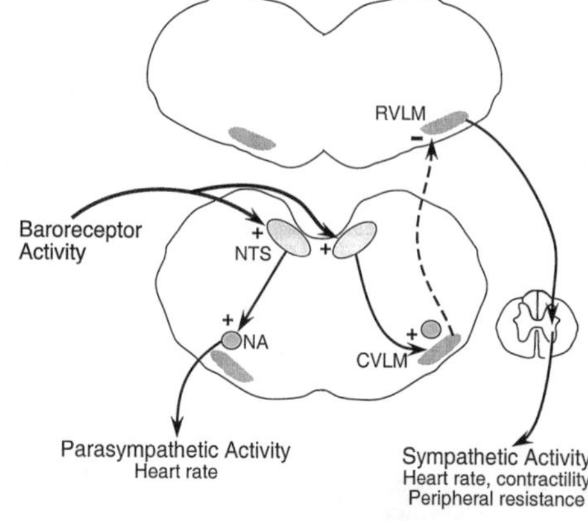

Diagram of the baroreceptor reflex pathway in the medulla. Baroreceptor afferent activity first synapses on neurons in the nucleus tractus solitarius (NTS). These neurons activate other neurons in either the nucleus ambiguus (NA) or caudal ventrolateral medulla (CVLM). Neurons in the NA are cell bodies for preganglionic nerve fibers that innervate the heart. Thus, increases in baroreceptor activity will increase parasympathetic drive to the heart. Neurons in the CVLM inhibit neurons in the RVLM, which activate cell bodies of preganglionic sympathetic nerve fibers in the spinal cord. Thus, increases in baroreceptor activity will decrease sympathetic drive to the heart and blood vessels. The net effect of increases in baroreceptor activity is a decrease in heart rate and peripheral resistance.

ity to the heart, which helps to slow heart rate. If blood pressure decreases, the level of baroreceptor activation decreases, and thus there is less excitation of neurons in the NTS. This results in less inhibition of sympathetic activity and less activation of parasympathetic activity. This results in increases in vasomotor tone and heart rate, which help to elevate blood pressure back to normal. Note that the sympathetic and parasympathetic nervous systems act reciprocally to control blood pressure, so that increases in one are accompanied by decreases in the other.

The baroreceptor reflex is highly effective at rapidly controlling blood pressure during short-term perturbations, such as postural changes. One important feature of this control mechanism is that it is rapidly adapting so that it is capable of normalizing blood pressure even if the long-term level of blood pressure is changed.

109. Are there other types of sensors that are important in the regulation of blood pressure?

Yes. Another important neural control mechanism involved in blood pressure control is peripheral **chemoreceptors**. Chemoreceptors are located primarily in carotid and aortic bodies. They are stimulated by low arterial PO_2 but also may be stimulated by arterial pressures that fall below approximately 60 mmHg. Stimulation of chemoreceptors leads to an increased sympathetic tone (vasoconstriction) and increased vagal tone (bradycardia). In addition, there are mechanoreceptors in the heart, primarily the left ventricle, that act much like baroreceptors and can contribute to regulation of pressure, although the gain of this reflex is much less than that of the arterial baroreceptors.

110. Summarize the nervous control of arterial pressure.

Nervous control of arterial pressure is accomplished primarily by baroreceptors, peripheral chemoreceptors, cardiac mechanoreceptors, and central nervous system ischemic response. It acts through changes of sympathetic and vagal tone (control of total peripheral resistance, MCFP, and alterations in cardiac function). Nervous control of the circulation acts quickly; however, these systems tend to adapt when exposed to extended periods of blood pressure changes.

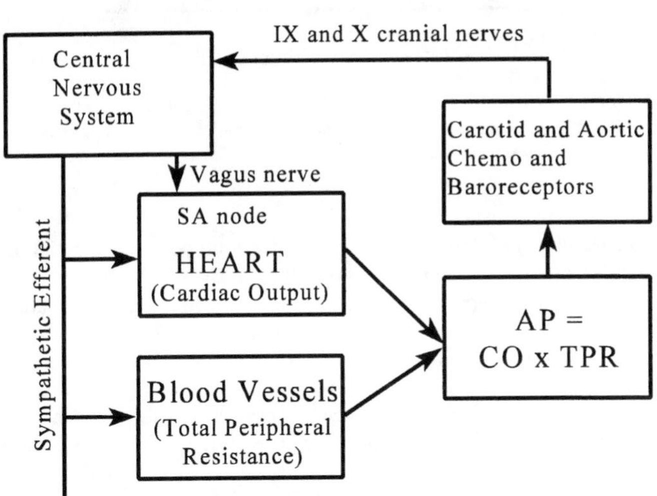

Diagram of the neural control of the circulation. IX = Glossopharyngeal nerve; X = vagus nerve; AP = arterial pressure; CO = cardiac output; TPR = total peripheral resistance.

111. If neural control systems are rapidly adapting, what are the mechanisms that are responsible for the long-term regulation of blood pressure?

Increases in blood volume cause increases in blood pressure by acting through cardiac output. Because blood volume is controlled primarily by renal excretory mechanisms, the kidney is the primary long-term controller of blood pressure in the body. The regulation of blood pressure by the kidney is referred to as the **pressure diuresis theory**.

112. What is the pressure diuresis theory?

The ability of the kidney to excrete sodium and water depends directly on the arterial pressure. As arterial pressure rises, urinary sodium and volume output increases (see figure), which results in a decrease in blood volume. This decrease in blood volume causes a reduction in cardiac output and therefore a reduction in blood pressure. As blood pressure is reduced, the excretory ability of the kidney is also reduced, restoring a steady state. The consequence of the pressure diuresis theory is that long-term blood pressure is controlled by the renal excretory ability, and the total peripheral resistance determines blood pressure only in the short term. Most importantly, this theory says that changes in renal vascular resistance or renal filtration and reabsorption are the only ways to alter blood pressure in the long term.

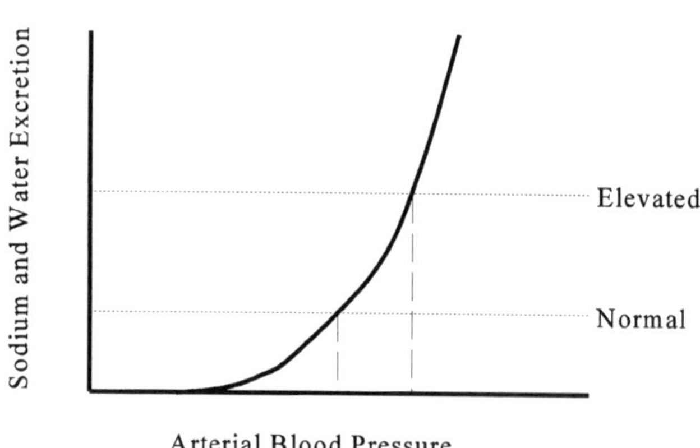

The relationship of renal perfusion pressure and sodium or water excretion. Dotted lines show normal or elevated sodium intake. Dashed lines show the resulting arterial blood pressure. The slope of this curve can be modified by angiotensin, aldosterone, and other factors.

113. What is the autoregulatory multiplier effect of total peripheral resistance?

Small increases in blood volume and cardiac output can have large effects on systemic vascular resistance (i.e., arterial or vasoconstriction) because increases in extracellular fluid volume and blood volume increase MCFP, which increases both venous return and cardiac output. Increases in cardiac output, acting through autoregulatory mechanisms, increase total peripheral resistance. Because arterial pressure equals cardiac output times total peripheral resistance, and because both cardiac output and total peripheral resistance are increased by increasing blood volume, the resulting increase in arterial pressure is referred to as a **multiplied effect**.

MICROCIRCULATION

114. What is the microcirculation?

The microcirculation is made up of the smallest blood vessels. It is generally defined as including the vessels with diameters less than 200 μ. These are the vessels that penetrate into the parenchymal tissue and are responsible for the primary control of blood pressure and fluid exchange in the circulation. The smallest vessels in the microcirculation are referred to as the **terminal microcirculation**. These are arterioles with diameters less than 100 μ, capillaries with diameters between 4 and 8 μ, and venules with diameters less than 150 μ.

115. What is the primary function of the microcirculation?

The microcirculation is responsible for exchange of nutrients, metabolites, oxygen, CO_2, ions, water, and heat. The exchange of materials between the circulatory system and the cells of the body takes place mainly in the capillaries. These vessels are small, averaging only 4–8 μ in diameter. The average capillary is approximately 500 μ in length.

116. How do substances move across the capillary wall?

- Transcellular—pathway for lipophilic substances
- Clefts—pathway for hydrophilic substances
- Fenestrae—pathway for large proteins
- Pinocytotic vessels—pathway for large hydrophilic molecules

117. Name the forces involved in the movement of water across the capillary wall.

The Starling forces:

- Hydrostatic pressure inside the capillary
- Hydrostatic pressure of the interstitial fluid
- Colloid osmotic pressure of the plasma
- Interstitial fluid colloid osmotic pressure

118. Explain how the Starling forces work.

The balance between hydrostatic (pressure) and osmotic forces determines the net movement of water from the capillary to the interstitial space. **Colloid osmotic pressure** is the pressure that occurs because of the presence of impermeable proteins in the plasma and interstitial fluid. The capillary membrane is nearly impermeable to protein. When the protein concentration is high on one side of the capillary membrane and low on the other, water moves in an attempt to equalize the concentrations. This pulling force on the water is colloid osmotic pressure. Most ions do not contribute to the forces across the capillary membrane because the membrane is freely permeable to them and they are in equilibrium. Under normal conditions, the balance of forces favors a net movement of water from the capillary to the interstitium. Nearly all of the fluid that enters the interstitial space is absorbed by lymphatic capillaries and moves into collecting lymphatics and into lymph vessels, where it is finally returned for blood circulation. Thus, **interstitial fluid volume** is the balance between capillary fluid filtration and lymphatic drainage.

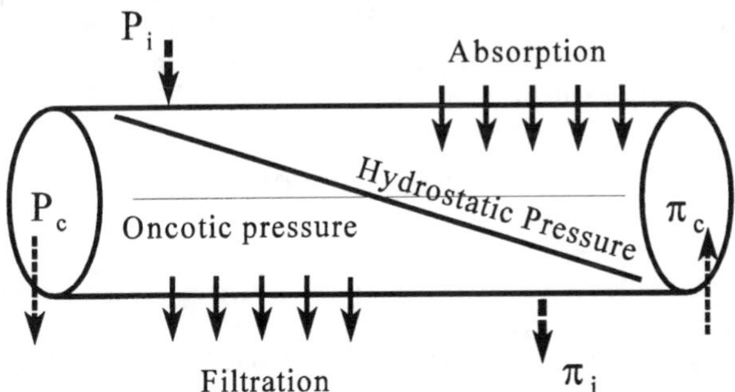

Schematic representation of the Starling forces acting on the capillary. P_c = capillary hydrostatic pressure; P_i = interstitial fluid pressure; π_c = capillary colloid osmotic pressure; π_i = interstitial fluid colloid osmotic pressure. Dashed arrows show direction in which force acts. Solid arrows show direction of fluid movement.

119. How are endothelial cells in a microcirculation involved in regulation of blood pressure?

Endothelial cells lining blood vessels experience deformational forces because of the velocity of blood flow and the viscosity of the blood. These endothelial cells in vascular beds, ranging from large muscular arteries to microvascular capillaries of specific organ systems, are capable of releasing mediators, which activate adjacent cell types. Responses of these cells depend on their differential recognition of the mediator signals and the functions coupled to a biochemical transduction system. For example, physical forces, hormones, cytokines, and coagulation products, which act on endothelial cells, can cause relaxation, contraction, proliferation, or chemotaxis in adjacent smooth muscle cells. Smooth muscle cells are not the only responder cells involved in endothelial responses; virtually all parenchymal cells can respond to mediators released by endothelial cells.

120. What type of vasoactive substances are released from endothelial cells?

Proteins
- Thrombin

Peptides
- Substance P
- Vasopressin
- Angiotensin

Kinins
- Bradykinin

Amines
- Serotonin
- Nucleotides
- Adenosine triphosphate (ATP)
- Adenosine diphosphate (ADP)

Metabolites of arachidonic acid
- Leukotrienes
- Prostaglandins

Hydroxy-eicosaetraenoic acids (HETEs)
- ETEs
- Nitric oxide

121. Describe the action of nitric oxide.

Nitric oxide is released from endothelial cells and causes a potent relaxation of vascular smooth muscle. When blood flow in the microcirculatory vessels is increased, shear forces acting on the endothelial cells cause the release of nitric oxide, which dilates the blood vessels. This flow-dependent dilation is an important regulator of shear stress and may be part of the mechanism by which flow is regulated during functional hyperemia.

SPECIAL CIRCULATIONS

122. What is the splanchnic circulation?

The splanchnic circulation is the blood supply to the liver, spleen, pancreas, stomach, and intestines. It is here that nutrients are absorbed from the gastrointestinal tract and enter the bloodstream. Major hemodynamic characteristics of this circulation are its large volume and high compliance.

123. What proportion of the cardiac output does the liver receive?

The liver receives about 25% of the cardiac output, or about 1250 mL/min. Of this total, approximately three-fourths comes from the portal vein, and about one-fourth comes from the hepatic artery. Portal venous blood reaches the liver from the intestinal circulation, where it has absorbed nutrients from the intestinal villi. Hepatic arterial blood is rich in oxygen and supplies the nutritive needs of the hepatic cells. A constant oxygen consumption in the liver is maintained by a variable and efficient extraction of oxygen by the hepatocytes.

124. What are the pressures in the hepatic circulation?

Portal venous pressure is about 10 mmHg, whereas the hepatic arterial pressure is about 90 mmHg. Because the resistance of the upstream vessels is much higher than the downstream vessels, the pressure in the sinusoids is quite low, only about 2–3 mmHg. The portal venous circulation is not autoregulated.

125. How does the liver contribute to the overall hemodynamics of the body?

The hepatic circulation is highly compliant. Because of this compliance and the large size of the organ, the liver serves as an important storage reservoir for blood. The liver normally contains approximately 15% of the total blood volume, which can be mobilized by increased sympathetic nerve activity in situations such as hemorrhage. In situations in which venous pressures are increased, large volumes of blood may be translocated to the liver, causing it to become enlarged.

126. What are the major characteristics of the intestinal circulation?

The vessels of the intestinal circulation are responsive to changes in sympathetic nerve activity as well as to circulating hormones. Both the resistance and the compliance of the intestinal circulation are under important sympathetic control. The intestinal circulation is highly compliant, so increased blood flow and volume in this vascular bed may cause reductions of blood flow to other organs. Because of the anatomic arrangement of the circulation in the intestinal villus, a countercurrent exchanger exists. This countercurrent blood flow may cause the tip of the villus to become ischemic during periods of low blood flow.

127. What is the blood flow to skeletal muscle?

Skeletal muscle blood flow is highly variable, depending directly on the metabolic activity of the tissue. At rest, intermittent contractions and relaxations of small arterioles cause a large percentage of the muscle capillary bed to be nonperfused at any given time. As a result, resting muscle has a low blood flow (approximately 2–3 mL/min/100 g). During exercise, arterioles within the muscle relax, and blood flow can increase dramatically (up to 100 mL/min/100 g in some muscles).

128. How is skeletal muscle blood flow controlled?

At rest, skeletal muscle blood flow is regulated by an interplay of extrinsic (sympathetic nerve activity) and local (metabolic) effects with the **sympathetic effects** dominating. During active muscle contraction, the local release of **vasodilator metabolites,** thought to include potassium, CO_2, lactic acid, or pH, provides the major control, completely overriding the sympathetic neural effects (functional hyperemia). The contraction of the muscle itself also plays a role in blood flow regulation in skeletal muscle, with maximal flow occurring during the periods between muscle contractions when the vessels are not being compressed by the muscle fibers.

129. What is unique about the cerebral circulation?

A constant blood supply to the brain is critical because even brief periods of ischemia can cause irreversible tissue damage. This constant blood flow is supported by an anatomic vascular pattern comprising many anastomoses, or alternative pathways for blood flow in the brain and strong local control of resistance. On a moment-to-moment basis, blood flow in the brain is maintained by this local autoregulation and under some extreme conditions by initiating powerful reflexes to maintain arterial blood pressure. Generally, total cerebral blood flow is maintained constant with blood being shunted to areas of high metabolic activity. For example, activation of visual cortex by a flashing light pattern on the retina increases blood flow only to areas associated with vision and not to other cortical areas.

130. How is cerebral blood flow regulated?

Cerebral blood flow is regulated almost exclusively by metabolic factors such as CO_2, K^+, and adenosine. Although cerebral blood vessels are innervated by sympathetic nerve fibers, their role in the control of blood flow is not clear.

131. What is the blood-brain barrier?

The capillaries of the cerebral circulation are significantly less permeable to proteins, peptides, and ions than capillaries in other areas of the body. This barrier to the movement of substances from the blood to the brain parenchyma protects the neurons from effects of substances being transported in the blood and is referred to as the **blood-brain barrier**. Anatomically, the blood-brain barrier results primarily from tight junctions between the endothelial cells of the cerebral capillaries.

132. What is the main function of the skin circulation?

In addition to supplying nutrients to the tissue, the skin circulation aids in the regulation of body temperature. When the body temperature is elevated, these vessels dilate to deliver more blood to the body surface, where it can be cooled. Under extreme conditions when heat must be conserved, skin blood vessels constrict, resulting in a nearly complete cessation of skin blood flow.

133. How is the skin blood flow controlled?

Blood flow to the skin is the most variable in the body. Skin blood vessels dilate directly in response to heat and constrict in response to cold. Most of the control occurs by sympathetic nerve activity evoked by neurons involved in temperature regulation. Blood flow to the skin can account for up to 25% of the cardiac output when body temperature is markedly elevated.

134. What are the factors that influence the blood flow to the heart?

Physical factors
Neural and neurohumoral factors
Metabolic factors

The **physical factors** include maintenance of blood pressure and the squeezing of the blood vessels during cardiac contraction. In contrast with other organs, the heart is responsible for maintaining arterial pressure. Because of this, decreases in cardiac function may be amplified by resulting falls in coronary artery perfusion pressure, which result in reductions in coronary blood flow and even further reductions in cardiac function due to cardiac ischemia. Most of the perfusion of the heart occurs during diastole because this is the period when the cardiac muscle relaxes, allowing passage of blood through the vessels. During systole, the contraction of the ventricles causes an extravascular compression, which can completely stop blood flow through the coronary vasculature.

135. What is the most important regulator of coronary blood flow?

The coronary circulation supplies the metabolic needs of the cardiac tissue. One of the most striking characteristics of the coronary circulation is the tight coupling between blood flow and metabolic activity. Thus, **metabolic autoregulation** and **functional hyperemia** play the most important role in the regulation of coronary perfusion. The mechanism for this link between cardiac metabolic rate and coronary blood flow is still not completely understood. What is known is that a decrease in the ratio of oxygen supply to oxygen demand causes the release of a potent vasodilator substance into the interstitial fluid of the heart, where it can relax coronary blood vessels in an attempt to normalize blood flow.

136. How important is the neural regulation of coronary blood flow?

Neural regulation of coronary blood flow is much less important than the metabolic regulation. Activation of cardiac sympathetic nerves, which increase heart rate and contractility, causes an increased rate of coronary metabolism and thus acts indirectly to increase blood flow.

BIBLIOGRAPHY

1. Berne RM, Levy MN: Cardiovascular Physiology, 7th ed. St. Louis, Mosby, 1997.
2. Guyton AC, Hall JE: Textbook of Medical Physiology, 9th ed. Philadelphia, W.B. Saunders, 1996.
3. Milnor WR: Cardiovascular Physiology. New York, Oxford University Press, 1990.
4. Roberts R (ed): Molecular Basis of Cardiology. Boston, Blackwell Scientific Publications, 1992.

5. RESPIRATORY PHYSIOLOGY

Marshall B. Dunning III, *Ph*.D., M.S.

STATIC PULMONARY MECHANICS

1. What is the primary function of the lung?

To maintain optimal levels of blood gases (i.e., oxygen and carbon dioxide) to meet metabolic demands.

2. Define static pulmonary mechanics.

Static refers to those properties of the lung (e.g., volume) that do not change acutely. **Mechanics** deals with the motions and forces acting on a body (i.e., the lung in this case). Thus, **static pulmonary mechanics** refers to the mechanical forces acting on the lung and chest wall that determine volume.

3. Name and define the various static lung volumes.

- **Vital capacity (VC)**—the amount of air that can be exhaled slowly and completely after a maximal inspiration. The VC is measured in liters and expressed at body temperature, pressure, saturated (BTPS).
- **Inspiratory capacity (IC)**—the amount of air that can be inhaled from the resting end-expiratory level expressed in liters at BTPS.
- **Inspiratory reserve volume (IRV)**—the amount of air that can be inhaled from the resting end-inspiratory level expressed in liters at BTPS.
- **Expiratory reserve volume (ERV)**—the amount of air that can be exhaled from the resting end-expiratory level expressed in liters at BTPS.
- **Tidal volume (V_t)**—the amount of air inhaled or exhaled during normal quiescent breathing expressed in milliliters at BTPS.
- **Residual volume (RV)**—the amount of air remaining in the lungs after a maximal expiration expressed in liters at BTPS.
- **Functional residual capacity (FRC)**—the amount of air in the lungs at resting end-expiratory level expressed in liters at BTPS.
- **Total lung capacity (TLC)**—the amount of air in the lungs at maximal inspiration expressed in liters at BTPS.

4. What is meant by the terms lung volumes or capacities?

Volumes are air-containing compartments of the lung that, although not visible on a chest radiograph, can be measured by various techniques. Lung **capacities** are two or more volumes added together:

$$TLC = VC + RV$$

$$FRC = ERV + RV$$

5. Define ATPS, BTPS, and STPD.

- **ATPS**—*a*mbient *t*emperature, *p*ressure, *s*aturated with water vapor (surrounding temperature, barometric pressure, and water vapor at that ambient temperature).
- **BTPS**—*b*ody *t*emperature, *p*ressure, *s*aturated with water vapor (37°C, current barometric pressure, 47 mmHg water vapor pressure).
- **STPD**—*s*tandard *t*emperature, *p*ressure, *d*ry (0°C, 760 mmHg, 0 mmHg water vapor pressure).

6. How does a person's age, height, sex, and ethnicity affect lung volumes or capacities?

A person's lung increases in size from birth to the late teens or early 20s, plateaus, then declines throughout life. With the **aging** process, there are natural lung tissue degenerative processes that reduce some of the lung volumes and increase others.

- RV increases with age (about 1% per year).
- VC decreases with age (about 0.5% per year).
- TLC decreases (about 0.2% per year).
- ERV decreases with age.
- FRC has no significant change.

Lung volumes are directly related to the **height** of an individual, and studies have demonstrated a 1–2% increase per centimeter in lung volumes when comparing age-matched and sex-matched subjects.

A **female** compared against her **male** counterpart (i.e., same age and height) has lung volumes 10–15% less, owing to differences in thorax-to-trunk ratios.

Different **ethnic groups** (e.g., African-Americans and Native-Americans) have been shown to be approximately 10–15% less than their white counterparts, again, apparently owing to differences in thorax-to-trunk ratio (i.e., longer legs, smaller trunk, and hence smaller lungs).

7. How is the RV measured?

The RV is not measured directly but determined mathematically by subtracting the ERV from the FRC:

$$\mathbf{RV = FRC - ERV}$$

8. What is the physiologic function of the FRC?

Breathing is **cyclic,** whereas blood flow through the pulmonary capillary bed is **continuous**. During the respiratory cycle, there are short periods of apnea (at end-inspiration and end-expiration) at which times there is no ventilation but continued blood flow. Without the FRC acting as a buffer for continued gas exchange during these apneic periods, this would, in effect, constitute an intrapulmonary shunt. This would lead to deoxygenated blood from the pulmonary capillaries emptying into the pulmonary veins (ordinarily rich in oxygen) and as a consequence lower arterial oxygen tension.

9. What are air trapping and hyperinflation?

Enlargement of the air spaces distal to the terminal bronchioles, as seen in the early stages of emphysema, is termed **air trapping**. With air trapping, there is an increase in the residual volume (RV) and functional residual capacity (FRC). As the emphysematous process worsens, there is further lung tissue and alveolar wall destruction as well as loss of elastic recoil, resulting in airway collapse and additional trapping and is now termed **hyperinflation**. With hyperinflation, there are increases not only in RV and FRC but also in the total lung capacity (TLC).

10. What is an obstructive ventilatory impairment?

The prolongation or impairment of airflow during expiration with concomitant air trapping and hyperinflation.

11. What is a restrictive ventilatory impairment?

The inability to expand the lung fully, the hallmark of which is a decrease in TLC.

12. List examples of conditions that result in a restrictive ventilatory impairment.

- Lung resection
- Thoracic cage deformities
- Scleroderma (progressive, leathery, induration of the skin of unknown etiology unknown; eventually, the skin becomes taut)

- Idiopathic pulmonary fibrosis (interstitial lung disease of unknown origin)
- Morbid obesity
- Asbestosis
- Third trimester of pregnancy

13. In a restrictive ventilatory impairment, which of the lung volumes or capacities are decreased?

Typically all volumes or capacities are proportionately decreased (see figure).

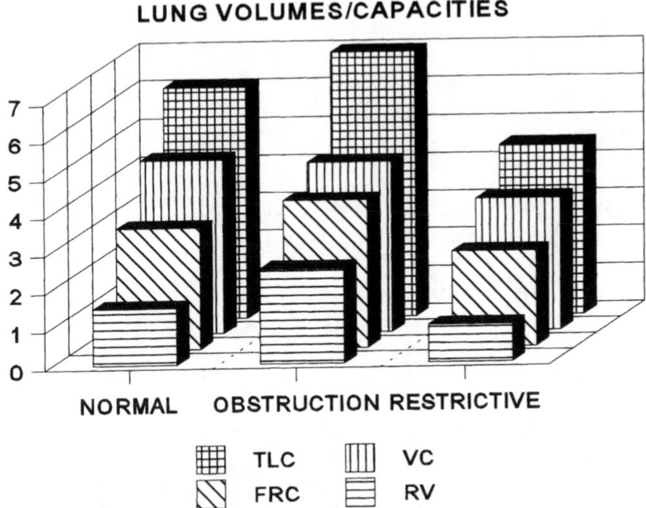

Relationship of the static lung volumes and capacities in normal, obstructive, and restrictive ventilatory impairments.

14. What determines the FRC?

The counterbalancing forces between the lung and the chest wall. The lung has a tendency to move inward and the chest wall outward.

15. Is there a disadvantage to a small FRC?

Too small of an FRC can cause wide fluctuations in the alveolar partial pressure of oxygen and lead to uneven distribution of ventilation.

16. Is there a disadvantage to a large FRC?

Although, at rest, a large FRC may buffer against wide fluctuations in alveolar oxygen levels, it is deleterious at increased minute volumes (e.g., during exercise). This is due to the need for rapid turnover of alveolar gases with increasing minute volumes, which cannot be achieved if the FRC is too large.

17. Does hyperinflation produce pulmonary disability?

Although hyperinflation indicates disease, it, in and of itself, does not produce disability. The major determinant is the amount of alveolar ventilation and gas exchange, which can be normal in patients with hyperinflation as evidenced by an increase in their FRC.

18. What factors give rise to an increase in the FRC resulting in hyperinflation?

- Increase in pulmonary compliance

- Expiratory airway obstruction
- Enlargement of the thorax

19. Define static pulmonary compliance and elastance.

Static pulmonary compliance is a measure of the elasticity of the lung expressed in liters per centimeter of water (L/cm H_2O). A high compliance infers increased elasticity and hence distensibility, whereas a low compliance implies a stiff lung. **Elastance** is the reciprocal of compliance and is therefore expressed as centimeters of water per liter (cm H_2O/L). Thus, a low elastance implies a high compliance or, in this case, an easily distensible lung:

$$C_L = \frac{\Delta V}{\Delta P}$$

$$E_L = \frac{\Delta P}{\Delta V}$$

ΔV = change in volume
ΔP = change in pressure
C_L = compliance of the lung; normal value 0.2 L/cm H_2O
E_L = elastance of the lung: normal value 5.0 cm H_2O/L

20. How is the static pulmonary compliance determined?

By measuring the change in transpulmonary pressure (alveolar pressure – pleural pressure) at the beginning and at the end of a change in lung volume. Because the intrapleural pressure is difficult to measure, intraesophageal pressure, which mimics intrapleural pressure, is monitored via an intraesophageal balloon during a change in volume, which is measured by a spirometer. Pressure and volume are plotted against one another, and the slope of the volume-pressure curve in L/cm H_2O is the static compliance.

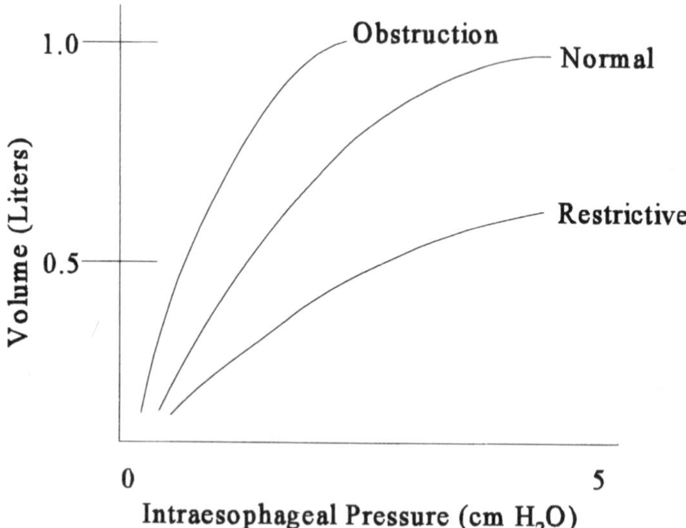

Static pulmonary compliance curves of normal, obstructive, and restrictive lungs.

21. A patient undergoing a static volume-pressure study showed an 8 cm H_2O intraesophageal pressure change during an inspiratory volume of 1.0 L. Determine the static pulmonary compliance and elastance.

$$C_L = \frac{\Delta V}{\Delta P} = \frac{1.0\ L}{8\ cm\ H_2O} = 0.12\ L/cm\ H_2O$$

$$E_L = \frac{\Delta P}{\Delta V} = \frac{8\ cm\ H_2O}{1.0\ L} = 8\ cm\ H_2O/L$$

The reduced compliance (normal 0.20 L/cm H_2O) and increased elastance (normal 5.0 cm H_2O/L) are consistent with a **stiff lung** (e.g., pulmonary fibrosis).

22. Define the law of Laplace.

The law of Laplace describes the relationship in a sphere between its radius and surface tension and their effect on pressure.

$$P = \frac{2T}{R}$$

Where P = pressure; T= surface tension (dynes/cm); and R = radius (cm).

23. Based on the law of Laplace, if two alveoli are side-by-side with radii of 75 and 150 m and surface tensions of 50 dynes/cm, which alveoli will collapse into the other?

$$P = \frac{2T}{R} = \frac{2(50\ dynes/cm)}{0.0075\ cm} = 13{,}333\ dynes/cm^2 \text{ or } 10\ mmHg \text{ or } 14\ cm\ H_2O$$

$$P = \frac{2T}{R} = \frac{2(50\ dynes/cm)}{0.0150\ cm} = 6{,}666\ dynes/cm^2 \text{ or } 5\ mmHg \text{ or } 7\ cm\ H_2O$$

($1\ \mu = 0.0001$ cm)
(1333 dynes/cm^2 = 1 mmHg)
(1 mmHg = 1.369 cm H_2O)

From this application of Laplace's equation, it is apparent that the smaller alveoli have a greater **collapse pressure** and will empty into the larger alveoli.

24. How is it possible that alveoli of varying sizes (i.e., diameters) can coexist without emptying into one another, based on the law of Laplace?

Type II alveolar epithelial cells secrete a substance called **pulmonary surfactant,** which has the unique ability not only to lower surface tension, but also to lower surface tension to a greater degree as the alveoli get smaller. The surface tension of pure water is about 72 dynes/cm, whereas the surface tension of alveoli with surfactant is lowered to between 5 and 30 dynes/cm.

Example: Alveolus 1 is 75 μ in diameter with a surface tension of 15 dynes/cm.
Alveolus 2 is 150 μ in diameter with a surface tension of 30 dynes/cm.

$$\text{Alveolus 1: } P = \frac{2T}{R} = \frac{2(15\ dynes/cm)}{0.0075\ cm} = 4000\ dynes/cm^2 \text{ or } 3\ mmHg \text{ or } 4\ cm\ H_2O$$

$$\text{Alveolus 2: } P = \frac{2T}{R} = \frac{2(30\ dynes/cm)}{0.0150\ cm} = 4000\ dynes/cm^2 \text{ or } 3\ mmHg \text{ or } 4\ cm\ H_2O$$

Thus, alveoli of different diameters can coexist because pulmonary surfactant lowers surface tension thereby equalizing collapse pressures among the alveoli.

25. Does the entire lung work on the same pressure-volume curve?

In the upright lung, there is an intrapleural pressure gradient from the top to the bottom owing to the effects of gravity. (See figure for example.) Thus, during an inspiration, although the change in transpulmonary pressure is the same from the top to the bottom, more air is directed toward the basilar alveoli as they are on different parts of the pressure-volume curve. This gives rise to regional differences in ventilation.

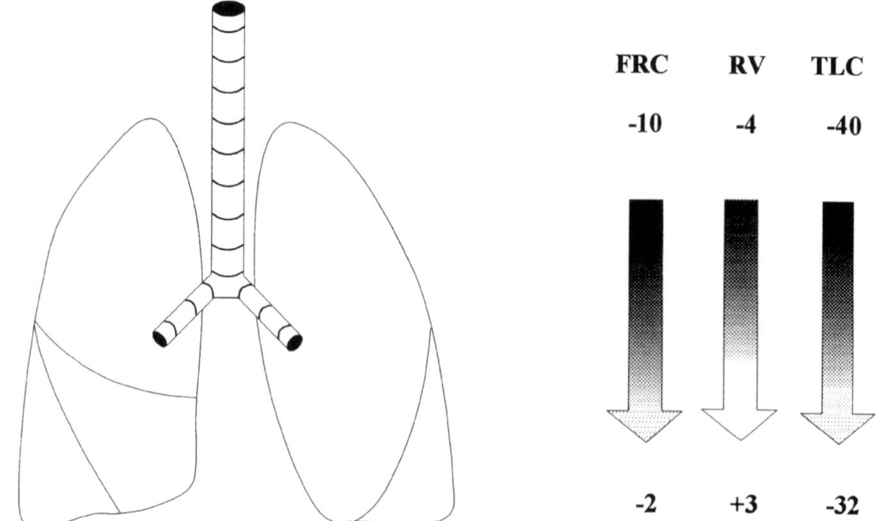

Intrapleural pressure gradient in cm H_2O from the top to the bottom of an upright lung at different lung volumes. This gradient accounts for differences in regional ventilation during inspiration owing to regional static lung compliance differences.

DYNAMIC PULMONARY MECHANICS

26. Define dynamic pulmonary mechanics.

Those properties of the lung (e.g., flow) that can vary from moment to moment and those mechanical forces that affect them.

27. Describe laminar and turbulent air flow.

In **laminar** or stream-lined **flow,** although the air moves faster in the center of the airway as compared with the sides, it moves parallel to the sides. In **turbulent flow,** eddies and vortices disrupt the air flow pattern, and as a result a higher driving pressure is required. Somewhere between laminar and turbulent is **transitional flow,** which has both laminar and turbulent flow patterns. For the most part, air flow in the tracheobronchial tree is laminar; however, there are turbulent flow patterns at the bifurcation of the airways.

28. What is the difference between ventilation and respiration?

Ventilation is a dynamic process that involves contraction of the respiratory muscles with subsequent changes in the size of the thorax and movement of air through the airways and into the alveoli.

Respiration, also a dynamic process, involves gas exchange (e.g., carbon dioxide and oxygen) either at the alveolar-capillary level or at the tissue-cellular level.

29. What is the difference between hyperventilation and hypoventilation?

Hyperventilation is ventilation in excess of metabolic needs and leads to an increase in arterial oxygen tension (Pa_{O_2}), a decrease in arterial carbon dioxide tension (Pa_{CO_2}), with a concomitant increase in the arterial pH (pHa). **Hypoventilation** is ventilation less than metabolic needs and results in a decrease in Pa_{O_2}, an increase in Pa_{CO_2}, with a concomitant decrease in the pHa:

Hyperventilation:	$Pa_{CO_2} < 35$ mmHg	pHa > 7.45
Hypoventilation:	$Pa_{CO_2} > 45$ mmHg	pHa < 7.35

Chronic hyperventilation or hypoventilation associated with abnormal $PaCO_2$ has near-normal pH.

30. Name the possible causes of hyperventilation.

Infections
Drugs
Hormones (e.g., progesterone)
Anxiety
Exercise

Increase in ventilation seen in infections and exercise may be appropriate to keep pace with the increased metabolic demands.

31. Name the possible causes of hypoventilation.

- Depression of the central nervous system (e.g., anesthesia, drugs, head trauma)
- Respiratory muscle disease
- Thoracic cage deformities
- Scleroderma
- Obstructive or restrictive ventilatory impairments

32. Which of the following have more of an effect on dynamic rather than static pulmonary mechanics: emphysema, pulmonary fibrosis, asbestosis, scleroderma, asthma, lung resection, bronchitis, morbid obesity, third trimester of pregnancy, and thoracic cage deformities?

Emphysema, asthma, and bronchitis are all classified as obstructive airways disease because they exhibit decreases in airway flow rates (**dynamic mechanics**) owing to loss of the structural integrity of the airway, decrease in airway patency, and as a consequence decrease in air flow. As these disease states worsen, there may also be changes in static pulmonary mechanics.

33. Why do individuals with emphysema tend to breathe slower with larger tidal volumes?

The mechanical work of breathing comprises an elastic component (lung tissue) and a non-elastic component (airway). To maintain their alveolar ventilation, emphysematous patients breathe at a slower respiratory rate to reduce air flow and hence the nonelastic (flow-resistive) component of mechanical work (see figure). They, however, need to increase their tidal volume to maintain normal alveolar ventilation.

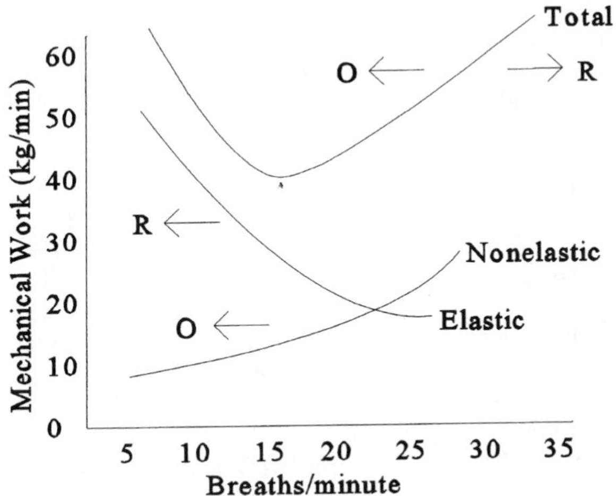

The effect of elastic and nonelastic work on total mechanical work and consequently the breaths/minute. The arrows indicate in which direction these curves are shifted from the normals in persons with either an obstruction (O) or a restriction (R).

34. What is the difference between alveolar volume and alveolar ventilation?

Alveolar (effective) **volume** is the amount of fresh inspired air that reaches the alveoli with each breath, whereas **alveolar ventilation** ($\dot{V}_A$) is the amount that reaches the alveoli per minute.

35. What is the difference between the tidal volume and minute ventilation?

Tidal volume (V_t) is the amount of air that is either inspired or expired during the respiratory cycle, whereas minute ventilation ($\dot{V}_E$) is the amount of air either inspired or expired each minute.

36. How are the V_t and $\dot{V}_E$ determined?

The subject is instructed to breathe quiescently through a mouthpiece/filter assembly with a nose clip attached into a spirometer for at least 1 minute, during which time the expired air is collected and respiratory rate measured. The V_t is determined by dividing the volume of air collected over the minute by the respiratory rate (i.e., frequency). The $\dot{V}_E$ is the total amount of expired air collected during the minute.

37. Calculate the V_t of a subject breathing with a respiratory rate of 12 and an exhaled $\dot{V}_E$ of 6 L.

$$V_t = \frac{\dot{V}_E}{f} = \frac{6\text{ L}}{12} = 0.5\text{ L (or 500 mL)}$$

38. Why is the expired volume not equal to the inspired volume during the respiratory cycle?

The expired volume is normally a little less than the previous inspired volume because at rest carbon dioxide production is normally a little less than oxygen consumption. Expired minute volume is about 60 mL less than inspired minute volume because oxygen **uptake** by the blood is greater than carbon dioxide **output** by the blood.

39. What is the anatomic dead space?

Anatomic dead space (ADS) refers to that portion of the breath that remains in the airways. The ADS does not contribute to gas exchange and is washed out on the next breath. This is also referred to as **wasted, ineffective,** or **useless** ventilation and typically is equal to 2.2 mL/kg of lean body weight. Surgical procedures such as a pneumonectomy or tracheostomy will reduce the ADS as will hyperextension of the neck or hypoextension of the jaw.

40. What is alveolar dead space?

Alveolar dead space is that portion of the breath entering alveoli that are not perfused as well as those alveoli receiving air in excess of their corresponding blood flow. (*Note:* There may be alveoli that are not receiving air with each breath, which, in effect, would also be contributing to the alveolar dead space; however, this volume is not included.)

41. What is physiologic dead space and what is its clinical significance?

Physiologic dead space is the ADS plus the alveolar dead space. Increases in physiologic dead space reflects poor match-up of alveolar ventilation and perfusion and as a consequence contributes to poor gas exchange.

42. If a 39-year-old, 68-kg man has a V_t of 500 mL and a breathing frequency of 14 breaths/minute, what is his $\dot{V}_E$ and alveolar ventilation?

$\dot{V}_E = V_t \times f = 500\text{ mL} \times 14 = 7000\text{ mL/min or } 7.0\text{ L/min}$

$\dot{V}_A = (V_t - \text{ADS}) \times f = (500\text{ mL} - 150\text{ mL}) \times 14 = 4900\text{ mL/min or } 4.9\text{ L/min}$

ADS (anatomic dead space) is equal to 2.2 mL/kg of lean body weight.

43. Define transpulmonary pressure.

Transpulmonary pressure (P_{tp}) is the pressure difference across the lung (alveolar pressure minus the pleural pressure). The net pressure difference determines whether the lung has a tendency to inflate or deflate. If P_{tp} is positive, the lungs tend to inflate, whereas a negative value results in a tendency for the lungs to collapse.

44. Define work in terms of the respiratory system.

Mechanical **work** is the product of the force applied to a body and the movement of that body in the line of force generally expressed in dynes per centimeter (dynes/cm). In the respiratory system, work is the product of pressure and volume also expressed as dynes/cm. The work of breathing includes compliance work, tissue resistance work, and airway resistance work (see figure in question 33).

45. What factors are important when considering the work of breathing?

- Total mechanical work
- Amount of alveolar ventilation
- Oxygen consumption by the respiratory muscles

46. What is meant by the term cost of ventilation (COV)?

That portion of total oxygen consumption used to drive the ventilatory muscles.

47. What portion of total oxygen consumption is used by the respiratory muscles?

Generally the COV in a normal subject at rest is approximately 2–5% of the total oxygen consumption up to minute volumes of about 50 L/min. It has been estimated that at minute volumes greater than 70 L/min (e.g., during severe exercise), the COV can exceed 30% of the total oxygen consumption. At rest, normal oxygen consumption is approximately 3.5 mL/min/kg of body weight or about 250 mL/min in a 70-kg person. Thus, the COV at rest is approximately 0.07–0.17 mL/min/kg or 5–12 mL/min in a 70-kg person.

48. Is the COV increased at rest in patients with emphysema?

At rest, the COV in patients with emphysema may be 4–10 times that of a normal. This increase in the COV is due to the increased work of the respiratory muscles to overcome the resistance to airflow seen in individuals with emphysema.

49. When is alveolar pressure equal to atmospheric pressure?

At end-expiration or end-inspiration, there is no air flow, and consequently the pressure within the alveoli, airways, and atmosphere is the same (i.e., 760 mmHg or 1034 cm H_2O at sea level). (*Note:* 1 mmHg = 1.36 cm H_2O.)

50. During V_t breathing, what forces determine direction of air flow?

During inspiration, contraction of the inspiratory muscles enlarges the thorax, lowering alveolar pressure to less than atmospheric pressure (subatmospheric), and as a consequence air flows inward. During expiration, the inspiratory muscles relax, and the thorax and lung recoil, increasing alveolar pressure above atmospheric pressure (supra-atmospheric), causing outward air flow.

51. What is a normal value for lung compliance and thoracic compliance?

Lung compliance (C_L) = 0.2 L/cm H_2O.
Thoracic cage compliance (C_T) = 0.2 L/cm H_2O.

52. Why is total (lungs and thorax) compliance less than either of its components alone?

Total compliance (C_{LT}) = 0.1 L/cm H_2O. As a single unit, the lungs have a tendency to pull inward, whereas the thorax has a tendency to pull outward. As a result, when acting together as a single unit, they require more force for a given volume change:

$$\frac{1}{C_{LT}} = \frac{1}{C_L} + \frac{1}{C_T} = \frac{1}{0.2} + \frac{1}{0.2} = \frac{2}{0.2} = \frac{1}{0.1} \text{ reciprocal} = 0.1 \text{ L/cm } H_2O$$

53. What determines the resting expiratory volume (i.e., the FRC)?

The resting expiratory level is determined by the counterbalance of the forces acting on the lung to pull it inward and those forces acting to distend the thoracic cage. The volume of air in the lung at resting end-expiratory level is the FRC.

54. Describe the phenomenon called lung hysteresis.

Hysteresis is a lag effect that occurs after the forces on a body are changed. In the lung, after a change in transpulmonary pressure, the volume change depends on the previous volume. As a result, when inflating or deflating the lung in 500-mL increments, the inspiratory and expiratory limbs of the volume-pressure curves are not the same.

55. If an emphysematous lung is more compliant than a normal lung, why does the individual have a more difficult time breathing?

Work of breathing (work of the respiratory musculature to overcome the elastic recoil of the lung and chest wall) studies have shown that although less work is required to inflate a more compliant lung, more work is required during the subsequent deflation (i.e., the lungs are much more distensible during inspiration but consequently much more collapsible during expiration, requiring a greater driving pressure). Therefore, the net effect is an increase in the work of breathing. Individuals with emphysema have an easier time getting air into the lung as compared with the normal; however, they have a much greater difficulty exhaling the air such that they have an increase in their work of breathing, which is manifested as shortness of breath (dyspnea).

56. Distinguish among pulmonary, airway, and tissue resistance.

Airway resistance is the impedance of air flow through the tracheal bronchial tree as a result of the friction of gas molecules:

$$\text{Airway resistance} = \frac{\text{change in pressure}}{\text{change in flow}}$$

$$R_{aw} = \frac{\Delta P}{\Delta \dot{V}} \quad \text{normal range: 0.6 to 2.4 cm } H_2O/L/s$$

Larger airways (> 2-mm inside diameter) account for about 80% and smaller airways (< 2-mm inside diameter) about 20% of total airway resistance.

Tissue resistance is the impedance to overcome the viscous forces within the lung parenchyma as they move during inspiration and expiration.

Pulmonary resistance is equal to the sum of airway and tissue resistance and is sometimes called total resistance. **Tissue resistance** comprises about 20% and airway resistance about 80% of total pulmonary resistance.

57. Show airway resistance curves for normal, obstructive ventilatory impairments, and restrictive ventilatory impairments.

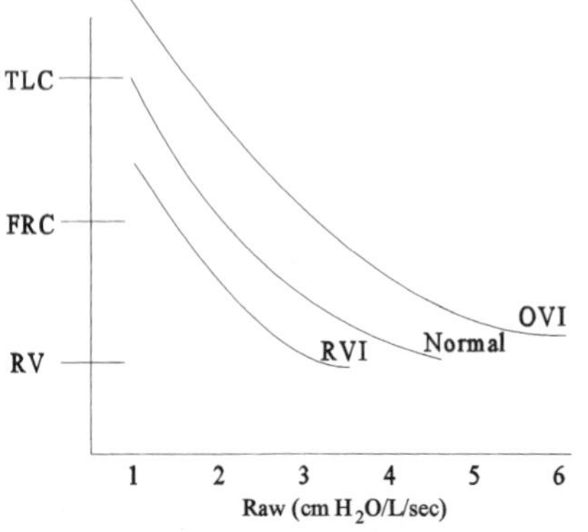

Airway resistance (R_{aw}) curves at various lung volumes for normal, obstructive ventilatory impairments (OVI), and restrictive ventilatory impairments (RVI).

58. Does nasal breathing contribute significantly to total airway resistance?

The upper airways (above the larynx) can contribute from 20% to 50% of total airway resistance. The nose can contribute as much as 50% of upper airway resistance in normal subjects.

59. Why is the airway resistance highest at low lung volumes (i.e., at or near RV) and lowest at high lung volumes (i.e., at or near TLC)?

Volume dependence of airway resistance is a result of two factors:

1. Alveolar wall tension
2. Airway caliber

At low lung volumes there is less tension in the alveolar walls and therefore a reduced parenchymal tethering (mechanical) effect on the airways. Also, there is less stretch in the airways, thereby decreasing the firing rate of airway stretch receptors with a subsequent increase in parasympathetic tone. Both of these lead to bronchial constriction and as a result an increase in airway resistance. At or near TLC, the reverse description is true, leading to a greater degree of airway patency (dilation) and consequently a reduction in airway resistance.

60. What is airway conductance?

Airway conductance (G_{aw}) is the reciprocal of airway resistance (R_{aw}) and is recorded in L/s/cm H_2O. A normal G_{aw}, inversely linear to lung volume, is between 0.42 and 1.67 L/s/cm H_2O.

61. During an inspiration, why is air flow turbulent in the trachea and not the terminal bronchioles, which have much smaller diameters?

Although the diameters of terminal bronchioles are much smaller than the trachea, less than 2 mm versus 20 mm, the total number of airways increases dramatically, and as a result the cross-sectional area also increases. Consequently the air is divided up among thousands of airways, velocity decreases, and air flow becomes laminar. As a matter of fact, air flow is almost never turbulent in the smaller airways of the lung, whereas it is turbulent in the larger airways (i.e., > 2 mm in diameter).

62. What is the Bernoulli effect?

The **Bernoulli effect** is seen as air passes into airways of smaller diameter with a concomitant increase in velocity or when air passes through a larger total cross-sectional area with a decrease in velocity. Thus, during exhalation, as air moves from many smaller airways with a combined larger total cross-sectional area toward fewer larger airways with a combined smaller cross-sectional area, there is an increase in velocity (i.e., air flow). Conversely, during inhalation, air moves from larger airways toward smaller airways with a concomitant pressure drop and deceleration of air flow.

63. What is a time constant?

A **time constant** = compliance × resistance within a given lung unit. Uneven distribution of ventilation in a lung unit can be accounted for by an increase (long) in the time constant. Thus, increasing compliance or resistance of a lung unit yields a long time constant and is consistent with maldistribution of air to that unit.

64. Define pendelluft.

Pendelluft is a phenomenon that occurs in the lung when there is uneven ventilation such that at end-tidal expiration, although there is no air flow at the mouth, there may still be flow within the lung. This is especially true in lung units that have long time constants (compliance × resistance) wherein gas moves from one unit to an adjoining unit.

65. In a normal subject, what limits exercise, the heart or the lungs?

A normal individual, trained or untrained, reaches maximal predicted heart rate long before maximal ventilatory capacity (resting minute ventilation 6–8 L/min can increase to 90–120 L/min during severe exercise) is reached. At maximal exercise, the minute ventilation is about 70% of its maximal capacity.

66. What are the various transmural pressures within the thorax?
Airway:

Airway transmural pressure = bronchial pressure – pleural (intrapleural) pressure

$$P_{aw} = P_{br} - P_{pl}$$

Transpulmonary:

Lung transmural pressure = alveolar pressure — pleural pressure

$$P_l = P_A - P_{pl}$$

Chest wall:

Chest wall transmural pressure = pleural pressure — atmospheric pressure

$$P_{cw} = P_{pl} - P_{atm}$$

Transthoracic:

Thoracic transmural pressure = alveolar pressure — atmospheric pressure

$$P_{thoracic} = P_A - P_{atm}$$

67. A decrease in forced expiratory flow is consistent with an underlying obstruction (e.g., emphysema). What limits air flow during a forced expiratory maneuver assuming maximal effort?

During a forced expiratory effort, intrathoracic pressures are increased 5–10 times above resting levels. These high intrathoracic pressures place the airway under considerable pressure, and if the airway is intact it remains patent. If, however, there has been loss of structural integrity because of a disease process, the airway undergoes dynamic compression reducing its caliber and consequently air flow as well. In extreme cases, the airway may actually collapse during the forced expiration trapping air distal to the point of airway collapse, resulting in not only a severe reduction in air flow, but also an apparent loss of volume.

GAS EXCHANGE

68. What is the percent of oxygen at sea level and at 18,000 feet (5486 m)?

Sea level: 21% (20.93%)
18,000 Feet: 21%

69. If the percent oxygen is 21% both at sea level and at 18,000 feet, why do we become short of breath at high altitudes?

Although the concentration of oxygen is the same at both sea level and 18,000 feet, the differences in partial pressure are responsible for hypoxemia at higher altitudes.

$$PO_2 = FO_2 \times P_B$$

PO_2 = partial pressure of oxygen in mmHg or torr (1 torr = 1 mmHg)
FO_2 = fractional concentration of oxygen; 0.2093

P_B = barometric pressure; 760 torr at sea level and 380 torr at 18,000 feet
$Po_2 = 0.2093 \times 760$ torr = 159 torr at sea level
$Po_2 = 0.2093 \times 380$ torr = 79 torr at 18,000 feet

Thus, at higher elevations (e.g., 18,000 feet), an individual is breathing lower partial pressures of oxygen (e.g., 79 torr). Normal arterial oxygen (Pao_2) levels are greater than 80 torr, which can be achieved while breathing at sea level where the Po_2 is about 159 torr but not at higher elevations where the Po_2 is much lower and in some cases less than a normal Pao_2.

70. State the gas composition and concentration of ambient, inspired, and expired air at sea level.

GAS	AMBIENT AIR (DRY)			INSPIRED AIR	EXPIRED AIR
	%	Fractional Concentration	Partial Pressure (mmHg)	Partial Pressure (mmHg)	Partial Pressure (mmHg)
Nitrogen	78.10	0.7810	593.5	556.8	566.3
Oxygen	20.93	0.2093	159.1	149.2	100.0
Carbon dioxide	0.03	0.0003	0.2	0.2	40.0
Trace gases*	0.95	0.0095	7.2	6.7	6.7
Water vapor	0.00	0.00	0.0	47.0	47.0

*Inert gases (e.g., argon, neon, helium).

71. What is the difference between hypoxemia and hypoxia?

Hypoxemia is below normal arterial oxygen tension, whereas **hypoxia** is the state of tissue oxygen deficiency. Hypoxemia does not necessarily imply hypoxia and vice versa.

72. What is the difference between external, internal, and cellular respiration?

- **External respiration** involves the exchange of gases (oxygen and carbon dioxide) between the alveoli and the pulmonary circulation at the level of the alveolar/capillary membrane.
- **Internal respiration** involves the exchange of oxygen and carbon dioxide between the systemic circulation and the tissues.
- **Cellular respiration** involves the process of oxygen exchange between the cell and its mitochondria to be used as an oxidizing agent resulting in the production of high-energy bonds.

73. What is a shunt?

There are two types of shunts: **venous-to-arterial** (V-A) and **arterial-to-venous** (A-V).

- In a V-A shunt, blood bypasses ventilated regions of the lung and is dumped back into the arterial system, thereby lowering the oxygen level.
- In an A-V shunt, arterialized blood is dumped into the venous system (e.g., atrial-septal defect).

74. What is a normal shunt fraction?

Approximately 2–5% of the cardiac output is shunted through the pulmonary circulation via the thebesian veins of the heart and branches of the bronchial circulation.

75. Define $C(a\text{–}v)O_2$ and give a normal range.

$C(a\text{–}v)O_2$ is the difference between the arterial oxygen content and venous oxygen content, which reflects the amount of oxygen extracted. The normal range is about 4.5–6.0 mL/100 mL of blood. This means on average that about 5.0 mL of oxygen is extracted for every 100 mL of blood passing through the tissues.

76. What are the causes of hypoxemia?

Hypoventilation
Gas diffusion defects
Pulmonary shunts
Ventilation/perfusion mismatching
High altitude

77. What is the normal oxygen consumption ($\dot{V}O_2$) of a person at rest?

Approximately 3.5 mL/min/kg body weight. Thus, a 70-kg person would have a $\dot{V}O_2$ of 245 mL/min (3.5 mL/min × 70 kg) at rest.

78. What is the normal carbon dioxide production ($\dot{V}CO_2$) of a person at rest?

Approximately 3.0 mL/min/kg body weight. Thus, a 70-kg person would have a $\dot{V}CO_2$ of 210 mL/min (3.0 mL/min × 70 kg) at rest.

79. What is the difference between RQ and the respiratory exchange ratio (RER)?

The **RQ** is the ratio between carbon dioxide production and oxygen consumption occurring at the cellular level, whereas the **RER** is the ratio of carbon dioxide output and oxygen uptake occurring in the lung. In steady state, the RQ and RER are equal.

80. Given a $\dot{V}O_2$ of 300 mL/min and a $\dot{V}CO_2$ of 250 mL/min, determine the RQ.

$$RQ = \frac{\dot{V}CO_2}{\dot{V}O_2}$$

$$RQ = \frac{250 \text{ mL/min}}{300 \text{ mL/min}} = 0.83$$

81. During transient hyperventilation, why does the RER increase and not the RQ?

The RER is determined by measuring oxygen uptake and carbon dioxide output from the lung. If an individual is transiently hyperventilating, there is an increase in carbon dioxide output from the lung, and as a result the RER increases. Transient hyperventilation does not affect cellular metabolism; therefore, carbon dioxide production does not change, and subsequently there is no change in the RQ.

82. What happens to the RER when an individual transiently hypoventilates?

During transient hypoventilation, there is a decrease in carbon dioxide output at the level of the lung, and as a result the RER decreases.

83. What is the difference between P_AO_2 and PaO_2?

- **P_AO_2** is the partial pressure of alveolar oxygen expressed in mmHg or torr. The normal value is about 100 mmHg or torr.
- **PaO_2** is the partial pressure of arterial oxygen expressed in mmHg or torr. The normal adult value is $>$ 80 mmHg or torr.

84. What is diffusion?

Diffusion is a process whereby a gas moves from an area of higher concentration to an area of lower concentration across a semipermeable membrane. In the lung, diffusion involves the movement of oxygen and carbon dioxide between the alveoli and the pulmonary capillary bed along their respective gradients across the alveolar-capillary membrane.

85. Describe the pathway for diffusion of oxygen from the alveolus to the red blood cell.

On reaching the alveolar-capillary membrane, an oxygen molecule must cross through the epithelium of a type I alveolar cell, basement membrane, and endothelium; into the plasma; and then into the red blood cell.

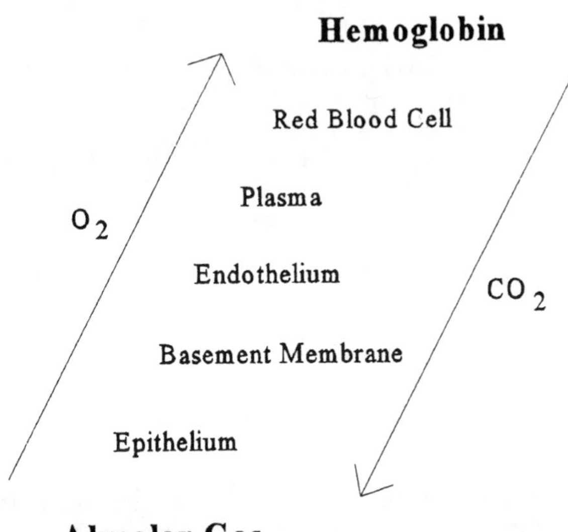

Pathway for diffusion of oxygen from the alveolus to the hemoglobin molecule and carbon dioxide in the opposite direction.

86. How thick is the diffusion pathway (i.e., from the alveolar surface to the surface of the red blood cell)?

About 0.1–0.3 μ (1 μ = 0.003 mm).

87. What factors increase the pathway for diffusion?

- Intra-alveolar edema
- Thickening of the alveolar wall
- Interstitial edema
- Thickened capillary endothelium
- Increased intracapillary path (capillary dilation)

88. How large is the surface area for diffusion in the lung?

The surface area available for gas exchange in the lung is approximately 70–90 m^2, about the size of one side of the playing surface of a tennis court (singles court is 189 m^2; doubles court is 252 m^2). In comparison, the skin has a surface area of about 1.5–2.0 m^2, and as such the lung has been referred to as the **environmental organ** because it has a surface area some 40 times larger than the skin.

89. What factors determine the rate of gas transfer across the alveolar-capillary membrane?

- Pressure difference of the gas between the alveoli and the blood

- Surface area available
- Membrane thickness
- Solubility of the gas
- Diffusion coefficient

90. How long is the transit time in the pulmonary capillary bed?

Under resting conditions, red blood cells move through the pulmonary capillary bed in approximately 0.75 seconds, although equilibration of oxygen and carbon dioxide takes place in about 0.25 seconds.

91. What are the normal partial pressures of oxygen and carbon dioxide in the pulmonary artery and vein?

Pulmonary Artery	Pulmonary Vein
Po_2 = 40 mmHg	100 mmHg
Pco_2 = 47 mmHg	40 mmHg

92. Define solubility.

The amount of gas (in milliliters) that must be dissolved in 100 mL of a liquid to increase the partial pressure by 1 torr.

93. What are the solubility coefficients for the major alveolar gases?

O_2 = 0.024
CO_2 = 0.570
N_2 = 0.012

94. If the solubility of carbon dioxide is more than 20 times greater than for oxygen, why is the rate of equilibration for these two gases the same?

Although the solubility of carbon dioxide is much greater than for oxygen, its larger diffusion coefficient offsets this, and the net effect is nearly the same equilibration.

95. What is the difference between diffusion limited and perfusion limited?

In a **diffusion-limited** gas exchange situation, the alveolar gas is still equilibrating with the blood cell at the end of its transit time. In a **perfusion-limited** gas exchange situation, the blood cell has reached equilibration with alveolar gas during its transit time. Carbon monoxide represents a diffusion-limited exchange, whereas oxygen and carbon dioxide are perfusion limited.

96. In the systemic circulation are oxygen and carbon dioxide diffusion or perfusion limited?

In contrast to the situation in the lung in which both oxygen and carbon dioxide reach equilibration during the transit time (i.e., perfusion limited), in the systemic capillaries, a longer transit time sees greater oxygen extraction and greater carbon dioxide unloading. Therefore, in the systemic circulation, oxygen and carbon dioxide are diffusion limited.

97. Describe Fick's law as it applies to the diffusion of gases across the alveolar-capillary membrane of the lung.

Fick's law states that the diffusion of a gas (e.g., oxygen or carbon dioxide) across a tissue (e.g., the alveolar-capillary membrane) is proportional to the surface area of the tissue and the pressure difference of the gas on either side of the membrane but inversely proportional to the thickness of the tissue:

$D_{gas} = A \times D_C/T \times (P_1 - P_2)$
D_{gas} = diffusion of a gas
A= surface area of the membrane (cm^2)

T= thickness of the membrane (cm)
D_C = diffusion constant of the gas (related to its solubility and molecular weight) (cm^2/mmHg/min)
$P_1 - P_2$ = pressure gradient of the gas between the two sides (mmHg)

98. The ability of the lungs to transport gas is dependent on what two primary factors?
Distribution of alveolar ventilation and perfusion, and the pulmonary diffusing capacity.

99. Is gas exchange more homogeneous in the standing or supine position?
Although gas exchange is somewhat heterogeneous throughout the lung because of differences in ventilation-perfusion match-up from the top of the lung to the bottom, the mismatching is more exaggerated in the vertical (standing position) lung as compared to the horizontal (supine position) lung. Thus, in assuming the supine position, gas exchange becomes more homogeneous.

100. List the factors that contribute to gas exchange being more homogeneous in the supine position.

- The apical-to-basilar distance is greater than from side-to-side, which contributes to more uneven distribution of ventilation and perfusion as a result of the gravitational pull on the lung in the standing versus supine positions.
- The vertical distance is less in the supine position, leading to better match-up between pulmonary blood flow and alveolar ventilation.

101. What is the clinical significance of the alveolar-arterial oxygen difference [$(A-a)Do_2$]?
$(A-a)Do_2$ provides an objective index for assessing the match-up of alveolar ventilation and pulmonary blood flow. Typically the $(A-a)Do_2$ should be less than about 10 mmHg.

102. What is the water vapor pressure (PH_2O) at body temperature and at the boiling point?

Body temperature (37°C):	47 mmHg
Boiling point (100°C):	760 mmHg

103. During strenuous exercise, the rate of gas diffusion can increase by a factor of three. What factors can account for this marked increase?

- Increase in the number of functional alveolar/capillary units, hence an increase in surface area
- Increase in ventilation/perfusion ratio (i.e., a better match-up of ventilation and perfusion) of alveolar/capillary units

PULMONARY CIRCULATION

104. Where does the pulmonary circulation start and end?
The pulmonary circulation encompasses those blood vessels (arteries, capillaries, and veins) that conduct blood from the right side of the heart (right ventricle) through the lungs and then return it to the left side of the heart (left atrium). The pulmonary circulation begins at the pulmonic valve and ends at the junction of the pulmonary veins with the left atrium.

105. Describe the three-compartment model of the lung as it relates to ventilation and perfusion.
The three-compartment model describes three types of lung units (alveolar/capillary) and their ventilation/perfusion ($\dot{V}_A/\dot{Q}$) relationships:

- **Compartment 1**—alveolar/capillary units receiving little to no ventilation but normal blood flow; $\dot{V}_A/\dot{Q} = 0$

- **Compartment 2**—alveolar/capillary units receiving normal ventilation and normal blood flow; $\dot{V}_A/\dot{Q}$ = 0.1 to 10
- **Compartment 3**—alveolar/capillary units receiving normal ventilation but little to no blood flow; $\dot{V}_A/\dot{Q}$ = infinity

106. What are the blood flow characteristics through compartments 1, 2, and 3 of the three-compartment model of ventilation/perfusion?

It has been estimated that 90% of pulmonary capillary blood flow is through compartment 2, and the remaining 10% is split between compartments 1 and 3.

107. Describe West's zones of the lung.

- **Zone 1** is found at the top or apical area of the lung, a region where alveolar pressure exceeds pulmonary arterial and venous pressures:

$$P_A > P_a > P_v$$

- **Zone 2** is found midway in the lung, a region where pulmonary arterial pressure is greater than alveolar pressure owing to the hydrostatic effect:

$$P_a > P_A > P_v$$

- **Zone 3** is found near the bottom or basilar area of the lung, a region where both pulmonary arterial and venous pressures exceed alveolar pressure owing to increased patency of the capillaries, which subsequently compresses the alveoli:

$$P_a > P_v > P_A$$

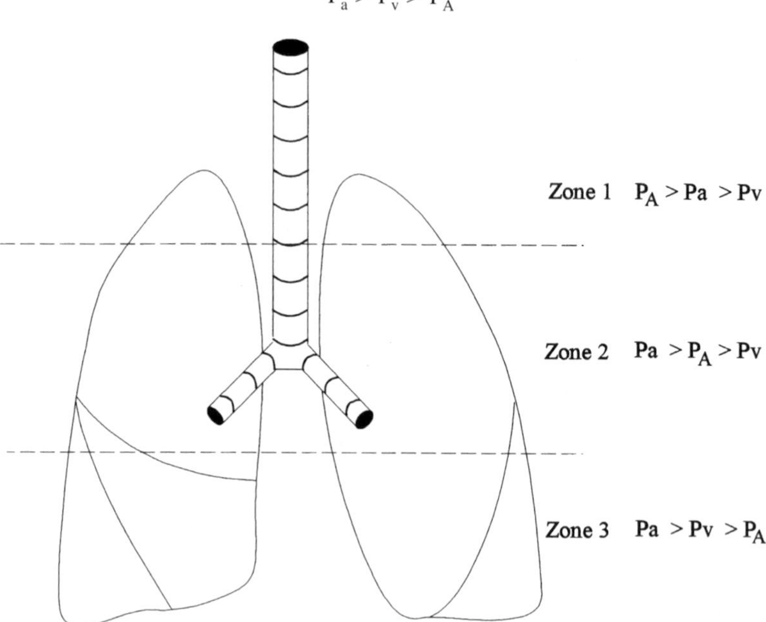

The alveolar (P_A), arterial (P_a), and venous (P_v) pressure gradients in the upright lung. In zone 1, there would be no flow; zone 2, intermittent blood flow; and zone 3, continuous blood flow through the pulmonary capillary bed.

108. What is the normal ventilation/perfusion ratio in healthy lungs?

Although a ventilation/perfusion ratio of 1.0 reflects equal distribution of ventilation and perfusion, there are, in fact, widely different ratios throughout the lung. This is due to both a ventilation and a perfusion gradient from the top of the lung to the bottom of the lung in the upright individual as a result of the effects of gravity on intrathoracic pressures. Not only does this gradient contribute to varying ratios, but also there are disproportionate ventilation and perfusion patterns to the lung units. Theoretically the ventilation/perfusion ratios can vary on a continuum from zero to infinity; however, the range is from 0.1 to 10. Approximately 90% of the pulmonary blood flow is to those areas with ventilation/perfusion ratios of about 1.0, and the remaining 10% is divided between ratios of 0.1 to 1.0 and 1.0 to 10.0 equally.

109. Show the relationship of ventilation and perfusion of an upright lung.

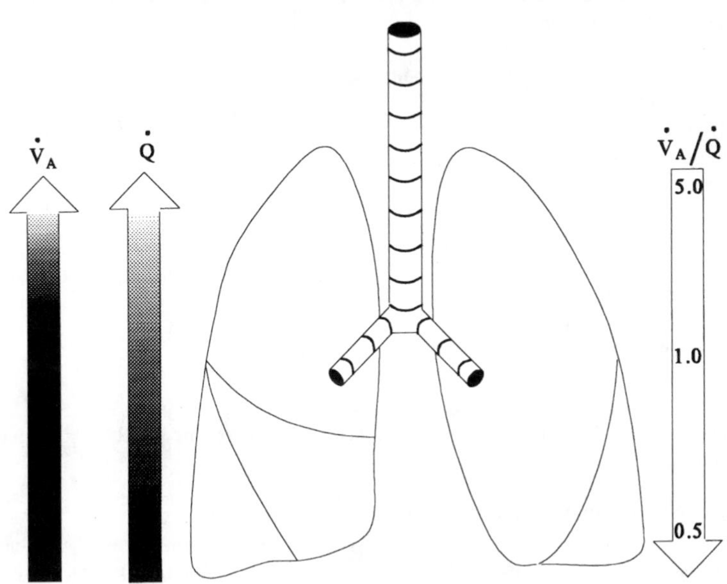

Relationship of ventilation ($\dot{V}_A$) and perfusion ($\dot{Q}$) from the top to the bottom of an upright lung.

110. Does the ventilation/perfusion ratio tell you anything about gas exchange?

The ventilation/perfusion ratio describes the relationship between ventilation and blood flow for the lung but provides no direct indication as to the gas exchange characteristics across the alveolar-capillary membrane.

111. Describe the ventilation/perfusion relationships of a ventilation/perfusion ratio of 0.6 versus a ratio of 8.0.

A ventilation/perfusion ratio of 0.6 implies poorly ventilated alveoli in relation to blood flow and as a result low arterial oxygen tension. A high ventilation/perfusion ratio of 8.0 implies overventilation in relation to blood flow and as a result normal arterial oxygen tension. Overventilation of alveoli does not make up for underventilated alveoli, and a ventilation/perfusion mismatch results.

112. What would be the ventilation/perfusion ratio of a single alveolus if the oxygen tension were equal to mixed venous oxygen tension?

The $\dot{V}_A/\dot{Q}$ ratio of the alveolar capillary unit would be approaching zero (e.g., in obstruction of a bronchus by a mucus plug).

113. Under what circumstances would mixed venous oxygen tension be equal to inspired oxygen tension?

As the ventilation/perfusion ratio approaches infinity, the capillary PO_2 approaches the inspired PO_2 (e.g., in hyperventilation).

114. What is extrapulmonary shunting?

Virtually all of the blood passes through the pulmonary circulation and hence participates in gas exchange. There are, however, several potential sites whereby blood bypasses the pulmonary circulation, and as a consequence mixed venous blood dumps back into the systemic circulation. Ultimately, extrapulmonary shunts dump **desaturated** venous blood into the pulmonary circulation downstream from the alveoli (arterialized blood), reducing the oxygen tension and content of the systemic arterial blood.

115. List examples of extrapulmonary shunting.

- Patent ductus arteriosus
- Atrial septal defect
- Thebesian venous blood flow
- Portion of the bronchial venous blood

116. What is intrapulmonary shunting?

Deoxygenated pulmonary capillary blood bypasses oxygenation and joins up with **arterialized** pulmonary blood, yielding an overall lower oxygen tension.

117. What are examples of intrapulmonary shunting?

A **capillary shunt** occurs when pulmonary blood does not come in contact with a ventilated alveolus (e.g., atelectasis or consolidated pneumonia).

A **venous admixture** occurs when pulmonary blood comes in contact with an alveolus that is underventilated.

118. Are extrapulmonary shunts refractory to supplemental oxygen?

Although supplemental oxygen increases alveolar and subsequently arterial oxygen tensions, the increase is generally not marked. This is due to the fact that although alveolar oxygen tension is increased, if pulmonary blood flow bypasses those alveoli, gas exchange does not take place, and consequently **deoxygenated** blood is still being dumped back into the **oxygenated** or **arterialized** blood, diluting it and rendering low arterial oxygen tensions.

119. Is supplemental oxygen of benefit in treating ventilation/perfusion mismatching?

In ventilation/perfusion mismatching, the pulmonary blood does come in contact with alveoli, and as such if alveolar oxygen is improved, so also are arterial oxygen tensions.

120. What is the difference between pulmonary and bronchial circulations?

The **pulmonary circulation** includes arteries, capillaries, and veins that function in gas exchange between the blood and the environment via the alveolar-capillary membrane. Pulmonary arteries are carrying mixed venous blood from the right side of the heart to the pulmonary capillaries where gas exchange takes place. The pulmonary veins carry **arterialized** blood back to the left side of the heart to be pumped out into the systemic circulation.

The **bronchial circulation** provides oxygenated blood to the tissues of the lung (parenchyma) and removes carbon dioxide. In contrast to the pulmonary arteries and veins, bronchial arteries are carrying **arterialized** blood, and bronchial veins are carrying **deoxygenated** blood.

Almost the entire cardiac output traverses the pulmonary circulation, whereas only about 1–2% of the cardiac output is directed through the bronchial circulation.

121. What is a bronchopulmonary arterial anastomosis?

A direct vascular connection between a pulmonary artery and a bronchial artery.

122. Define venous-admixture–like perfusion.

When poorly ventilated alveoli are well perfused, giving rise to a low ventilation/perfusion ratio, a venous-admixture–like perfusion occurs. The pulmonary capillary blood remains relatively poorly oxygenated and somewhat hypercapnic and subsequently mixes with arterialized blood, the net effect of which is lowering of arterial oxygen tension.

123. What is a true venous admixture?

When pulmonary blood flow bypasses ventilated alveoli, a true venous admixture occurs. In the healthy lung, about 2–3% of pulmonary blood flow is mixed directly with arterialized blood having not taken part in gas exchange.

124. Under normal conditions, how much blood is contained within the pulmonary capillary bed?

At any given time, the total blood volume of the pulmonary circulation is approximately 900 ml, 75–100 ml of which is in the pulmonary capillaries.

125. What is pulmonary vascular resistance and what is a normal value?

The resistance to blood flow through the pulmonary bed. A normal value is 1.5 mmHg/L/min. The pulmonary circulation is a high-compliance, low-resistance vascular bed that contributes to low pressures as compared to the systemic circulation.

126. What are the pressures within the pulmonary vasculature?

Pulmonary artery	25/8 mmHg (mean 15 mmHg)
Pulmonary capillaries	7 mmHg
Pulmonary veins	5 mmHg

127. What mechanisms are available to reduce pulmonary vascular resistance when pulmonary artery pressure increases?

- **Recruitment** involves the addition of either closed or underperfused capillaries to increase the cross-sectional area of the vascular bed, thus reducing the burden of increased pressure in the rest of the system.
- **Distention** involves the increase in capillary caliber primarily via a change in their shape (i.e., from a near-flattened to a circular shape).

128. Define hypoxic pulmonary vasoconstriction.

When the **alveolar** oxygen tension is reduced (< 70 mmHg), there is active vascular smooth muscle contraction in the precapillary pulmonary blood vessels. This shifts blood flow away from the area(s) of reduced oxygen tension to area(s) of normal oxygen tension. The underlying mechanism is not clearly understood but appears to be a local effect mediated by the alveolar epithelial cells. The hypoxic vasoconstriction seen in the lungs is unique, in that systemic hypoxia results in vasodilation.

129. What is the net mean filtration pressure at the pulmonary capillary membrane?

The balance of forces tending to cause movement of fluid outward is approximately +29 mmHg, whereas the balance of forces tending to cause absorption of fluid is approximately –28 mmHg. Thus, the **net mean filtration pressure** is +1 mmHg, which leads to a continuous flow of fluid out of the pulmonary capillaries and into the interstitial space.

	mmHg
Outward forces	
Mean capillary pressure	+7
Interstitial fluid colloid osmotic pressure	+14

(*Table continued on following page.*)

	mmHg
Outward forces (*cont.*)	
Negative interstitial fluid pressure	+8
Total	+29
Inward force	
Plasma fluid osmotic pressure	−28
Total	−28
Net force	**+1**

130. What happens to the fluid that is continually leaking from the pulmonary capillaries?

Under normal circumstances, the capillary fluid is picked up by the pulmonary lymphatic system and returned to the systemic circulation. (Lymph flow in the lung is only a few milliliters per hour.)

131. State Starling's equation for transvascular fluid movement.

$$\text{Flux} = K_{fc}[(P_{iv} - P_{is}) - r_c(C_{iv} - C_{is})]$$

Flux = flow (mL/min)
K_{fc} = capillary filtration coefficient (1/resistance)
P_{iv} = intravascular hydrostatic pressure
P_{is} = interstitial hydrostatic pressure
r_c = reflection coefficient (permeability of the membrane to the proteins exerting the oncotic pressure, averages about 0.75)
C_{iv} = intravascular colloid osmotic pressure
C_{is} = interstitial colloid osmotic pressure

132. What is the significance of negative flux and positive flux?

From Starling's equation, it becomes apparent that P_{iv} and P_{is} are tending to force fluids out of the capillary, and C_{iv} and C_{is} are tending to pull fluids into the capillary. Thus, a **negative flux** indicates fluid reabsorption, and a **positive flux** indicates fluid movement out of the capillary.

133. What is the pulmonary edema safety factor?

Because the net filtration pressure is positive in the pulmonary circulation, there is the tendency for fluid accumulation in the pulmonary interstitium as well as the potential for alveolar edema. In addition to the pulmonary lymphatics, there is a **pulmonary edema safety factor** that guards against the aforementioned. This safety factor requires the pulmonary capillary pressure to increase from 7 to 28 mmHg before pulmonary edema would occur.

134. What is the difference between high-pressure pulmonary edema and high-permeability pulmonary edema?

In **high-pressure** pulmonary edema, there is an increase in pulmonary hydrostatic pressure and as a result an increase in fluid leaking into the interstitial space and alveoli. This can occur in left heart failure.

In **high-permeability** pulmonary edema, there is an increase in capillary permeability to protein and as a result an increase in alveolar fluid. This can occur as a result of damage to the capillary endothelium by chemicals, drugs, or bacterial toxins.

135. What role does nitric oxide play in the control of pulmonary circulation?

Nitric oxide, derived from the endothelium, causes relaxation of vascular smooth muscle. The effects of nitric oxide are modulated via activation of guanylate cyclase and the subsequent production of cyclic guanosine monophosphate. Inhalation of 20 ppm nitric oxide attenuates the hypoxic pulmonary vasoconstriction.

136. Discuss metabolic functions of the lung and pulmonary circulation.

The pulmonary circulation is involved with activation and inactivation of many substances. For example, angiotensin I is converted to angiotensin II by angiotensin-converting enzyme during its passage through the pulmonary circulation. Angiotensin-converting enzyme is found on the surface of the pulmonary capillary endothelial cells. Angiotensin-converting enzyme has also been shown to inactivate bradykinin partially, whereas other substances (e.g., serotonin) are inactivated by uptake and storage. The lung can also secrete immunoglobulins (e.g., IgA) and heparin.

137. How does a deep inspiration affect pulmonary vascular resistance?

As an individual inhales from RV to TLC, there are changes in both alveolar and intrapleural pressures (see figure). The resistance in the extra-alveolar and corner vessels progressively decreases owing to the aforementioned pressure changes, whereas the resistance of intra-alveolar vessels increases as the lung volume increases. Overall the pulmonary vascular resistance decreases from RV to FRC, then increases to TLC as the volume in the lung is progressively increased.

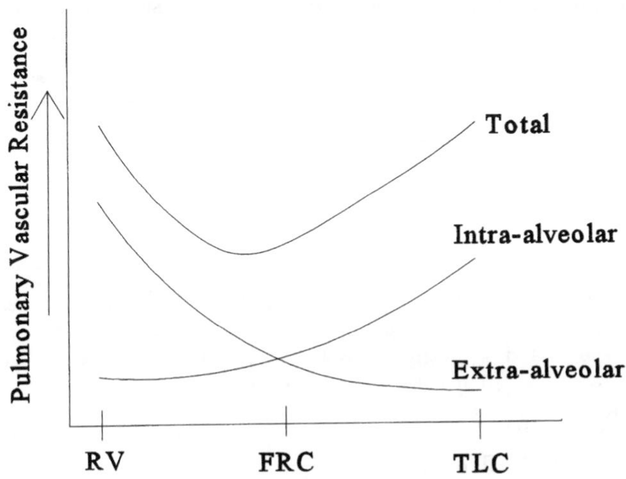

Changes in pulmonary vascular resistance at different lung volumes.

138. What are the neural controls of pulmonary vascular resistance?

- **α-Adrenergic stimulation** causes vascular constriction and hence an increase in PVR.
- **Stimulation of the β-adrenergic receptors** causes dilation and hence a decrease in PVR.
- **Increased sympathetic nerve activity** results in pulmonary vasculature constriction.

GAS TRANSPORT IN BLOOD

139. How are O_2 and CO_2 carried in the blood?

Oxygen is carried in the blood either dissolved (0.003 ml O_2/torr Po_2) or bound to hemoglobin (1.34 ml O_2/g Hb).

Carbon dioxide is carried in three ways

1. Dissolved (2.4 ml/100 ml of blood)
2. As carbamino compounds (5–10%), which are chemical combinations of carbon dioxide to the terminal amine groups of blood proteins (e.g., hemoglobin)
3. As bicarbonate ions (80–90%)

140. What is the function of carbonic anhydrase?

In the red blood cell and on the vascular endothelial surface of the lung, carbonic anhydrase

(CA) is involved in the CO_2 hydration reaction that converts CO_2 to carbonic acid, which subsequently dissociates into hydrogen and bicarbonate ions. Inhibition of CA would require a significant increase in cardiac output to ensure adequate CO_2 exchange.

$$CO_2 + H_2O \overset{CA}{\leftrightarrow} H_2CO_3 \leftrightarrow H^+ + HCO_3^-$$

141. Describe the Bohr and Haldane effects.

The **Bohr effect** states that increasing P_{CO_2} reduces the affinity of hemoglobin for oxygen, thus facilitating the release of oxygen. The Bohr effect aids in the unloading of O_2 from the blood at the level of the tissues.

The **Haldane effect** states that decreasing the O_2 saturation causes a leftward shift in the CO_2 dissociation curve thus facilitating the uptake of CO_2. The Haldane effect helps the loading of CO_2 into the blood at the level of the tissues as the blood gives up O_2 to the tissues.

142. Define respiratory and metabolic acidosis and alkalosis in terms of arterial blood gases.

	ACIDOSIS	ALKALOSIS
Respiratory	Increased Pa_{CO_2} Decreased pHa	Decreased Pa_{CO_2} Increased pHa
Metabolic	Normal Pa_{CO_2} Decreased pHa Decreased bicarbonate	Normal Pa_{CO_2} Increased pHa Increased bicarbonate

Respiratory acidosis and alkalosis are caused by hypoventilation and hyperventilation respectively. Metabolic acidosis is caused either by the loss of bicarbonate ions (e.g., diarrhea) or an increase in acid load in the blood (e.g., ketoacids in uncontrolled type 1 diabetes mellitus). Metabolic alkalosis is caused by either an excess in bicarbonate (e.g., excessive antacid intake) or loss of acid (e.g., severe and prolonged vomiting).

143. Describe the relationship between Pa_{CO_2} and pHa.

The relationship between the arterial CO_2 and pH can be described by a derivation of the Henderson-Hasselbalch equation.

$$pHa = pk + \log \frac{[HCO_3^-]}{s \times Pa_{CO_2}}$$

pk = pH value at which the solute is 50% dissociated (6.1)
s = solubility coefficient (0.0301)

The ratio of the bicarbonate ion to CO_2 determines the pHa. If the Pa_{CO_2} increases, then the pHa decreases and, conversely, if the Pa_{CO_2} decreases, then the pHa increases. Starting with a normal Pa_{CO_2} of 40 mmHg, for every 20 mmHg increase, the pHa will decrease by 0.10, and for every 10 mmHg decrease, the pHa will increase by 0.10. Thus, there is an inverse relationship between Pa_{CO_2} and pHa.

144. How much oxygen can hemoglobin carry?

Each molecule of hemoglobin can bind four oxygen atoms. Thus, each gram of hemoglobin can carry 1.39 mL of oxygen (1 mmol of hemoglobin can carry 14 mmol of oxygen).

1mmol of hemoglobin = 64.5 g
1mmol of O_2 = 22.4 mL

$$\frac{4 \times 22.4 \text{ mL/mmol } O_2}{64.5 \text{ g of Hb}} = \frac{89.6 \text{ mL/mmol}}{64.5 \text{ g Hb}} = 1.39^* \text{ mL } O_2\text{/gram of Hb}$$

*Typically, 1.34 is used because 1.39 represents chemically pure hemoglobin.

145. John suffered acute carbon monoxide poisoning, which resulted in a carboxyhemoglobin level of 50%. Frank, diagnosed with an anemia, had a hemoglobin of 7 g/dL. In terms of oxygenation, which of the patients is in a more critical situation?

In both cases, the hemoglobin available for oxygen transport is in effect reduced by one-half. In the case of the acute carbon monoxide poisoning, one-half of John's hemoglobin is bound to carbon monoxide (COHb = 50%), thereby reducing his arterial oxygen content:

$$\text{Oxygen content} = 1.34\,(\text{hemoglobin} \times \text{Sa}O_2) + (\text{Pa}O_2 \times 0.003)$$

$$O_2 \text{ content} = 1.34(14 \text{ g/dL} \times 50\%) + (80 \text{ mmHg} \times 0.003)$$

$$O_2 \text{ content} = 9.38 \text{ g/dL} + 0.24 = 9.62 \text{ mL/100 mL of blood}$$

Likewise, because Frank's hemoglobin is reduced by one-half of normal, if we assume a normal hemoglobin of about 14 g/dL, his oxygen content is reduced to the same level as John's:

$$O_2 \text{ content} = 1.34(7 \text{ g/dL} \times 100\%\ O_2 \text{ saturation}) + (80 \text{ mmHg} \times 0.003)$$

$$O_2 \text{ content} = 9.38 \text{ g/dL} + 0.24 = 9.62 \text{ mL/100 mL of blood}$$

Although their arterial oxygen contents are reduced to the same level, John is in a more critical situation because carbon monoxide poisoning not only reduces the oxygen-carrying capacity of the blood but also shifts the oxyhemoglobin dissociation curve to the left, altering the affinity of hemoglobin for oxygen. Studies have demonstrated that as the carboxyhemoglobin increases, the affinity of hemoglobin for oxygen increases, which results in less availability of oxygen to the tissues. Evidence has also shown that carbon monoxide can diffuse into cells and bind to myoglobin and cytochromes. An increase in carboxymyoglobin may produce a functionally hypoxic state at the level of the mitochondria despite oxygen delivery at the capillary level. Inhibition of cytochrome C oxidase by carbon monoxide may interfere with transport of adenosine triphosphate across the mitochondrial membrane according to recent studies.

146. At what partial pressure of carbon monoxide (PCO) and oxygen (PO_2) is hemoglobin maximally saturated?

PCO of 1 mmHg (0.14%) saturates hemoglobin to 100% (carboxyhemoglobin).

PO_2 of > 150 mmHg (> 21%) saturates hemoglobin to 100% (oxyhemoglobin).

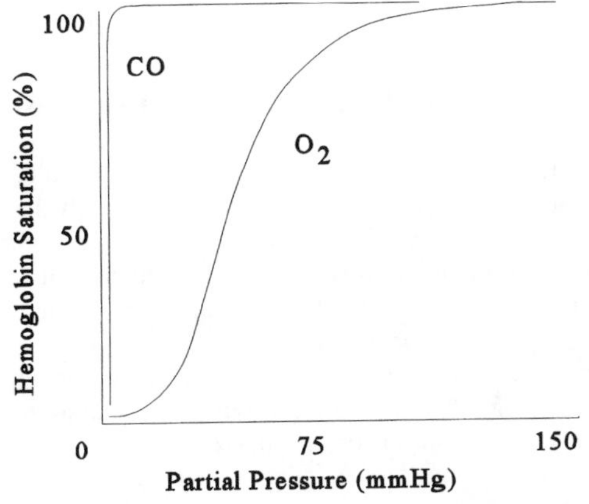

The dissociation curves for oxyhemoglobin and carboxyhemoglobin.

CONTROL OF BREATHING

147. Define control of breathing.

The control of breathing involves mechanisms that work together to generate, regulate, and adjust ventilation to match metabolic needs, whether it be during quiet breathing, sleep, or severe exercise (see figure).

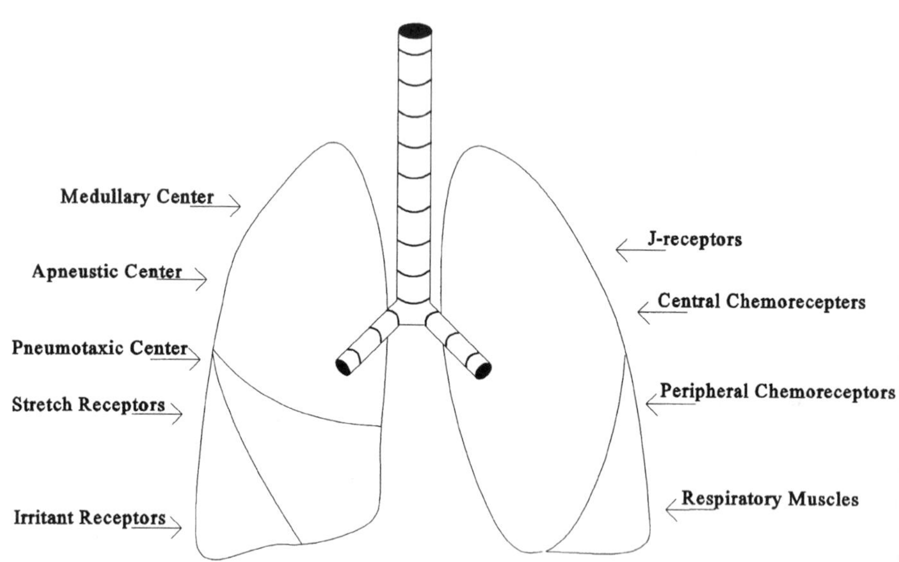

Schematic overview of the functional (not anatomic) control of breathing.

148. What are the mechanisms that control breathing?

- Neural medullary and pontine centers
- Central and peripheral chemosensors
- Lung receptors
- Respiratory muscles

149. What are the functions of the medullary, apneustic, and pneumotaxic respiratory centers?

The **medullary center** (located in the reticular formation of the medulla) is responsible for the coarse control of breathing. It has been divided into two anatomically discrete areas: A dorsal respiratory group of neurons located within the nucleus of the tractus solitarius is associated with inspiration, and a ventral respiratory group of neurons located in the nucleus ambiguus and retroambiguus is associated primarily with expiration. The medullary center has been identified as the site for the inherent rhythmicity of breathing.

The **apneustic center** is found in the lower portion of the pons and appears to retard the switch-off of inspiration. Although there is some question as to whether or not the apneustic center plays a role in human respiration, it has been associated with prolonged inspiratory gasps.

The **pneumotaxic center,** located in the nucleus parabrachialis of the upper pons, is responible for switching off inspiration (i.e., it limits inspiration). A strong signal from the pneumotaxic center causes a short inspiration (0.5 seconds) and increases breathing frequency up to 30–40 breaths/min, whereas a weak stimulus prolongs inspiratory effort for 5 seconds or more, decreasing the breathing rate to just a couple of breaths per minute. The pneumotaxic center does contribute to regulation of inspiratory volume.

150. What is meant by the term inspiratory ramp signal?

During normal breathing, the nerve impulse pattern sent to the inspiratory muscles exhibits a weak signal followed by a progressively stronger signal (i.e., a ramp signal) over a 2-second duration and then a 3-second termination. The pattern of the inspiratory ramp signal allows for a smooth inspiration rather than an abrupt inspiration.

151. Where are the central and peripheral chemoreceptors located?

- Central chemoreceptors—within the ventrolateral surface of the medulla
- Peripheral chemoreceptors—in the carotid bodies (located at the bifurcation of the common carotid arteries) and in the arch of the aorta

152. To what do the peripheral chemoreceptors respond?

The peripheral chemoreceptors respond to changes in PaO_2, $PaCO_2$, and the arterial pH by changing their rate of nerve firing to the central nervous system. Specifically, either a decrease in PaO_2 or arterial pH or an increase in the $PaCO_2$ alters the rate of firing. For example, a change in the rate of nerve firing in response to PaO_2 begins at about 500 mmHg and reaches its maximum when the arterial oxygen drops below 50–60 mmHg. The increase in response to hypoxemia is largely as a result of the peripheral chemoreceptors.

153. Outline the nerve pathway of the peripheral chemoreceptor system.

From the carotid bodies, afferent nerve fibers pass through Hering's nerve to the glossopharyngeal nerves and then to the dorsal respiratory neurons of the medulla. From the aortic bodies, afferent nerve fibers pass through the vagi and then to the dorsal respiratory neurons.

154. What is the normal response to breathing increasing F_ICO_2?

Normal individuals increase their ventilation by a factor of four when breathing 5% carbon dioxide or approximately 1.5–2.5 L/min per mmHg increase in $PaCO_2$. (See figure, top of next page.)

155. How is the response to oxygen measured?

There are both steady-state and rebreathing techniques available to test an individual's ventilatory response to decreasing F_IO_2. So as not to confound the results, the gas mixture must be maintained with near-normal alveolar carbon dioxide levels.

156. To what do the central chemoreceptors respond?

The central chemoreceptors, because of their location, respond to changes in the pH of the extracellular fluid of the brain. The makeup of the extracellular fluid is determined by the cerebrospinal fluid, local blood flow, and local metabolism. Although the blood-brain barrier is impermeable to the hydrogen ion (H^+), carbon dioxide diffuses across it easily. An increase in the $PaCO_2$ leads to an increase in cerebrospinal fluid carbon dioxide, thereby increasing H^+, which, in turn, stimulates the central chemoreceptors, resulting in an increase in ventilation. The central chemoreceptors are responsible for about 60% of the ventilatory response to carbon dioxide.

157. What is the normal pH of the cerebrospinal fluid?

7.32.

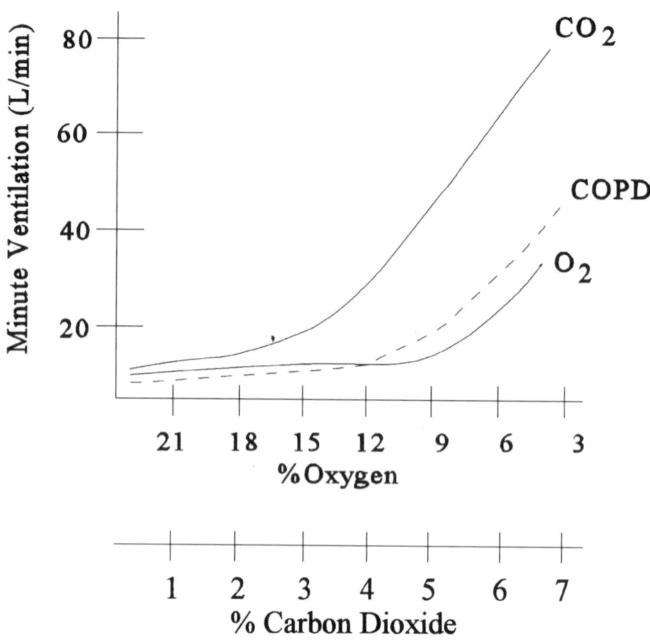

The normal ventilatory responses to decreasing inspired oxygen (O_2) and increasing inspired carbon dioxide (CO_2). The chronic obstructive pulmonary disease (COPD) curve represents the blunted CO_2 response in a person with emphysema.

158. How does a change in $Pa{CO_2}$ affect cerebrospinal fluid pH as compared with arterial pH?

Because it has less protein than arterial blood, the cerebrospinal fluid pH has lower buffering capacity than the arterial blood. Therefore, a small change in $Pa{CO_2}$ results in a larger change in cerebrospinal fluid pH as compared with arterial pH.

159. Can a reduction in arterial pH without a concomitant increase in $Pa{CO_2}$ stimulate a change in ventilation?

In the face of a decrease in arterial pH alone, ventilation increases under isocapnic conditions (see figure). The increase in ventilation seen in response to a decrease in arterial pH (e.g., meta-

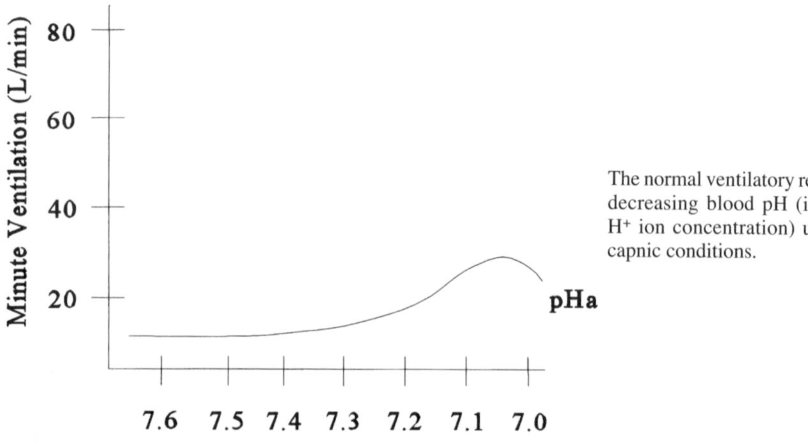

The normal ventilatory response to decreasing blood pH (increasing H^+ ion concentration) under isocapnic conditions.

bolic acidosis) is less than under hypercapnic conditions. The peripheral chemoreceptors have been implicated in the primary response, although a secondary effect from the central chemoreceptors may also play a role.

160. Identify the different types of lung receptors and discuss their function.

1. **Pulmonary stretch receptors** are located in the smooth muscle of the airway and respond to lung distention, subsequently increasing expiratory time and thereby decreasing respiratory rate. Two types of pulmonary stretch receptors have been identified, slowly adapting (SAR) and rapidly adapting (RAR) receptors. The SARs lie in the smooth muscle of both intrathoracic and extrathoracic airways and are activated by increases in V_t. The SARs may be responsible for increased expiratory time (T_E). Although the SARs are mechanoreceptors, evidence has demonstrated that they may also respond to changes in carbon dioxide. Airway hypercarbia decreases SAR discharge and subsequently increases respiratory drive to reduce airway levels of carbon dioxide. The RARs are associated with airway epithelial cells near the carina and large bronchi of the lung and respond to both mechanical and chemical stimuli. Both hyperinflation and hypoinflation stimulate the RARs and may be responsible for the deflation reflex. Reports have also demonstrated response of the RARs to smoke and ammonia.
2. **Juxtacapillary or juxta-alveolar receptors** are located in the capillary or alveolar walls. They respond to pulmonary capillary congestion and increases in interstitial fluid, thereby resulting in tachypnea and dyspnea. There is also an associated reflex bradycardia and hypotension.
3. **Irritant receptors** are located in the epithelial cells of the nose and upper airways. They respond to smoke, dust, cold air, and noxious gases, resulting in hyperpnea and bronchoconstriction.
4. **Upper airway receptors** are located in the nose, larynx, nasopharynx, and trachea. They respond to both mechanical and chemical stimuli, causing coughing, sneezing, and bronchospasm.

161. What is the short-term response to breathing at high altitudes?

On ascending to a high altitude (e.g., 10,000 feet [3048 m]), the resulting decrease in PaO_2 is sensed by the peripheral chemoreceptors with a concomitant increase in alveolar ventilation. As a result of this hyperventilation, there is a decrease in arterial and cerebrospinal fluid CO_2. This reduction in cerebrospinal fluid PCO_2 leads to an increase in pH, which inhibits the central chemoreceptors.

162. What happens after several days at high altitude?

Although the bicarbonate (HCO_3^-) level is decreased, restoring the cerebrospinal fluid pH and eliminating the alkalemia, hyperventilation continues.

163. What are the mechanisms involved in high-altitude acclimatization?

With high-altitude acclimatization, there is observed an increase in alveolar ventilation, capillarity, gas diffusion, and oxygen extraction (i.e., wider arteriovenous oxygen content difference). Concomitant increases in red blood cell content (hematocrit may rise to 60%) and hemoglobin (may rise to 20 g/dL) will result in an increase in the oxygen-carrying capacity. There is also a leftward shift in the oxyhemoglobin dissociation curve, which increases the affinity of hemoglobin for oxygen.

164. During the normal course of the day, what factor is the most important in the control of breathing?

Under normal circumstances, the $PaCO_2$ is the major determinant of breathing being held to within ± 3 mmHg. A 1–2 mmHg increase in the $PaCO_2$ evokes a 30–40% increase in minute ventilation.

165. What is the hypoxic drive?

Because of chronic carbon dioxide retention, patients with chronic obstructive pulmonary disease have lost their sensitivity to pH changes in the cerebrospinal fluid and remain dependent on the response of peripheral chemoreceptors to arterial oxygen changes. Thus, arterial hypoxemia and not hypercapnia provides their stimulus to breathe (i.e., the hypoxic drive or low oxygen stimulus). This drive can be dampened by supplemental oxygen, and thus, when titrating oxygen it is best to monitor the $PaCO_2$ as well as the PaO_2.

166. In carbon monoxide poisoning, will the hypoxic drive be triggered?

Although the oxygen content and saturation are low, the PaO_2 is within normal limits and thus the hypoxic drive will not be triggered.

167. What is Kussmaul breathing?

In diabetic ketoacidosis, there is a decrease in arterial pH, which leads to an increase in V_t and $\dot{V}_E$ that has been termed **Kussmaul breathing**. Kussmaul breathing leads to hypocapnia and a subsequent decrease in the extracellular bicarbonate content.

168. What is the difference between apnea and apneustic breathing?

- **Apnea** is the cessation of breathing with or without a concomitant decrease in arterial oxygen
- **Apneustic breathing** is characterized by prolonged inspirations followed by brief periods of expiration.

169. What is Cheyne-Stokes breathing?

Cheyne-Stokes breathing is a form of periodic breathing characterized by a waxing-waning tidal volume with interspersed periods of apnea lasting 10–20 seconds. The underlying mechanism of Cheyne-Stokes breathing is a lag time between hyperventilation, which increases PaO_2 and decreases $PaCO_2$ and chemosensor detection. The respiratory center responds by decreasing ventilation, and consequently the PaO_2 decreases and $PaCO_2$ increases. This results in a cycle that repeats itself about every 40–60 seconds.

170. Describe the Hering-Breuer reflex.

The Hering-Breuer reflex, also referred to as the **inspiratory-inhibitory** or **inflation reflex,** is triggered by large inspiratory efforts. The subsequent increase in lung volume causes increased rate of firing from the airway stretch receptors and switching off of the inspiration. It is thought that the Hering-Breuer reflex becomes active when the V_t is greater than 1.5–2.0 L.

171. What is the deflation or excito-inspiratory reflex?

The deflation reflex is initiated by collapse of areas of the lung, which elicits a rapid inspiration and an increase in frequency of breathing.

172. At what level of respiratory muscle force does fatigue set in?

The respiratory muscles can work at about 40% of their maximal force for indefinite periods. Above this level, respiratory muscle fatigue becomes a major factor and can contribute to ventilatory failure.

173. What is the duty cycle?

A **duty cycle** is not a list of jobs a worker is to complete by the end of his or her shift that repeats itself every day. The duty cycle is an objective measurement to assess respiratory muscle function. It is the ratio of inspiratory time to the duration of the respiratory cycle (both inspiratory and expiratory times) and is seen to increase in respiratory muscle fatigue:

$$\text{Duty cycle} = \frac{T_I}{T_I + T_E} = \frac{T_I}{T_{tot}}$$

T_I = inspiratory time
T_E = expiratory time
T_{tot} = total duration of one respiratory cycle

174. What is meant by the term air hunger?

As the $PaCO_2$ increases above 50–60 mmHg, the individual's minute ventilation is nearing maximum, and he or she experiences a sensation of labored breathing or **air hunger**. If the $PaCO_2$ exceeds 80–100 mmHg, the individual can become semicomatose, and at levels greater than 120 mmHg, death occurs. Air hunger is also referred to as **dyspnea**.

175. What is the gamma system?

The **gamma system** has been implicated in the sensation of dyspnea that occurs when there is an increase in respiratory effort as a result of respiratory disease. The intercostal muscles and the diaphragm contain receptors in their muscle spindles, innervated by gamma motoneurons, which are stimulated by muscle elongation and hence control the strength of contraction.

176. What factors account for the sensation of dyspnea?

Dyspnea, or labored breathing, is a subjective feeling experienced by an individual who is having a difficult time breathing deep or fast enough to keep up with the increasing metabolic demands of oxygen consumption and carbon dioxide production. The primary factors associated with the feeling of dyspnea include:

Hypercapnia
Hypoxia
Increase in the mechanical work of breathing
A psychogenic component

177. During exercise, there is an increased metabolic demand that is met by a concomitant increase in ventilation. This increase in ventilation is as a result of changes in V_t and respiratory rate. What is the appropriate response in terms of V_t and respiratory rate?

Changes in ventilation can be accomplished by increasing V_t, respiratory rate, frequency, or a combination. The normal response is a linear increase in both $\dot{V}_E$ and V_t until about half the individual's VC. Beyond that, increases in $\dot{V}_E$ are accomplished by significant increases in respiratory rate. Up to about twice the V_t, T_I (inspiratory time) remains constant with concomitant decreases in T_E. Further increases in V_t are inversely related to T_I. Thus, increases in $\dot{V}_E$ are now a result of decreases in both T_I and T_E.

178. What is the pre-Botzinger complex?

A region located in the ventrolateral medulla model that contains a group of pacemaker neurons responsible for respiratory rhythmogenesis.

179. Discuss the model of respiratory rhythm generation.

Evidence has suggested that the respiratory cycle is made up of three phases, which has been proposed as a model for respiratory rhythm:

- **Phase 1**—inspiratory phase, which is terminated by late-inspiratory inhibitory interneurons
- **Phase 2**—postinspiratory phase, which inhibits inspiratory neurons
- **Phase 3**—expiratory phase, which promotes active expiration

180. What is the mechanism of chemotransduction by the cells of the carotid body in response to decreased PaO_2?

Although the mechanism has not been clearly elucidated, it has been suggested that in response to low arterial oxygen (below 50–60 mmHg), there is a reduction in potassium (K^+) channel activity and an increase in calcium (Ca^{++}) from intracellular stores. A reduction in cell membrane bound K^+ channel activity would lead to depolarization and subsequent propagation of action potentials. This would lead to opening of voltage-gated Ca^{++} channels, allowing Ca^{++} to enter the cell and subsequent release of neurotransmitter.

181. A reduction in cerebrospinal fluid pH results in an increase in ventilation. Is the hydrogen ion itself a unique chemical stimulus to the observed change in ventilation?

There is a greater increase in ventilation owing to reduction in cerebrospinal fluid pH as a result of hypercapnia than isocapnic acidemia. These results suggest that a reduction in cerebrospinal fluid pH, although a stimulus to increased ventilation, is not the unique stimulus because there is a difference in the ventilatory response to a metabolic acidosis or a respiratory acidosis.

182. What limits how long you can hold your breath?

The break point for breath hold occurs at about a $Pa{CO_2}$ of 50 mmHg. At this point, the stimulus to breathe overwhelms any voluntary effort to hold your breath.

183. What is the synergistic effect between carbon dioxide and oxygen?

It has been shown that the ventilatory response to an increased $Paco_2$ combined with a decreased PaO_2 is augmented. The combined effect is a greater stimulus to an increased ventilation than the sum of each separately (i.e., synergism).

184. Is the inspired oxygen tension less in a commercial airplane than at sea level?

The cabins of commercial aircraft are pressurized to about 5000–6000 feet above sea level. As a result, although the fractional concentration of oxygen is the same as at sea level, the barometric pressure is less, yielding a lower oxygen tension.

Example: Given the following data, calculate the inspired oxygen tension (P_IO_2) in the cabin of an airplane:

$P_B = 600$ mmHg

$P_{H2O} = 47$ mmHg

$F_IO_2 = 0.2093$ (21%)

$P_IO_2 = F_IO_2 \times (P_B - P_{H_2O}) = 0.2093(600 \text{ mmHg} - 47 \text{ mmHg}) = 116 \text{ mmHg}$

This translates to a lower arterial oxygen tension in the passenger owing to a lower inspired oxygen tension. At sea level, the inspired oxygen tension is 149 mmHg.

BIBLIOGRAPHY

1. American Thoracic Society: Single-breath carbon monoxide diffusing capacity (transfer factor). Am J Respir Crit Care Med 152:2185–2198, 1995.
2. Cherniack RM: Pulmonary Function Testing, 2nd ed. Philadelphia, W.B. Saunders, 1992.
3. Cherniack RM, Cherniack L, Naimark A: Respiration in Health and Disease, 3rd ed. Philadelphia, W.B. Saunders, 1983.
4. Forster RE, Dubois AB, Briscoe WA, Fisher AB: The Lung: Physiologic Basis of Pulmonary Function Tests, 3rd ed. Chicago, Year Book Medical Publishers, 1986.
5. Guyton AC, Hall JE: Textbook of Medical Physiology, 10th ed. Philadelphia, W.B. Saunders, 2001.
6. Hlastala MP, Berger AJ: Physiology of Respiration, 2nd ed. Oxford, Oxford University Press, 2001.
7. Levitzky MG: Pulmonary Physiology, 5th ed. New York, McGraw-Hill, 1999.
8. Murray JF, Nadel JA: Textbook of Respiratory Medicine, vol 1, 3rd ed. Philadelphia, W.B. Saunders, 2001.
9. Ruppel G: Manual of Pulmonary Function Testing, 7th ed. St. Louis, Mosby, 1998.
10. Shapiro BA, Peruzzi WT, Templin R: Clinical Application of Blood Gases, 5th ed. St. Louis, Mosby, 1994.
11. West JB: Respiratory Physiology: The Essentials, 6th ed. Philadelphia, Lippincott Williams & Wilkins, 2000.

6. RENAL PHYSIOLOGY

David L. Mattson, Ph.D.

BODY FLUIDS

1. How much of the body is composed of water?

By weight, the body is composed of 50–70% water. This percentage varies depending on the individual body type because the water content of fat (approximately 20%) is much less than that of muscle (approximately 70%). In general, an average person has a total body water (TBW) of approximately 60% of body weight. The average 70-kg man would then have approximately 42 L of TBW (70 × 0.6 [1 L of water has a mass of 1 kg]). In contrast, an extremely lean, muscular individual would have a TBW that is close to 70% of total body weight, and an obese person would have a TBW that is nearer to 50% of total body weight.

2. Where in the body is the TBW located?

TBW is distributed between two major compartments, the **intracellular** and the **extracellular compartments,** which are separated by the cell membranes. The fluid volumes in these compartments are known as the **intracellular fluid** (ICF) and the **extracellular fluid** (ECF). The ICF is the fluid found within the cells, and the ECF is the fluid outside of cells, including the interstitial fluid, lymph, and plasma.

3. What proportion of TBW is in the intracellular and extracellular compartments?

In general, the ICF comprises two-thirds of TBW, whereas the ECF constitutes one-third of TBW. The average 70-kg man with approximately 42 L of TBW would then have approximately 28 L (42 L × ⅔) in the ICF and approximately 14 L (42 L × ⅓) in the ECF.

4. How is the ECF distributed?

The ECF is distributed into two major compartments, the **interstitial fluid** and the **plasma**. The barrier between these two compartments is composed of the highly permeable systemic capillaries. The interstitial fluid volume is approximately four-fifths of ECF, and the plasma volume is approximately one-fifth of ECF volume. The average 70-kg man with 14 L of ECF volume would therefore have approximately 11.2 L in the interstitial fluid (14 L × ⅘) and approximately 2.8 L of plasma (14 L × ⅕).

5. Calculate the normal blood volume.

The normal plasma volume is approximately 2.8 L, and the hematocrit (packed red blood cell fraction of blood) averages 0.38 to 0.42; therefore, the average individual has a blood volume of approximately 4.7 L (plasma volume/[1 – Hct] = 2.8 L/[1 – 0.4]).

6. What is osmolarity?

Osmolarity is a function of the total number of particles in solution, independent of mass, charge, or chemical composition. The dissolved particles (osmolytes) exert a force that tends to pull water across semipermeable membranes (osmotic pressure). Dissolved particles in biologic solutions are expressed in terms of milliosmoles (mOsm). For substances that do not dissociate into smaller particles when dissolved (i.e., urea, glucose, inulin), 1 mole = 1 osmole and 1 mmole = 1 mOsm. For substances that dissolve into two particles (sodium chloride [NaCl]) or three particles (calcium chloride [$CaCl_2$]), the osmolarity is double or triple the molarity (1 mmole NaCl = 2 mOsm). Osmolarity is therefore the concentration of osmotically active particles in solution and is expressed in terms of mOsm/L of water. In the body, the osmolarity of the ECF and ICF averages 280–300 mOsm/L.

7. What is osmolality?

An alternative notation used to express the concentration of dissolved particles is **osmolality,** which is expressed in terms of mOsm/kg of water. In relatively dilute solutions, such as those found in the body, the difference between osmolarity and osmolality is so small that the two terms are used interchangeably.

8. Define osmosis.

Osmosis is the movement of water across a semipermeable membrane owing to differences in osmolarity (an osmotic pressure gradient). Osmosis occurs from a fluid compartment in which the solute concentration is lower to a second compartment in which the solute concentration is higher until the osmolarity on each side of the membrane is equal. A semipermeable membrane (such as a cell membrane) is one that is permeable to water but not solutes. It is critical to recognize that a dissolved particle can exert an osmotic force only if it is not permeable in the membrane.

9. What is tonicity?

The total concentration of solutes in a solution that are not permeable in the cell membrane. Because these solutes exert an effective osmotic pressure in cells, the tonicity of a solution determines the effect of the solution on water movement into or out of cells.

10. Explain the influence of hypotonic, isotonic, and hypertonic solutions on cell volume.

- When a cell is placed in an **isotonic** solution, the cell volume will be unaltered.
- When a cell is placed in a **hypotonic** solution, the cell will swell.
- When a cell is placed in a **hypertonic** solution, the cell will shrink.

11. Is there a difference in the total osmolarity of the ICF and ECF?

No, under normal steady-state conditions, the total concentration of dissolved particles in the intracellular and extracellular compartments is equal because the cellular membranes are highly permeable to water, and any differences in osmolarity between these compartments are quickly corrected due to osmosis. Because the total concentration of substances that are osmotically active is the same in the ECF and ICF, the osmolarity of the ECF and ICF is equal (280–300 mOsm/kg).

12. Are there differences in the ionic composition of the fluid found in the ECF and ICF?

Over 90% of the ions in the extracellular fluid are sodium, chloride, and bicarbonate; the concentration of other ionic species in the ECF is relatively low. In contrast, the intracellular fluid is high in potassium and phosphate, whereas the ions abundant in the extracellular fluid (sodium and its anions) are relatively low within the cells.

Concentration of Selected Ions (mEq/L), pH, and Osmolarity (mOsm/L) in the ECF and ICF

	ECF	ICF (MUSCLE)
Sodium	145	10
Potassium	4	155
Calcium	5	0
Chloride	110	2
Bicarbonate	24	8
Phosphate	2	140
pH	7.4	7.15
Osmolality	290	290

13. Why are there differences in the concentration of the individual ions in the ECF and ICF?

The primary reason for the difference observed in the ECF and ICF is the cell membrane and the Na^+, K^+-ATPase pump which is found in the cell membranes. Cell membranes are highly permeable to water but the permeability to most electrolytes is relatively low. The Na^+, K^+-ATPase pump also plays a critical role in the regulation of intracellular concentration by actively transporting sodium out of cells (against this ion's electrochemical gradient) and pumping potassium into cells. Although sodium is driven by its electrochemical gradient into the cells, the sodium that diffuses into cells is actively extruded from the cells to maintain a low intracellular sodium concentration, whereas potassium is actively transported into cells.

14. Are there differences in the composition of the plasma and the interstitial fluid?

There is a slight difference in the ionic composition of plasma when compared to the interstitial fluid. This difference is due to plasma protein (approximately 6 g/dL), which is mostly in the form of albumin. The plasma proteins are effectively trapped in the plasma because the capillary membranes in most tissues are relatively impermeable to protein. The albumin carries a net negative charge, which tends to hold extra amounts of cations in the plasma. This property, known as the **Donnan effect,** slightly alters the distribution of other ions between the plasma and the interstitial space and leads to slightly greater concentration of cations (3–4 mEq/L) and slightly decreased concentration of anions in the plasma relative to the interstitial fluid.

15. Does water move from one body compartment to another?

Yes, as a result of differences in hydrostatic pressure, osmotic pressure, or both.

16. What regulates the distribution of water between the plasma and the interstitial fluid?

Fluid exchange between the plasma and the interstitial fluid is governed by **Starling's law** for capillary fluid exchange. That is, the net flux of fluid into or out of capillaries is determined by the algebraic sum of the hydrostatic and osmotic forces on either side of the capillaries. As a result of the pumping action of the heart, a systemic capillary has a relatively high hydrostatic pressure (25 mmHg) that favors movement of fluid out of the capillaries. Forces opposing movement of fluid out of the capillaries include the plasma oncotic pressure (the osmotic pressure exerted by proteins) and interstitial fluid hydrostatic pressure. Without forces opposing capillary hydrostatic pressure, primarily the plasma oncotic pressure, the plasma volume would rapidly be transferred to the interstitial fluid. These forces can be expressed in the simple equation:

$$\text{Flux} = K_f\,[(P_{cap} + \Pi_{int}) - (\Pi_{cap} + \Pi_{int})]$$

K_f = Ultrafiltration coefficient
P_{cap} = Capillary hydrostatic pressure
Π_{int} = Interstitial oncotic pressure
Π_{cap} = Plasma oncotic pressure
P_{int} = Interstitial hydrostatic pressure

In general, the forces favoring filtration slightly exceed those opposing filtration. This leads to a net filtration out of the capillaries, which is collected as lymph and returned to the circulation.

17. How is fluid exchanged between the ECF and ICF?

The movement of fluid between the ECF and ICF is governed by osmotic forces. The cell membranes are highly permeable to water and semipermeable to most solutes. Any change in ionic composition in one compartment is reflected in the osmolarity of that compartment (provided that the ion is not permeable in the cell membrane), and water quickly crosses the cell membranes until osmolarity is equal in both compartments.

18. How can the different body fluid compartments be measured?

The volume of different body compartments can be measured most easily by determining the volume of distribution of compounds known to be freely distributed within a certain compartment. In this technique, a known quantity of a substance that is distributed in the body fluid compartment of interest is administered. After a sufficient amount of time is allowed for equilibration, a sample of the fluid from that compartment is taken. By dividing the original amount injected (A_X) by the concentration of substance X at equilibrium (C_X), the volume of distribution (V_{DX}) is calculated ($V_{DX} = A_X/C_X$).

19. Describe the ideal substance for measuring volume of distribution.

- Nontoxic
- Mixes well in and is not removed from the targeted compartment
- Is not metabolized or synthesized in the body
- Rate of excretion easily quantified
- Easily and accurately measurable

Example: A 70-kg man is injected intravenously with 4×10^6 cpm of tritiated water (^3H_2O); 15 minutes later, a blood sample is taken, and the blood contains 100 cpm/mL ^3H_2O. The calculated volume of distribution of ^3H_2O in this individual is therefore 40 L (4×10^6 cpm/100 cpm/mL = 40,000 mL = 40 L). In cases in which compounds are excreted, the amount that has been excreted must be subtracted from the amount originally injected to determine an accurate volume of distribution.

20. Name some compounds used to measure volume of distribution of different body fluid compartments.

Body Fluid Compartment	Compound
Total body water	H_2O (^3H_2O)
Extracellular volume	Sodium (^{22}Na)
	Inulin (^3H-inulin)
	Iothalamate (^{125}I-iothalamate)
Plasma volume	Albumin (^{125}I-albumin)
	Evans blue dye

21. How can the volume of the interstitial fluid and ICF compartments be determined?

The ICF and interstitial fluid volumes can be calculated using the measured volumes of TBW, ECF volume, and plasma volume:

- The **ICF volume** can be determined by subtracting the ECF volume from TBW (ICF = TBW – ECF).
- **Interstitial fluid volume** can be calculated by subtracting plasma volume from extracellular volume (ISF = ECF – PV).

22. What will happen to the different body volume compartments after the intake of isotonic saline solution?

Isotonic NaCl (0.9%, 290 mOsm/L) has an osmolarity equal to that found in the ECF and ICF. Both NaCl and water are freely permeable throughout plasma and the interstitial space, so an isotonic NaCl load will be **equally distributed** throughout the ECF. Because sodium can enter the cells but is actively excluded by the Na^+, K^+-ATPase, any added sodium will be effectively trapped in the ECF. Since isotonic saline has the same osmolarity as the ECF and ICF, there will be no osmotic effect leading to a fluid shift between the ECF and ICF. The intake of isotonic NaCl will thus **increase TBW and ECF but will not appreciably alter ICF volume;** osmolarity of both the ECF and the ICF will be **unaltered** from the original value.

23. What will happen to the different body volume compartments after the intake of hypertonic saline solution?

A hypertonic NaCl load (osmolarity > 290 mOsm/L) will also initially be distributed equally throughout the ECF. The difference between the isotonic and hypertonic load is the final osmolarity that is attained in the ECF and ICF. Because the osmolarity will initially be increased in the ECF owing to the hypertonic saline, water will move freely down its concentration gradient out of the cells until a new osmolarity is achieved. A hypertonic NaCl load will therefore **expand TBW, increase ECF,** and **decrease ICF volume**. A new level of osmolarity will be attained that will be equal throughout the ECF and ICF but will be **elevated from the value before the hypertonic load**.

24. What will happen to the different body volume compartments after the intake of hypotonic saline solution?

A hypotonic NaCl load (osmolarity < 290 mOsm/L) will also initially be distributed equally throughout the ECF. The major difference between the isotonic and hypotonic loads is the final osmolarity that is attained in the ECF and ICF. Because the ECF osmolarity initially will be decreased, water will move down its concentration gradient out of the ECF into the cells until a new osmolarity is achieved. A hypotonic NaCl load will therefore **expand TBW, increase ECF volume,** and **increase ICF volume**. The new level of osmolarity will be **equal** throughout the ECF and ICF and will be **decreased from the original value**.

25. How are clinical abnormalities in body fluid status evaluated?

The most commonly used clinical index of body fluid is the measurement of plasma or serum sodium. Because sodium and its anions are the major ionic species of the ECF, **plasma sodium** (P_{Na}) is used as a clinical indication of volume status. Under normal conditions, P_{Na} is 145 mEq/L. When P_{Na} exceeds this value, the patient is said to be **hypernatremic;** when a patient's P_{Na} is less than this value, the individual is **hyponatremic**.

26. What conditions lead to hypernatremia?

- Conditions in which thirst is impaired (coma, neurologic abnormality, or drug effects)
- Situations with no access to drinking water
- Loss of extracellular water (increased ECF sodium concentration with decreased ECF volume)
- Sodium retention or excess sodium intake (increased ECF sodium concentration with normal or elevated ECF volume)
- Selective loss of ECF fluid (e.g., owing to lack of secretion of antidiuretic hormone [ADH] or the inability of the kidneys to respond to ADH)
- Excessive evaporative losses (such as those that occur in individuals with extensive second-degree and third-degree burns)
- Conditions in which excessive amounts of sodium-retaining hormones (such as aldosterone) are secreted into the blood

It is important to distinguish the cause of hypernatremia in patients to select the correct therapeutic measures to be taken.

27. Name some conditions that lead to hyponatremia.

- Excess retention or intake of water (hyponatremia with increased ECF volume): Inappropriate or uncontrolled secretion of ADH (kidney retains excess amounts of water and leads to expansion of extracellular water and hyponatremia)
- Increased excretion or decreased intake of sodium (hyponatremia with reduced ECF volume)
  Kidney disease
  Inappropriate use of diuretics
  Conditions in which there is decreased secretion of sodium-retaining hormones (aldosterone)

28. What is edema?

Edema is a condition in which excess fluid accumulates in the body tissues, usually in the interstitial spaces. This condition occurs when an alteration in Starling's forces for systemic capillary exchange occurs.

29. List some causes of edema.

- Increased systemic capillary hydrostatic pressure
- Decreased plasma oncotic pressure (owing to decreased plasma protein)

- Increased systemic capillary permeability
- Blockade of lymphatic return to the venous circulation (leading to edematous build-up of fluid in the interstitial spaces)

30. Why is the kidney important in regulating the body volumes?

In the most basic terms, the primary function of the kidneys is to maintain the composition of the ECF and ICF. To understand the impact of altered renal function on body fluid volumes, it is critical to understand not only the processes by which the kidneys operate, but also the relationship between the different body fluid compartments. The kidneys regulate body fluid volume and composition by controlling the rate of excretion of various substances. This is accomplished through a complex and integrated relationship between the kidney, the endocrine system, the nervous system, and the cardiovascular system.

31. List the three main processes by which the kidneys maintain homeostasis of the body fluids.

1. **Bulk filtration:** The blood flow to the kidney is approximately 1200 mL/min or 20% of cardiac output. About 20% (100 mL/min) of the plasma that flows to the kidney is filtered out of the glomerular capillaries into the renal tubules in the process known as **glomerular filtration**. This is the initial step in the formation of urine.
2. **Reabsorption:** This is the mechanism whereby the renal tubules reabsorb the solutes and fluid that were filtered. This process is normally responsible for the return of approximately 99% of the glomerular filtrate to the ECF.
3. **Secretion:** This is a tubular transport process in which substances are transported by an individual tubular segment from the extracellular space into the tubular fluid to be excreted in the urine.

RENAL HEMODYNAMICS

32. Briefly describe the gross anatomy of the kidney.

The kidneys are paired organs found against the dorsal wall of the abdomen just beneath the diaphragm and behind the peritoneum. The renal tissue can be grossly divided into three major zones: cortex, outer medulla, and inner medulla.

33. What is a nephron?

A nephron is the basic unit of the kidney. Each normal human kidney has approximately 1 million nephrons. (See top figure on next page.)

34. Describe the path blood travels as it passes from the renal artery to the renal vein.

Blood enters the kidney through the renal artery; then flows through the interlobar artery, arcuate artery, interlobular artery, afferent arteriole, glomerular capillaries, efferent arteriole, peritubular capillaries, and interlobular, arcuate, and interlobar veins; and finally the renal vein. Of note, glomerular ultrafiltration occurs in the glomerular capillaries, and uptake of solute and water that has been reabsorbed by the epithelial cells occurs in the peritubular capillaries.

35. Are there different types of nephrons?

There are two general types of nephrons: **cortical** (superficial) and **juxtamedullary** (deep) nephrons. (See bottom figure on following page.)

36. How are different types of nephrons distinguished?

Number	Tubular structure
Location	Vascular structure

(See bottom figure on page 129.)

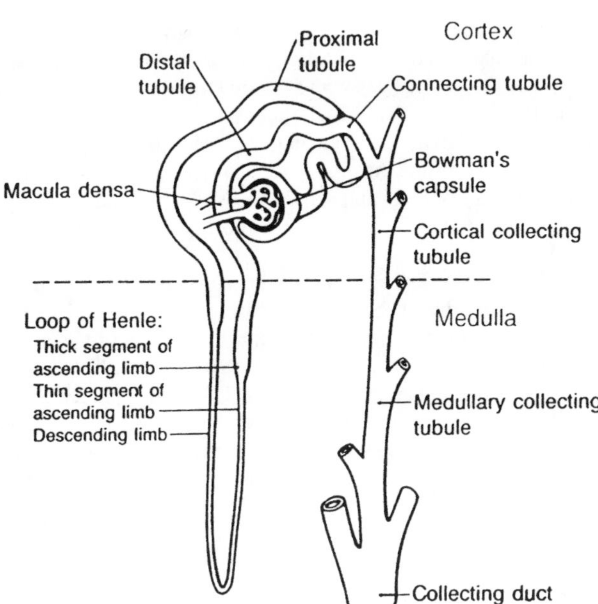

Tubular segments of a nephron. (Reproduced with permission from Guyton AC, Hall JE: Textbook of Medical Physiology, 9th ed. Philadelphia, W.B. Saunders, 1996.)

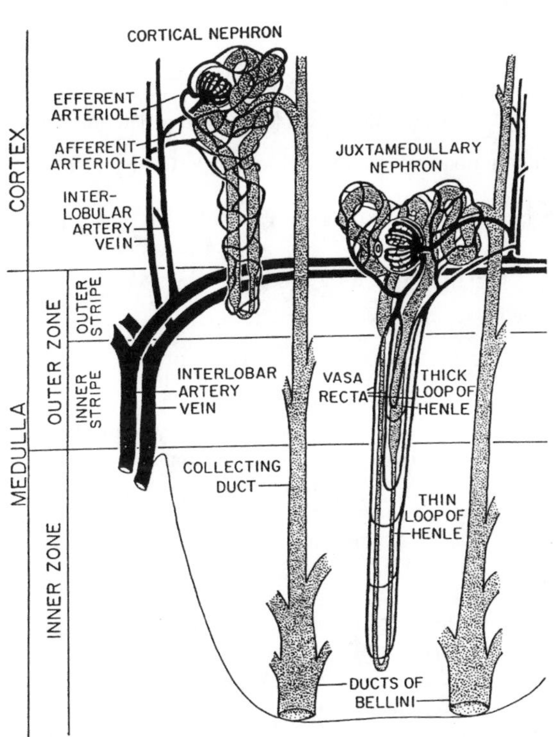

Anatomy and vasculature of cortical (superficial) and juxtamedullary (deep) nephrons. (Reproduced with permission from Pitts RF: Physiology of the Kidneys and Body Fluids, 3rd ed. St. Louis, Mosby, 1974.)

37. What are the distinguishing characteristics of a superficial nephron?

Superficial cortical nephrons (see bottom figure, page 129) comprise approximately 90% of all nephrons and are located with the glomerulus near the surface of the kidney. The tubular structure differs in the medulla, where these nephrons have a short thin descending limb of Henle, which turns within the outer medulla and leads to the thick ascending limb. The postglomerular vasculature of the superficial nephron consists of an efferent arteriole, which gives rise to peritubular capillaries. Fluid and solutes reabsorbed from tubular segments located in the renal cortex are taken up into the blood in these postglomerular capillaries.

38. What are the distinguishing characteristics of the deep or juxtamedullary nephrons?

Juxtamedullary nephrons (see bottom figure, page 129) make up 10% of all nephrons with glomeruli found deep in the cortex near the junction of the cortex and medulla. Juxtamedullary nephrons have long thin descending limbs of Henle, which descend deep into the inner medulla, turn back as the thin ascending limb, and become the thick ascending limb at the border of the outer and inner medulla. The postglomerular vasculature of the deep nephrons is also an efferent arteriole, but this vessel gives rise to the vasa recta capillaries, which are found in the medulla and are responsible for the uptake into the ECF of fluid absorbed by the nephron segments in the renal medulla.

39. How is the glomerular filtrate formed?

The glomerular filtrate is the total flux of fluid across the glomerular capillaries. The glomerular filtrate is formed by the sum of the hydrostatic and oncotic pressures in the glomerular capillaries and Bowman's space. These forces, along with the hydraulic permeability and surface area of the glomerular capillary membranes, determine the net flux of fluid known as the glomerular filtration rate (GFR).

40. What forces govern glomerular filtration?

The following equations express all the forces involved in determining GFR:

$$\text{GFR} = (\text{ultrafiltration coefficient}) \times (\text{forces opposing and favoring filtration})$$

$$\text{GFR} = (\text{ultrafiltration coefficient}) \times [(\text{forces favoring filtration}) - (\text{forces opposing filtration})]$$

$$\text{GFR} = K_f \times [(P_{GC} + \Pi_{BS}) - (\Pi_{GC} + P_{BS})]$$

Because Π_{BS} is negligible under normal conditions:

$$G_{FR} = K_f \times (P_{GC} - \Pi_{GC} - P_{BS})$$

Where:

K_f = Ultrafiltration coefficient: the product of the hydraulic permeability (L_p) and the surface area (SA) of the glomerular capillary membranes
P_{GC} = Glomerular capillary hydrostatic pressure
Π_{GC} = Glomerular capillary oncotic pressure
P_{BS} = Bowman's space hydrostatic pressure
Π_{BS} = Bowman's space oncotic pressure

41. What are the pressures favoring and opposing filtration?

- **Glomerular capillary hydrostatic pressure** (P_{GC}): P_{GC} averages approximately 60 mmHg at the afferent end of the glomerular capillaries and falls to 58 mmHg at the efferent end of the glomerular capillaries.
- **Bowman's space oncotic pressure** (Π_{BS}): Normally, this force is negligible because minimal amounts of protein are filtered.
- **Hydrostatic pressure in Bowman's space** (P_{BS}): P_{BS} is approximately 20 mmHg and remains constant from the afferent to the efferent end of the glomerular capillaries.

- **Glomerular capillary oncotic pressure** (Π_{GC}): Π_{GC} averages 25 mmHg at the afferent end of the glomerular capillaries.

42. Do the pressures favoring and opposing filtration change over the length of the glomerular capillaries?

Because fluid is filtered out of the plasma in the glomerular capillaries while plasma proteins are left behind in the blood, the plasma protein concentration and oncotic pressure increase as blood proceeds from the afferent to the efferent end of the glomerular capillaries. The change in Π_{GC} has a major impact on the net force for glomerular filtration. At the beginning (afferent end) of the glomerular capillaries, the sum of the forces for glomerular filtration greatly favors net filtration. The net pressure favoring glomerular ultrafiltration (P_{UF}) can be approximated as follows: $P_{UF} = [(P_{GC} + \Pi_{BS}) - (\Pi_{GC} + P_{BS})] = [(60 + 0) - (25 + 18)] = 17$ mmHg. At the distal (efferent) end of the glomerular capillaries, the plasma oncotic pressure rises by as much as 15 mmHg, which drastically alters the forces for filtration: $P_{UF} = [(P_{GC} + \Pi_{BS}) - (\Pi_{GC} + P_{BS})] = [(58 + 0) - (40 + 18)] = 0$ mmHg. The concentration of protein in the glomerular blood therefore has a marked impact on the forces that favor glomerular filtration.

43. What is the GFR in a normal human?

120 mL/min (172.8 L/day) (average).

44. Explain the concept of clearance.

Clearance is the hypothetical volume of plasma from which the kidney removes all of a substance per unit time. The clearance of substance X (C_X) can be calculated by multiplying the urine-to-plasma concentration ratio of substance X by the urinary flow rate:

$$C_X = UF \times (U_X/P_X)$$

U_X = Urine concentration of compound X (mg/dL)
UF = Urine flow rate (mL/min)
P_X = Plasma concentration of compound X (mg/dL).

Because urinary and plasma concentration of substance X must be in the same units, the clearance value will have the same dimensions (i.e., volume/time) as urinary flow rate.

45. How can GFR be measured?

Ideally, substances that are freely filtered at the glomerulus and neither reabsorbed nor secreted by the renal tubules are ideal markers for the measurement of glomerular filtration. One substance commonly used to measure GFR in experimental situations is **inulin,** a polysaccharide (molecular weight = 5500), which is infused intravenously. Because the kidney removes inulin from the body by filtration and does not secrete, reabsorb, or metabolize this compound, the clearance of inulin (C_{inulin}) equals GFR:

$$GFR = C_{inulin} = UF \times U_{inulin}/P_{inulin}$$

C_{inulin} = Inulin clearance
UF = Urinary flow rate
U_{inulin} = Urine inulin concentration
P_{inulin} = Plasma inulin concentration

In this equation, the plasma and urine inulin concentrations must be expressed in the same units (i.e., mg/dL) and cancel each other out in the calculation. The units of GFR are then the same as the units of urinary flow rate (i.e., mL/min).

46. Can GFR be evaluated clinically?

Although inulin is the compound of choice for the measurement of GFR in experimental situations, this compound must be infused intravenously before any measurements can be made. In the clinical setting, creatinine clearance is used to measure GFR. Creatinine is an endogenous substance formed by creatine metabolism in skeletal muscle; it is produced at a relatively constant rate, is freely filtered by the glomerulus, and is not appreciably reabsorbed or secreted.

47. How is creatinine clearance used to evaluate GFR clinically?

Creatinine clearance (C_{creat}) can be used as an index of GFR:

$$C_{creat} = GFR = UF \times (U_{creat}/P_{creat})$$

U_{creat} = Urine concentration of creatinine (mg/dL)
UF = Urine flow rate (mL/min)
P_{creat} = Plasma concentration of creatinine (mg/dL)

If we assume a state of constant creatinine production, urinary excretion of creatinine can be considered a constant K. Because creatinine is excreted only by the process of glomerular filtration, we can then say that:

$$\text{Creatine production} = \text{creatinine excretion} = K = (U_{creat} \times UF)$$

Because $GFR = (U_{creat} \times UF)/P_{creat}$, substituting K into the equation gives $GFR = K/P_{creat}$. Therefore, GFR α $1/P_{creat}$

Because P_{creat} normally equals 1 mg/dL, if we divide 100 by P_{creat}, we get an estimate of the percentage of normal GFR in this patient.

48. What are the possible concerns in the use of plasma creatinine to estimate GFR?

1. Creatinine can be secreted by the renal tubules, which leads to an overestimation of GFR even if creatinine clearance is determined.

2. The use of serum creatinine as an index of GFR assumes that all individuals have the same production rate of creatinine and therefore the same serum concentration.

3. Although changes in serum creatinine can indicate alterations in renal function, a relatively slight increase in serum creatinine from 1.0 mg/dL to 1.5 mg/dL would correspond to a decrease in GFR from 100% (1/1 × 100) to 67% (1/1.5 × 100) of normal.

49. What is contained in the glomerular ultrafiltrate?

The glomerulus is composed of the glomerular capillaries with endothelial cells covered by a basement membrane. The capillaries are surrounded by epithelial cells known as **podocytes**. Although the endothelial layer contains fenestrations of approximately 1000 Å diameter that are freely permeable to water and most small solutes, the podocytes have foot processes that form filtration slits (approximately 40 × 140 Å), which retard the filtration of macromolecules based on size. In addition, the surface of the endothelial cells, the basement membrane, and the podocytes all contain negatively charged glycoproteins, which inhibit filtration of negatively charged molecules (such as plasma protein). In general, the largest molecules that can be effectively filtered are less than 25 Å in diameter, although positively charged molecules can still be filtered at sizes as large as 40 Å.

50. Why isn't protein filtered in the glomerulus?

The glomerular ultrafiltrate is an ultrafiltrate of plasma excluding plasma protein and any substances bound to protein. Protein is excluded from the glomerular ultrafiltrate because of the specialized structure of the glomerular membranes.

51. What is the level of renal blood flow (RBF) in a normal human?

1.0–1.25 L/min to both kidneys (average).

52. Can renal blood flow be measured?

In experimental animals, RBF can be measured directly using electromagnetic flowmetry of other devices used to measure blood flow invasively. This is not the case in patients, but a good index of RBF can be gained by determining the clearance of para-amino-hippuric acid (PAH). PAH clearance can be used to quantitate renal plasma flow (RPF) because this compound is freely filtered at the glomerulus and secreted by the organic acid transporter in the proximal tubule, but it is not reabsorbed by any nephron segments. The clearance of PAH can be calculated as:

$$C_{PAH} = RPF = UF \times (U_{PAH}/P_{PAH})$$

U_{PAH} = Urine concentration of PAH (mg/dL)
UF = Urine flow rate (mL/min)
P_{PAH} = Plasma concentration of PAH (mg/dL)

The value obtained for RPF can then be converted to RBF by dividing RPF by the fraction of blood that is plasma: RBF = RPF/(1 – Hct).

53. What is the filtration fraction?

The fraction of RPF that is filtered at the glomerulus.

54. How is the filtration fraction (FF) calculated?

FF = GFR/RPF.

55. How can RPF be calculated?

RPF is the fraction of RBF that is plasma. If RBF and the hematocrit (Hct) are known, RPF can be calculated as: RPF = RBF × (1 – Hct).

56. Describe what is meant by renal vascular resistance.

Resistance is generally defined by Poiseuille's law, in which resistance is proportional to $(8\eta l)/(\pi \times r^4)$, where r = the radius of the vessel, η = viscosity of the blood, and l = length of the vessel. Although Poiseuille's law is applicable only to steady flow of an ideal fluid through cylindrical tubes and is not correct for pulsatile flow of blood through blood vessels, it is a useful equation to understand the factors that can alter vascular resistance. Because the viscosity of the blood and the length of the renal vessels can be considered constant, alterations in resistance are generally attributed to changes in vessel radius. As the resistance is inversely proportional to the radius raised to the fourth power, small changes in vessel radius can have profound effects on vascular resistance.

57. What are the preglomerular blood vessels?

Those found before the glomerulus:

- Renal artery
- Interlobar artery
- Arcuate artery
- Interlobular artery
- Afferent arteriole

58. What are the postglomerular blood vessels?

Those found after the glomerulus:

- Efferent arteriole
- Peritubular (or vasa recta) capillaries
- Renal vein

59. Which blood vessels in the kidney provide for the greatest resistance to blood flow?

Efferent and **afferent arterioles**. This is indicated by a large decrease in intravessel pressure from the beginning to the end of these vessels. Intravascular hydrostatic pressure falls from approximately 100 mmHg to 60 mmHg from the beginning to the end of the afferent arteriole and from approximately 60 mmHg to 15 mmHg across the efferent arteriole.

60. Do selective changes in preglomerular and postglomerular renal vascular resistance lead to similar changes in RBF?

RBF is equal to the driving pressure (ΔP) divided by the renal vascular resistance (RVR): RBF = ΔP/RVR. An increased renal vascular resistance at any location in the renal vascular network leads to a decrease in RBF. Conversely, decreased renal vascular resistance at any location in the renal vascular tree leads to increased RBF. Increases or decreases in preglomerular or postglomerular resistance have the same general effect on renal blood flow.

61. How would selective changes in preglomerular or postglomerular renal vascular resistance alter GFR?

In general, GFR increases when the driving force for filtration (glomerular capillary pressure) is increased, and GFR decreases when glomerular capillary pressure is decreased. Because elevated resistance in preglomerular vessels leads to a decrease in pressure in all vessels downstream (including the glomerular capillaries), increased preglomerular resistance decreases GFR (as well as RBF). In contrast to the effects of increased preglomerular vascular resistance, increased postglomerular resistance leads to increased hydrostatic pressure in upstream segments (including the glomerular capillaries) causing an increase in GFR despite a decrease in RBF.

62. How do selective changes in renal preglomerular and postglomerular resistance alter filtration fraction?

In general, alterations in preglomerular resistance do not alter filtration fraction, whereas changes in postglomerular resistance do alter filtration fraction.

63. Summarize the influence of changes in preglomerular and postglomerular renal vascular resistance on RBF, GFR, and filtration fraction.

PREGLOMERULAR RESISTANCE	POSTGLOMERULAR RESISTANCE	RBF	GFR	FILTRATION FRACTION
⇑	=	⇓	⇓	=
=	⇑	⇓	⇑	⇑
⇓	=	⇑	⇑	=
=	⇓	⇑	⇓	⇓

64. Explain how fluid and solutes reabsorbed by the renal tubules are taken back up into the plasma.

The uptake of reabsorbed solute and water into the ECF is the primary role of the postglomerular peritubular and vasa recta capillaries. These capillaries are extremely effective for the uptake of reabsorbed substances for two reasons:

1. Hydrostatic pressure in these capillaries is fairly low—on the order of 15 mmHg in the peritubular capillaries and 6–10 mmHg in the vasa recta capillaries.
2. Oncotic pressure in these capillaries is relatively high.

Because 20% of the plasma is filtered at the glomerulus, the blood entering the efferent arteriole and continuing to the postglomerular capillaries has an elevated protein concentration and oncotic pressure (approximately 35–40 mmHg), which favors reabsorption. The balance of Starling forces for capillary exchange in these vessels is in favor (low capillary hydrostatic pressure and high capillary oncotic pressure) of net uptake of fluid back into the vasculature and the ECF.

65. Briefly describe the physiologic regulators of GFR and RBF.

A number of different systems are involved in the physiologic regulation of RBF and GFR. Hormones or autacoids that constrict the renal vasculature and **decrease RBF and GFR:**

- Endothelin
- Norepinephrine (released by sympathetic nerve stimulation)
- Angiotensin II

Factors that can **increase GFR and RBF:**

- Nitric oxide
- Bradykinin
- Prostaglandins

66. What is meant by autoregulation of GFR and RBF?

Autoregulation of GFR and RBF refers to the constancy of GFR and RBF when renal perfusion pressure is increased from 80 to 160 mmHg. To understand how autoregulation occurs, it is helpful to consider the response of tubes with a fixed resistance and those that are distensible during changes in perfusion pressure. If the renal vasculature functioned as a set of rigid tubes (fixed resistance), RBF would be predicted to increase directly with arterial pressure. Recall that blood flow (F) is directly proportional to perfusion pressure (P) and inversely proportional to resistance (R): F α P/R. A direct increase in pressure with no change in resistance would thus lead to a proportional increase in flow. In contrast to the circumstance with rigid tubes, if the renal vasculature functioned as a set of distensible vessels, the increased perfusion pressure would dilate the vessels, and vascular resistance would decrease. Combined with the increased perfusion pressure, the fall in resistance would lead to even greater changes in flow than would be seen with rigid tubes. Instead of either of these two types of responses, RBF and GFR are maintained constant as perfusion pressure is increased.

67. How must vascular resistance change during autoregulation?

Renal vascular resistance must increase (vessel diameter must decrease) as pressure is increased to maintain GFR and RBF constant over the wide range of perfusion pressure.

68. Describe the mechanisms that lead to the autoregulation of GFR and RBF.

Autoregulation of GFR and RBF is thought to be mediated by two mechanisms:

- Myogenic response
- Tubuloglomerular feedback

The **myogenic response** is an intrinsic property of blood vessels whereby stretch of the vessel leads to a reflex contraction of the vascular smooth muscle. The myogenic response can also be observed in many vascular beds in addition to the renal vasculature. In **tubuloglomerular feedback,** increased tubular flow rate and increased NaCl transport rate in the macula densa cells initiate a feedback signal that is sent to the afferent arteriole to constrict in order to maintain a constant level of GFR and therefore tubular flow rate. In combination, the myogenic response and tubuloglomerular feedback are capable of maintaining GFR and RBF fairly constant over a wide range of arterial pressures.

69. Are GFR and RBF altered in pathologic conditions?

Any number of pathologic conditions can lead to alterations in GFR or RBF. GFR and RBF are usually decreased in both **acute** and **chronic renal failure**.

70. Define acute renal failure.

An abrupt impairment or interruption of renal function that is indicated by abnormally low or absent urinary excretion; this condition is often reversible. Acute renal failure can be caused by many conditions:

- Decreased blood supply to the kidney
- Acute injury to glomeruli or blood vessels

- Damage to renal tubules or the renal interstitium
- Obstruction of the lower urinary tract

71. Define chronic renal failure.

An irreversible and progressive loss of nephrons over an extended period of time.

72. What are the changes in GFR and RBF that occur in acute renal failure?

The rapid decrease in nephron function brought about acute renal failure is indicated by a fall in GFR, which can be determined clinically by increased serum or plasma creatinine.

73. List the types of renal vascular injury or abnormalities that can lead to acute renal failure.

Decreased blood flow to the kidney that leads to acute renal failure is known as **prerenal failure** or **acute ischemic renal failure**. Prerenal failure can be caused by the following:

- Hemorrhage
- Major surgery
- Diagnostic radiology techniques
- Severe vomiting, diarrhea, or other conditions that lead to severe dehydration, hypotension, or decreased blood volume

74. Describe glomerulonephrotic syndrome in acute renal failure.

Acute renal failure owing to glomerulonephrotic syndromes usually occurs 1–3 weeks after a **streptococcal** or **gram-negative infection**. This condition develops as a result of the deposition of antibody-antigen complexes in the glomerulus. These complexes, along with white blood cells, become entrapped in the glomeruli, reducing GFR and increasing the permeability of the glomerulus to protein. The glomerulonephrotic syndrome is therefore associated with decreased GFR and increased proteinuria. The acute glomerulonephrotic syndrome usually lasts 1–2 weeks, and renal function gradually returns to normal in the next few weeks to months.

75. Is GFR altered in chronic renal failure?

In chronic renal failure, the number of nephrons is progressively and irreversibly decreased. Although the remaining nephrons hypertrophy in an attempt to compensate for the loss of other nephrons, chronic renal failure eventually is associated with a reduction in GFR. This condition can be detected clinically as a gradual increase in serum or plasma creatinine that occurs over time (months to years).

TRANSPORT IN NEPHRON SEGMENTS

76. Name the different methods by which the kidney handles ions, nutrients, and water.

Normal renal function requires the movement of ions, essential nutrients, and water both into and out of the plasma compartment. These functions are accomplished by 3 major mechanisms:

1. Bulk filtration into the glomerulus
2. Reabsorption from the tubule into the plasma along nephron segments
3. Secretion from the plasma into the tubule at specific sites along the nephron

77. What different types of substances undergo these transport functions along the nephron?

The major **compounds** that must be transported along the nephron after filtration include glucose, proteins, and amino acids. Because ions are freely soluble in plasma, they are also freely filtered. All ions need to be reabsorbed along the nephron back into the plasma. The most critical of these **ions,** however, include Na^+, Cl^-, K^+, HCO_3^-, Ca^{++}, and Mg^{++}. Other nonessential waste products must predominantly remain in the tubular fluid, such as urea, uric acid, ammonia, and creatinine. Most of these nonessential waste products are filtered freely, which is one of the mechanisms by which the kidneys clear the body of these compounds. In addition, **organic acids** and **bases** are transported (secreted) from the plasma into the tubular fluid as yet another mechanism for excreting substances into the urine. This function is particularly important for the removal of drugs and other pharmacologic substances from the plasma.

78. What is the filtered load of a substance?

The mass of any substance that is filtered at the glomerulus per unit time. This filtered load is critical to the tubular transport functions and ultimate renal handling of ions and filtered solutes. The **filtered load** is expressed simply as:

$$\text{Filtered load} = \text{GFR} \times [\text{P}]_x$$

where GFR = glomerular filtration rate and $[\text{P}]_x$ = the plasma concentration of any compound. (Theoretically, this equation should also factor a coefficient of filtration (k) for each compound, but for purposes of clinical use we can ignore this constant).

79. Give an example using the filtered load of Na^+ in humans.

Filtered load = GFR × $[\text{P}]_{Na^+}$
and GFR = 0.125 L/min; $[\text{P}]_{Na+}$ = 140 mM/L
Filtered Na^+ load = (0.125 L/min) × 140 mM/L
= 17.5 mM/min or approximately 25,200 mM Na^+/d

Therefore, it becomes readily apparent that the nephrons of the kidneys must have a large capacity to transport and reabsorb Na^+ because the daily filtered Na^+ load exceeds 10 times the total body Na^+.

80. Describe the filtered loads of some common plasma constituents and their percentages of tubular reabsorption into the plasma before urinary excretion.

*Quantities Involved in Urine Formation in the Human**

Fluid: Renal blood flow (RBF) = 1200 mL/min (20–25% of cardiac output)
Renal plasma flow (RPF) = 660 mL/min
Glomerular filtration rate (GFR) = 125 mL/min
Fraction of plasma flow filtered (GFR/RPF) = 0.18–0.20

Solutes:

	PLASMA CONCENTRATION (MM)	FILTERED/DAY		EXCRETED/DAY		PERCENT REABSORBED
		mmoles	g	mmoles	g	
Sodium	140	25,200	570	103	2.3	99+
Chloride	105	18,900	660	103	3.7	99+
Bicarbonate	25	4,500	275	2	0.1	99+
Potassium	4	720	30	100	4.2	86+
Glucose	5	900	160	trace		100
Urea	5	900	50	360	20.0	60
Urate	0.3	54	9	4	0.7	93
Water		180L		1–1.5 L		99+

*Average values for a man weighing 70 kg.

81. What are the types of reabsorption that take place in the proximal convoluted tubules (PCT)?

Large amounts of fluid and solutes are reabsorbed by both passive and active mechanisms. It is the major segment of the nephron where reabsorption occurs.

82. How much of the filtered load is reabsorbed in the PCT?

The PCT is the nephron segment for **bulk** reabsorption of water and other substances back into the plasma. This segment reabsorbs approximately 67% of the filtered water, Na^+, Cl^-, K^+, and urea. Other important substances such as glucose, amino acids, and small filterable proteins are completely (100%) reabsorbed by the PCT.

67% REABSORBED	100% REABSORBED*
Filtered water	Glucose
Na^+	Amino acids
CL^-	Small filterable proteins
K^+	
Urea	

*To achieve 100% reabsorption, both passive and active processes must be involved.

83. If bulk reabsorption occurs in the PCT, is this nephron segment highly permeable to water and solute?

The PCT is often referred to as a **leaky** epithelium. In other words, both water and solutes easily cross this tubular segment, and the tight junctions between PCT cells do not afford much of a barrier to fluid movement either at the apical or at the basolateral membranes.

84. If the PCT is a leaky epithelium, what is the osmolality of tubular fluid at the end of this tubular segment?

The PCT undergoes isosmotic reabsorption, which is consistent with the leaky nature of the tubular cells in this nephron region. Thus, if the ultrafiltrate of the plasma at Bowman's capsule is isosmotic and provides tubular fluid with an osmolality of 290 mOsm/kg, the osmolality of the tubular fluid at the end of the PCT will also be 290 mOsm/kg. In other words, as solutes are reabsorbed in the PCT, water passively follows the solutes, thereby maintaining an isosmotic fluid in the tubular lumen.

85. Is filtration the only way the nephron gets substances into the tubular fluid?

No. Some substances enter the tubular fluid by active secretion from the basolateral cell membrane to the tubular lumen. These substances reach the basolateral membrane of the PCT by passive movement at the peritubular capillaries into the interstitial fluid surrounding the PCT and proximal straight tubules (PST). In addition to active secretion of substances, passive **back leak** of soluble ions is known to occur. This passive back leak from the basolateral to the apical sides of the PCT occurs only when either the concentration or electrochemical gradients favor movement in this direction. Because the PCT is leaky, water passively follows during ionic back leak, thereby maintaining isosmotic fluid in the tubular lumen.

86. What are the major classes of compounds secreted into the PCT and PST?

The major transport systems in this tubule segment for secretion are specific to organic anions and organic cations. These are the same systems that function for the secretion of PAH (organic acid). The active transport sites for these organic anions and cations are located on the basolateral membranes of the late PCT and throughout the PST.

87. What are the major mechanisms for Na^+ reabsorption in the PCT?

The most critical mechanism for reabsorbing Na^+ in the PCT is **active transport by Na^+, K^+-ATPase** located on the basolateral membrane of the tubular cell. This is the same active transport mechanism that is responsible for maintaining cell volume in cells throughout the body. The active removal of Na^+ from the cells establishes a low intracellular Na^+ and a negative intracellular electrical potential, which favors the facilitated movement of Na^+ down its electrochemical gradient from the tubular lumen into the cells. Na^+ enters the PCT cell on the apical membrane through a number of facilitated transport processes. The PCT is particularly well suited for net reabsorption processes into the cell because of the large surface area on the brush border membrane of the apical surface. The active Na^+, K^+-ATPase extrusion of Na^+ from the cell into the interstitial compartment across the basolateral membrane produces the required concentration gradient for Na^+ between the tubular lumen and the intracellular compartment. Thus, despite the isotonic nature of the PCT tubular fluid, active transport of Na^+ out of the cell on the basolateral membrane establishes an effective concentration gradient for the movement of Na^+ from the tubular lumen into the cell across the apical membrane.

88. How important is Na^+, K^+-ATPase in the reabsorption of Na^+, Cl^-, and water in the PCT?

The active transport of Na^+ out of the cell at the basolateral membrane is essential to the reabsorption of Na^+ from the PCT. In the absence of active Na^+, K^+-ATPase at the PCT, delivery of Na^+ out of this nephron segment is approximately 65% of the filtered Na^+ load. Thus, at least two-thirds of the filtered Na^+ load is reabsorbed via mechanisms dependent on the Na^+, K^+-ATPase enzyme. This requirement is particularly important in clinical states in which severe damage is done to the proximal tubule, and the Na^+, K^+-ATPase no longer functions efficiently. These clinical manifestations are observed in conditions of renal ischemia or following exposure to certain nephrotoxic drugs that cause severe damage to PCT cells. Under these circumstances, delivery of Na^+ out of the PCT is greatly increased, and unless other tubular mechanisms downstream from the PCT are able to compensate in their reabsorption of Na^+, severe natriuresis and Na^+ loss occur.

89. What are the major anions that get reabsorbed across the PCT?

Cl^-
HCO_3^-
Anionic amino acids

90. Why is the reabsorption of these anions critically dependent on the active transport of Na^+, K^+-ATPase?

When the PCT no longer possesses the ability to extrude Na^+ from the inside of the cell, the reabsorption of major anions is greatly decreased. This is particularly noticed in various kidney diseases in which the PCT is damaged and the Na^+, K^+-ATPase activity is reduced, leading to natriuresis. This Na^+ loss is associated with significant proteinuria and increased excretion of HCO_3^- and Cl^-. These losses may lead to significant decreases in plasma oncotic pressure, hypochloremia, and alkalosis.

91. How are Na^+ and HCO_3^- reabsorption linked in the PCT?

The reabsorption of sodium bicarbonate ($NaHCO_3$) is critical to the net reabsorption of Na^+ in the proximal tubule as well as to the understanding of the regulation of urinary acidification. In addition to the Na^+, K^+-ATPase located on the basolateral membrane, the **apical** membrane possesses a Na^+-H^+ cotransporter which utilizes the electrochemical gradient favoring the movement of Na^+ into the cell from the tubular lumen in exchange for secretion of H^+ from inside the cell into the lumen. This electroneutral transporter is not only responsible for one-third of proximal tubule sodium reabsorption in the PCT, but also provides the driving force for coupled HCO_3- reabsorption (see figure). The lumenal brush border of the PCT contains large amounts of carbonic anhydrase, which catalyze the production of carbonic acid (H_2CO_3). H_2CO_3 then dissociates into CO_2 and water, and the CO_2 diffuses into the cell down its concentration gradient. Inside the cell, an abundance of carbonic anhydrase catalyzes the synthesis of carbonic acid in the reverse direction, producing intracellular H^+ and HCO_3^-. The HCO_3^- is reabsorbed across the basolateral membrane and into the interstitium while the free H^+ becomes available to the Na^+-H^+ cotransporter for further secretion of H^+ into the tubular lumen. In this way, the PCT is able to reabsorb both Na^+ and HCO_3^-.

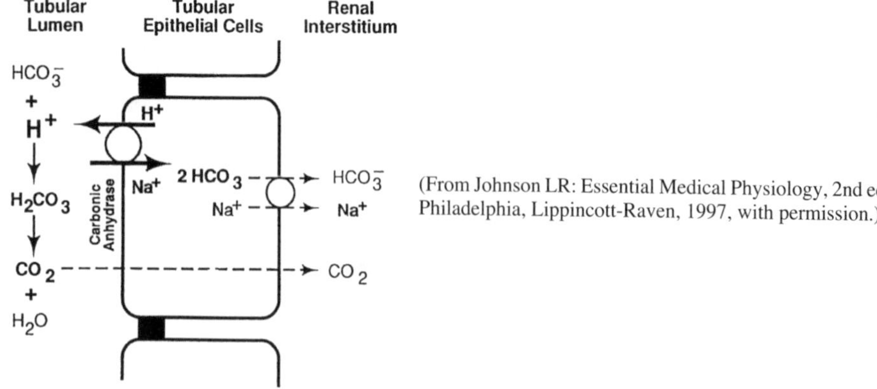

(From Johnson LR: Essential Medical Physiology, 2nd ed. Philadelphia, Lippincott-Raven, 1997, with permission.)

92. Why is it necessary to reabsorb HCO_3^- in the form of CO_2 and water rather than by simply allowing passive HCO_3^- diffusion across the apical membrane down its concentration gradient?

Passive HCO_3- reabsorption across the apical membrane would certainly be the simplest mechanism for the dual reabsorption of $NaHCO_3$. To acidify the urine effectively, the apical membrane must maintain a relative impermeability to HCO_3-. (This process is best shown by the high reflection coefficient of the PCT apical membrane to HCO_3^-.) All cell membranes are highly permeable to dissolved gases such as CO_2. Thus, the brush border of the apical membrane of the PCT cell contains carbonic anhydrase, which helps catalyze the formation of CO_2 and H_2O from HCO_3-.

93. Does inhibition of HCO_3^- transport affect Na^+ reabsorption in the PCT?

Inhibition of HCO_3^- transport has been used as an effective "diuretic and natriuretic" agent for many years. Inhibition of carbonic anhydrase using acetazolamide (Diamox) effectively increases urinary Na^+ and HCO_3^- excretion and alkalinizes the urine. Other physiologic mechanisms of altering the PCT Na^+-H^+ exchanger may also affect tubular $NaHCO_3$ reabsorption. In this regard, metabolic or respiratory acidosis increases Na^+-H^+ exchange and increases secretion of H^+ in the PCT, whereas metabolic or respiratory alkalosis decreases the activity of the Na^+-H^+ exchange mechanism and thereby decreases urinary acidification.

94. Is Na^+ reabsorption linked to any other substances in the PCT?

A number of facilitated transport mechanisms are coupled with Na^+ in the reabsorptive process of the PCT. These Na^+-coupled transport mechanisms are located on the apical membrane of the PCT and include:

- Na^+–amino acid transporter
- Na^+–PO_4^- transporter
- Na^+–glucose transporter

Coupled Na^+-glucose Na^+–amino acid transport accounts for the complete reabsorption of the filtered load of glucose and amino acids in the PCT under normal physiologic conditions.

95. If glucose is 100% reabsorbed by the PCT, how does glucose get into the urine in diseases such as diabetes?

Because glucose undergoes a **facilitated** diffusion process, the glucose reabsorption is dependent on a fixed number of transport proteins located on the apical membrane. The relationship among plasma glucose and the rates of glucose filtration, reabsorption (via the facilitated diffusion transporter), and urinary excretion is shown in the figure. Under normal conditions, plasma glucose concentrations are less than 200 mg/dL. As plasma glucose concentrations increase, the filtration rate (or filtered load) of glucose also increases in a linear manner. The reabsorption capacity of the glucose transport mechanism is able to match the filtered glucose load up to about 200 mg/dL plasma glucose concentration. At that point, the reabsorptive capacity of the glucose transporter can no longer equal the delivery of glucose from the filtered load, and glucose begins to spill into the urine. Urinary glucose excretion begins to rise such that at any plasma glucose concentration above 200 mg/dL, the sum of the excretion rate and reabsorption rate must equal the filtered load. This point where filtered load of glucose equals the reabsorptive rate of glucose is called the **transport maximum** (T_m). In pathologic conditions such as diabetes mellitus, plasma glucose often increases beyond the 200 mg/dL level because of an inability of cells throughout the body to transport glucose properly into the intracellular compartment. Under these conditions, glucose then appears in the urine as glucosuria because the filtered load of glucose exceeds the T_m for glucose.

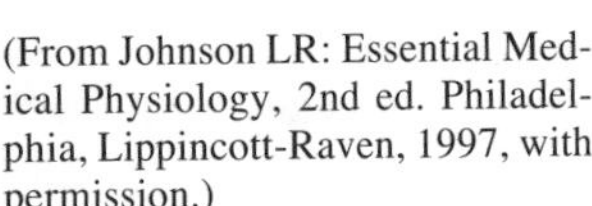
(From Johnson LR: Essential Medical Physiology, 2nd ed. Philadelphia, Lippincott-Raven, 1997, with permission.)

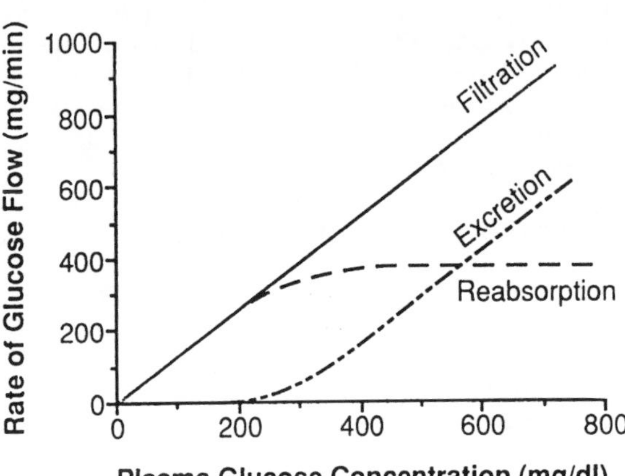

96. If a transport maximum (T_m) exists for facilitated glucose reabsorption, do similar types of T_m exist for the secretion of organic acids and bases into the tubular lumen?

All kidney transporters exhibit a T_m at a specific plasma concentration for their substrate, including transporters that are located on the basolateral membrane of the PCT such as the organic acid and organic base transporters. The relationships between plasma PAH concentrations (organic acid) and the rates of PAH excretion, secretion, and filtration are shown in the figure. Similar to glucose, as plasma concentrations of PAH are increased, the filtration rate or filtered load of PAH increases in a linear fashion. Similarly, the secretion rate of PAH increases as plasma PAH concentration increases. Because PAH is being transported from the blood into the nephron, the increase in the rate of excretion of PAH is rapid, and this excretion rate equals the sum of the secretion rate and the fil-

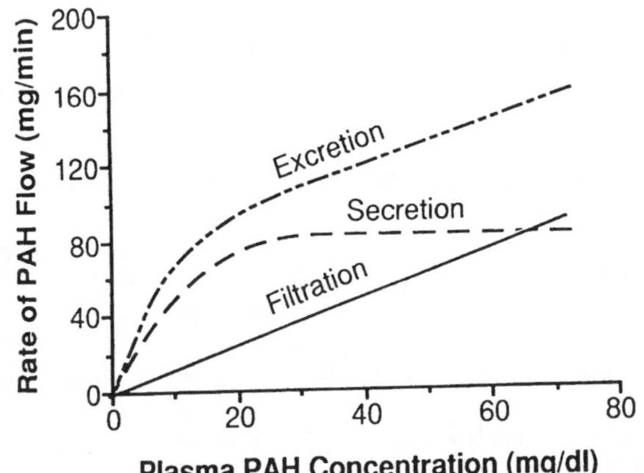

(From Johnson LR: Essential Medical Physiology, 2nd ed. Philadelphia, Lippincott-Raven, 1997 with permission.)

tered load. Once the organic acid secretory capacity of the PCT is saturated (i.e., the T_m for organic acid secretion is reached), there is no further increase in the secretion rate of the compound, and as further elevations in plasma PAH concentration occur, the increases in excretion are equal to the rise in filtered load. In this example for the organic acid PAH, the T_m exists at a plasma PAH concentration of approximately 20 mg/dL, and the T_m for PAH secretion is approximately 80 mg/min.

97. What are the characteristics of the thin descending limb of the loop of Henle for water and solute movement?

The thin descending loop of Henle is relatively impermeable to Na^+, Cl^-, and urea but readily permeable to water. As the thin descending limb descends into the inner medulla, the interstitial solute concentration increases to as much as 1200 mOsm/L. There is, therefore, a strong osmotic driving force favoring the reabsorption of water in the thin descending limb. As tubular fluid moves from the end of the PST to the tip of the loop of Henle, the osmolality of the tubular fluid increases because water is reabsorbed by osmosis while NaCl is trapped in the tubular lumen. This increase in tubular Na^+ and Cl^- concentration in the thin descending loop of Henle is critical for the urinary concentration and dilution mechanism.

98. How are water and solutes handled by the thin ascending limb of the loop of Henle?

The changes in tubular fluid in the thin ascending limb are related to the relative impermeable state of this nephron segment for water compared with that of NaCl. Thus, in this segment of the nephron, there is a passive diffusion of NaCl out of the tubular lumen and into the interstitium, leaving water behind. This movement of NaCl occurs **down** its concentration gradient, which has been created from the thin descending limb (i.e., water permeability in thin descending limb exceeds that of NaCl). These differential permeabilities are important for helping to establish an effective concentration gradient between the tubular lumen and renal medullary interstitium.

99. Why are there no active transport mechanisms in the thin descending and ascending loops of Henle for reabsorption of ions?

The thin loops of Henle contain only simple squamous types of cells. These cells have few mitochondria, function primarily with anaerobic metabolism, and produce only small amounts of ATP required for active transport.

100. What are the most important transport characteristics of the thick ascending loops of Henle?

The medullary thick ascending limbs (MTAL) have two major functions in the reabsorption of water and solutes:

1. These cells are quite impermeable to water.
2. The cells contain a unique Na^+-K^+-$2Cl^-$ transporter that is capable of transporting large quantities of NaCl from the tubule lumen into the medullary interstitium. Because NaCl is being selectively reabsorbed in this segment with water remaining in the tubular lumen, the osmolality of the tubular fluid decreases and may even become **hypotonic** with respect to plasma by the end of the MTAL.

101. How do the transport mechanisms in the early distal tubule contribute to the reabsorption of NaCl?

The early distal tubule is impermeable to water but contains an Na^+/Cl^- cotransporter that is sensitive to thiazide diuretic agents. The selective reabsorption of solute (NaCl) in this segment further dilutes the tubular fluid.

102. How does the late portion of the distal convoluted tubule contribute to the tubular reabsorption of Na^+?

Reabsorption of Na^+ in the principal cells of the late distal tubule is dependent on the electrochemical gradient for Na^+ established by the Na^+, K^+-ATPase in the basolateral membrane.

Lumenal membrane Na^+ channels permit reabsorption down the electrochemical gradient and into the cells; the Na^+, K^+-ATPase in the basolateral membrane then removes the reabsorbed Na^+ from the cells. In addition to the reabsorption of Na^+, these cells are also important in the secretion of K^+. The Na^+, K^+-ATPase in the basolateral membrane moves K^+ into the cells and K^+ exits the cells through channels in the apical membrane.

103. How is Na^+ reabsorption controlled in the principal cells of the distal convoluted tubule (DCT) and cortical collecting duct?

Aldosterone (a steroid) affects distal convoluted tubules primarily by increasing Na^+, K^+-ATPase activity in the basolateral membrane and by increasing the apical membrane permeability for Na^+. After combining with its specific receptor in the cell cytoplasm, aldosterone moves to the nuclear membrane, where it activates the transcription and translation of specific apical membrane Na^+ channels. Insertion of these Na^+ channels into the apical membrane allows increased flux of Na^+ into the cell from the tubular lumen down the concentration gradient, which is continually maintained by the activity of the basolateral Na^+, K^+-ATPase. The increased substrate for the ATPase enzyme (Na^+) provides active transport of Na^+ out of the cells and into the interstitium. The reabsorption of sodium is completed by the movement of sodium into the peritubular capillaries and plasma. In contrast to the MTAL cells, the principal cells of the late distal tubule are water permeable in the presence of antidiuretic hormone, and the reabsorption of Na^+ in this nephron segment can be associated with water reabsorption as well. Thus, water is reabsorbed in distal convoluted tubules under conditions when the body needs to conserve water.

104. Is Na^+ the only critical ion controlled at the DCT?

No. Because Na^+ reabsorption in the distal convoluted tubule is highly coupled to the Na^+, K^+-ATPase, Na^+ reabsorption is associated with K^+ movement into the cell from the extracellular space. In this regard, K^+ secretion (K^+ movement from basolateral to apical membranes) is heavily controlled in distal convoluted tubules by the presence or absence of aldosterone. Thus, although simultaneously stimulating Na^+ reabsorption at the basolateral membrane, the concentration gradient for K^+ is created, which favors K^+ movement from inside the cell into the tubular lumen. Aldosterone, therefore, is known not only for its critical ability to stimulate Na^+ reabsorption, but also for its direct effects to enhance K^+ removal from the plasma and excretion into the urine.

105. What are the functions of the cortical collecting tubule (CCT) in determining the final composition of the tubular fluid (urine)?

The CCT provides reabsorption of small amounts of remaining Na^+ in the tubular fluid. The **primary function of the CCT** is the **reabsorption of water**. These tubular cells specifically express a family of **water channels** called **aquaporins** at both the apical (aquaporin 2) and the basolateral (aquaporin 4) membranes. The insertion of the aquaporins in the apical membrane are under the control of ADH. The aquaporins are a unique family of proteins with selective and specific structures that provide passive water movement across cell membranes. Water movement through aquaporin channels occurs only as a function of osmotic gradients, and these channels function in a bidirectional fashion.

106. What are the primary purposes of the medullary collecting duct in the regulation of urinary composition?

- Regulate the final urinary osmolality
- Control water reabsorption and excretion

Similar to the CCT, the medullary collecting duct promotes water reabsorption by expressing aquaporins. These segments express aquaporin 2 in the apical membranes in the presence of ADH, also known as arginine vasopressin (AVP). The medullary collecting duct cells are normally impermeable to water. In the presence of ADH, these cells increase their expression and insertion of aquaporin into the apical membranes, thereby increasing the cells' permeability to water. During states of dehydration, the osmolality of the medullary and papillary interstitium is high, providing a strong osmotic gradient for the movement of water across the cell membrane and into the interstitium. This **reabsorbed** water is then removed by the ascending vasa recta and returned to the circulation.

URINARY CONCENTRATION AND DILUTION

107. What are some of the different abilities of species to concentrate their urine?

The relative urinary concentrating capacity of different animals depends on the availability of water in their environments and habitats as well as the composition of the diet of each respective species. For example, humans exist in an environment of plentiful water availability and, therefore, concentrate their urine to a maximal level of only 1200 mOsm/kg. This degree of urinary concentrating ability in humans is contrasted to numerous desert-dwelling rodents that may concentrate their urine from 5000 to 7000 mOsm/kg during severe dehydration. Dilution of the urine (i.e., excretion of water loads) is effective in all species. The ability to excrete large quantities of water in a short period of time is provided by the rapid ability of animals to reduce their urine osmolality to 50 Osm/kg or less.

108. Is the excretion of a hypertonic or hypotonic urine necessary for the maintenance of homeostasis?

The ability of the mammalian kidney to produce a dilute or concentrated urine enables our bodies to excrete or conserve water while maintaining a relative constancy of solute excretion. In conditions when excess fluids have been ingested, the kidney can form a dilute or hypotonic urine to excrete excess water. In contrast, in conditions when total body water must be conserved, our kidneys produce a concentrated or hypertonic urine, which enables the conservation of water with the normal excretion of solute. Some examples of conditions that lead to a loss of total body water are listed in the table:

SECONDARY TO NORMAL FUNCTIONS (INSENSIBLE WATER LOSSES)	SECONDARY TO EXCESS WATER LOST AFTER ENVIRONMENTAL REINTUBATIONS
Breathing	Excessive heat exposure
Sweating	Prolonged exercise
	Fever
	Diarrhea

109. Does the kidney have a constant interstitial fluid osmolality from the cortex to the papilla?

Interstitial osmolalities range from 290 mOsm/kg in the cortex (essentially equivalent to plasma) to potentially high interstitial fluid osmolalities equivalent to the maximal urinary concentrating ability in the inner medulla. In humans, interstitial osmolality can increase to approximately 1200 mOsm/kg after 24 hours of water restriction.

110. How does the medullary interstitial concentration gradient contribute to the final concentration of the urine?

The concentration gradient found in the interstitial space from the cortex to the medulla of the kidney is absolutely essential for the production of both a concentrated and a dilute urine. Under normal circumstances, the body loses water because of respiration and sweat. Thus, the kidney is constantly being presented with a condition that requires the reabsorption and preservation of water. The presence of a hypertonic renal interstitium allows the appropriate movement of water **from** the tubular lumen **to** the interstitial fluid and back into the blood. Under these normal conditions in which water reabsorption is of primary importance, the final concentration of the urine is determined by the concentration of the renal interstitium within the deepest portions of the kidney (i.e., the inner medulla). As discussed below, the movement of water out of the late distal tubule and the cortical and medullary collecting duct is entirely dependent on the presence of ADH.

111. Does the PCT contribute to the final urinary concentration?

The PCT is responsible for the **bulk** reabsorption of water via isotonic transport mechanisms. Thus, in the PCT, the reabsorption of water is an **isosmotic** bulk flow of fluid. If the reabsorption in these segments is isosmotic, the osmolality of the tubular fluid is not changed and, therefore, is not concentrated further above that of plasma. Thus, although these nephron segments are extremely important for the bulk reabsorption of NaCl, water, and other ions, they do not contribute directly to producing a concentrated urine.

112. If the PCT provides bulk reabsorption, does urea get reabsorbed in the PCT as well?

Urea is reabsorbed in the PCT in the same bulk manner as all other filtered substances. Approximately 67% of the filtered urea in the PCT is reabsorbed back into the interstitium.

113. Is the PCT important in water reabsorption even though it does not participate in forming the final concentration of the urine?

The PCT is absolutely essential to the net reabsorption of water. Approximately two-thirds of the filtered load of water is reabsorbed in the PCT along with the other bulk reabsorbed filtered substances. In pathologic conditions in which the reabsorptive processes of the PCT are damaged (e.g., acute renal failure), there may be water loss via lack of the necessary reabsorption in this nephron segment. The contribution of the PCT to overall water reabsorption is therefore **critical to maintaining net water balance of the organism,** even though this nephron segment does not provide a mechanism for specifically changing the osmolality of the urine.

114. What are the major ionic components responsible for generating hypertonic urine?

A concentrated renal inner medullary interstitium is required to create an osmotic gradient for the reabsorption of water from the lumen of the collecting duct into the interstitial spaces. This concentration gradient is established by the excess concentration of NaCl and urea in the interstitial space of the inner medulla. This creates a hypertonic environment in the interstitial space surrounding the medullary collecting ducts and provides a driving force for water reabsorption in these distal tubular segments.

115. With the creation of a hypertonic inner medulla, how does water then get reabsorbed?

Under circumstances of water loading, the late distal tubule and collecting ducts are relatively **impermeable** to water. Therefore, the tubular fluid remaining within the nephron at the late distal tubule is excreted into the urine with an osmolality that is hypotonic to plasma. In the presence of ADH, the late distal tubule and collecting ducts become permeable to water; under these circumstances, water will be reabsorbed by osmosis from the tubular lumen into the interstitial space. Because the interstitial osmolality is hypertonic in the renal medulla, the urine excreted is hypertonic.

116. How does the kidney establish a differential concentration gradient from the cortex to the inner medulla during water deprivation?

The kidney generates a hypertonic inner medullary interstitium by both passive and active transport mechanisms. The degree of hypertonicity achieved is directly proportional to the length of the loop of Henle, such that the longer the loop of Henle, the greater the capacity to concentrate solutes in the inner medulla and consequently to concentrate the urine. The passive mechanisms reside primarily in the thin descending and ascending limbs of the loop of Henle. The thin descending limb is relatively impermeable to NaCl and urea with respect to water, whereas the thin ascending limb is relatively impermeable to water compared with the reabsorption of NaCl. Thus, in the thin descending limb, water is reabsorbed by osmosis leading to the concentration of solutes and the formation of hypertonic tubular fluid at the tip of the loop of Henle. In the thin ascending limb, the concentrated NaCl in the tubular lumen then moves out of the lumen down its concentration gradient. The active mechanism for creating a concentration of solutes in the renal medulla is the Na^+-K^+-Cl^- cotransporter of the thick ascending limb. The thick ascending limbs are impermeable to water. When Na^+ and Cl^- are actively reabsorbed in this segment in the absence of water reabsorption, the tubular fluid becomes dilute with osmolalities decreasing to levels as low as 100 mOsm/kg or less. The close proximity of the thin descending and ascending limbs provides the perfect juxtaposition of nephron segments for establishing a **countercurrent exchange** of solutes (see figure) and, in essence, for **trapping** the ions within the renal medulla and papilla.

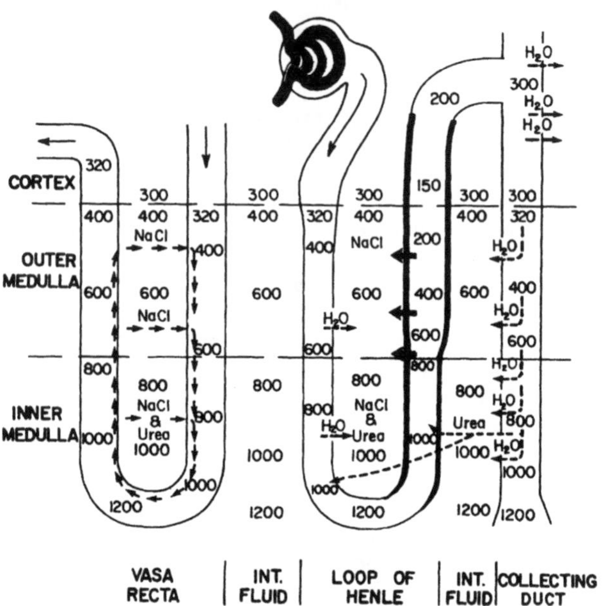

(From Guyton AC, Hall JE: Textbook of Medical Physiology, 9th ed. Philadelphia, W.B. Saunders, 1996, with permission.)

117. What is the role of the vasa recta capillaries?

The function of the vasa recta capillaries is to deliver nutriti` e substances to the structures of the renal medulla and to reabsorb water and solutes reabsorbed in the loop of Henle and collecting ducts. The descending and ascending vasa recta are positioned within the inner medulla and papilla in close juxtaposition with the descending and ascending limbs of the loop of Henle as well as the medullary and papillary collecting ducts. These groups of tubules and capillaries are closely associated into bundles called **medullary rays**.

The vasa recta are capillaries that allow free exchange between the blood and interstitial compartments. In essence, they provide the conduit for returning reabsorbed water back to the renal vein and central circulation. When water is reabsorbed from the collecting duct (in the presence of ADH) down the concentration gradient that has been established in the hypertonic renal interstitium, the gradient may be lost because of dilution of the Na^+, Cl^-, and urea. Because the osmolarity of blood within the vasa recta equilibrates with the interstitial space, the reabsorbed water equilibrates with the blood in the ascending vasa recta. This is where the circuit of water reabsorption is then completed with water moving into the ascending vasa recta and returning to the central circulation.

118. Is urea absorption critical to the overall concentrating ability of the renal papilla?

Urea contributes to the medullary interstitial concentration gradient by being reabsorbed from the tubular fluid in the collecting duct. Reabsorption at the collecting duct is wholly dependent on the presence of ADH; this nephron segment remains impermeable to urea in the absence of ADH. Reabsorption of urea is important to the overall ability of the kidney to produce a concentrated urine. In the absence of urea reabsorption in the inner medulla, the ability of the kidney to reabsorb water and hence concentrate the urine is greatly impaired.

119. How does the MTAL contribute to the overall cortical-papillary concentration gradient?

The MTAL can be thought of as the engine that drives the concentration of urine. The reabsorption by the Na^+-K^+-$2Cl^-$ transporter on the apical membrane is driven by the electrochemical gradient for Na^+, which is established by the Na^+, K^+ ATPase on the basolateral membranes of this segment. The critical nature of this transporter in the generation of a concentrated urine is best demonstrated by the use of **loop diuretics,** such as furosemide and bumetanide. These diuretics block the MTAL cotransporter and prevent the reabsorption of NaCl in these segment of the nephron. These drugs not only cause profound natriuresis, but also prevent water reabsorption because the medullary interstitial concentration gradient is effectively abolished by these compounds. Thus, the urinary osmolality is not increased beyond that of plasma, even in the presence of sufficient ADH, because the medullary interstitial space no longer contains sufficient solutes to provide an adequate gradient for the reabsorption of water from the collecting ducts.

120. What is meant by countercurrent multiplication?

This general physiologic term describes the physical juxtaposition of fluids flowing in close proximity to one another but in opposite directions. In the case of the kidney, **countercurrent multiplication** is used in both the loop of Henle segment of the nephron and in the vasa recta capillaries, both of which descend deeply into the renal medulla. In each of these structures, there is flow of fluid in opposite directions and in close proximity to one another. In the case of the loop of Henle, the descending limb maintains different permeability properties compared with the ascending limb. This allows the creation of different concentration gradients in each of these limbs and creates the continual flow of ions out of the ascending limb, thereby effectively **concentrating** those ions secondary to the **countercurrents** of tubular fluid flow in close proximity to one another. Thus, the countercurrent multiplier is essential for the maintenance of an effective interstitial concentration gradient between the cortex and papilla.

121. How does the kidney produce a dilute urine?

Dilution of the urine is equally critical for the appropriate maintenance of plasma volume and water balance. Several factors account for the effective production of a dilute urine and **washout** of the cortical papillary concentration gradient.

1. Water ingestion decreases plasma ADH; therefore, the late distal tubule and collecting duct become relatively impermeable to water and urea. In the absence of ADH, water reabsorption in the distal segments of the tubule is minimal, and the final urine will have an osmolality similar to that of the hypotonic tubular fluid found in the early distal tubule.

2. The loss of urea reabsorption at the collecting duct decreases the osmotic concentration of the medullary interstitium. The dilution of the plasma by the ingested water creates a gradient in the ascending vasa recta for movement of NaCl and urea into the blood and out of the medullary interstitium. This loss of osmotic activity in the inner medulla effectively **washes out** the cortical-medullary concentration gradient. In the absence of a concentration gradient, any remaining permeability of the collecting duct cells does not result in the reabsorption of water because the medullary osmotic gradient has been diminished.

122. What is the time frame for washout of the cortical-papillary concentration gradient during the elimination of a water load?

After ingestion of 1 L of water in a normal adult over a 30-minute period, the concentration gradient is effectively eliminated within 20 minutes, and the urine osmolality decreases from concentrated values of 600–1000 mOsm/kg to 300 or less. Within 1 hour after ingestion of this load, urine osmolality can be as low as 50 mOsm/kg, which is significantly less than that of plasma. Thus, the kidney's osmotic gradient is effectively removed, the urine osmolality is more dilute than plasma, and the body is effectively eliminating free water from the circulation.

REGULATION OF PLASMA OSMOLALITY

123. What is the normal range of plasma osmolality (P_{osm}) in humans?

The normal range of P_{osm} in humans is 260–310 mOsm/kg. This range represents the extremes from overhydration (260 mOsm/kg) to severe dehydration (310 mOsm/kg). Under normal states of hydration, the P_{osm} is approximately 290 mOsm/kg.

124. What is the primary hormone responsible for the control of P_{osm}?

The regulation of water balance and P_{osm} is under unique control by ADH, which is synthesized in the hypothalamic regions of the brain by magnocellular neurons located predominantly in the supraoptic and paraventricular nuclei. These nuclei provide neural projections into the hypophyseal stalk with terminals located in the neurohypophysis.

125. How is ADH release from the neurohypophysis controlled?

The exact cellular mechanisms responsible for the control of ADH release remains unknown. What is known and well documented is that specialized cells within the anteroventral region of the hypothalamus, a portion of the brain that lacks the blood-brain barrier, sense the change in P_{osm} and function as an osmoreceptor. When P_{osm} is elevated, indicating relative dehydration, the cells shrink and send neural signals to the supraoptic and paraventricular nuclei, resulting in the release of ADH from granulated nerve terminals. When P_{osm} is reduced from normal values, the cell bodies of these neurons are thought to expand or swell and inhibit the release of ADH from their neuronal projections. The relationships between P_{osm} and plasma ADH concentrations are shown in the figure. These data show that the entire range of P_{osm} is essentially regulated over a narrow range of plasma concentrations of ADH (i.e., 0–12 pg/mL). (See figure.)

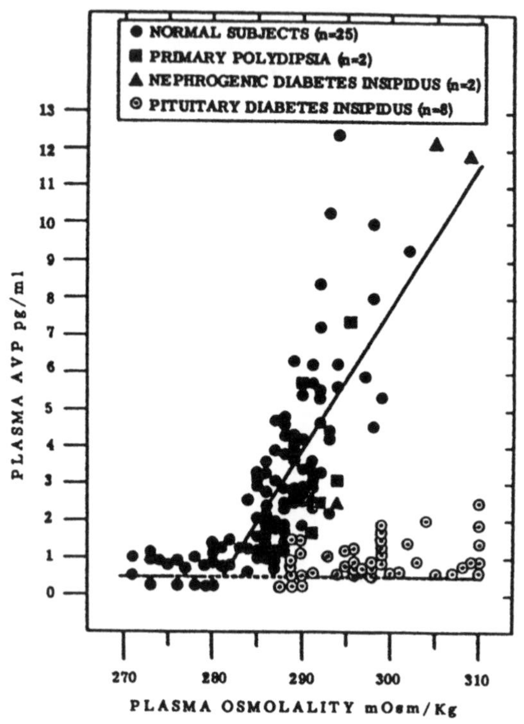

(From Robertson GL, Mahr EA, Athar S, Sinha T: Development and clinical application of a new method for the radioimmunoassay of arginine vasopressin in human plasma. J Clin Invest 52: 2340–2352, 1973, with permission.)

126. If regulation of total body water is critical for the maintenance of life, are there sensors for body fluid volumes that may also affect ADH release?

The other major sensors of body fluid volume are the low-pressure baroreceptors located in the right and left atria and in the vena cava just outside the right atrium. These are called **low-pressure baroreceptors** because they function in regions of the cardiovascular system where the vascular pressure is relatively low and does not undergo wide variations on a beat-to-beat basis. These baroreceptors sense the relative **stretch** or volume of blood entering the heart from the body and from the pulmonary circulation. The neural projections from these volume sensors enter the central nervous system via cranial nerve X (vagus) and reflexively regulate the release of ADH from the neurohypophysis. In this regard, when plasma volume is elevated (i.e., overhydration and low P_{osm}), stimulation of these receptors by excess stretch invokes an inhibitory reflex to decrease the release of ADH from the neurohypophysis. Conversely, when plasma volume is reduced (i.e., dehydration and increased P_{osm}), the reduced stretch on these low-pressure volume receptors decreases the inhibitory nerve fiber activity to the central nervous system and increases ADH release.

127. How does ADH increase or decrease plasma osmolality?

The release of ADH increases the permeability of the collecting duct to water and therefore increases water reabsorption and urine osmolality (see figure). The reabsorption of water from the collecting ducts directly enters the blood. ADH controls water independently of other ions and solutes. The nephron site of ADH's major effect is the late distal tubule and collecting duct. At this point in the nephron, nearly all of the solutes and osmotically active particles have already been reabsorbed. Thus, free water enters the bloodstream, diluting other ions and osmotically active particles, which decreases the P_{osm}. In contrast, when ADH release is decreased, the medullary and papillary collecting ducts remain relatively impermeable to water, and the net excretion of water is increased. Again, this water loss occurs in the absence of appreciable loss of ions; therefore, a net loss of free water occurs. This process provides a critical pathway for increasing the net concentration of ionic and osmotically active particles in the plasma compartment, thereby providing a net increase in P_{osm}.

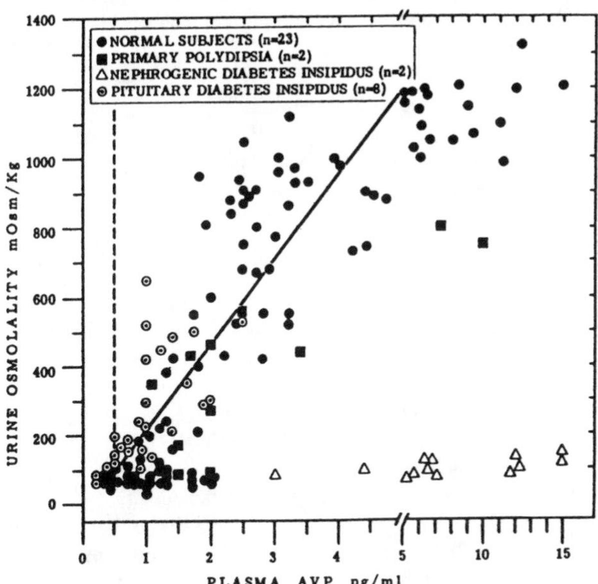

(From Dunn FL, Brennan TJ, Nelson AE, Robertson GL: The role of blood osmolality and volume in regulating vasopressin secretion in the rat. J Clin Invest 52:3212–3219, 1973, with permission.)

128. How is the relative clearance of water determined?

The clearance of water is termed **free water clearance** (C_{H_2O}) (i.e., the water that is cleared from the plasma that is free of osmotically active particles). C_{H_2O} must be equal to the urine flow less the osmolar clearance or clearance of osmotic substances:

$$C_{H_2O} = UF - C_{osm}$$

Because $C_{osm} = V \times U_{osm}/P_{osm}$, by simple substitution:

$$C_{H_2O} = UF - [V \times (U_{osm}/P_{osm})]$$

In most cases, the value for C_{H_2O} is a negative value. For example, during normal states of hydration:

U_{osm} = 700 mOsm/kg
UF = 1 mL/min
P_{osm} = 290 mOsm/kg

C_{H_2O} calculates to be –1.40 mL/min. This means that 1.40 mL/min of water that is free of osmotically active particles is being **reabsorbed** or returned from the tubular fluid back into the plasma every minute. When C_{H_2O} is positive, the organism is in a state of overhydration, and there is a net excretion of **free** water into the urine.

129. What is water balance?

The relationship between water intake and water loss. Although water loss is regulated primarily by controlling water excretion into the urine, it also includes the removal of water from the body as a result of other sources that are not easily regulated: respiration, sweating, and fecal water. On the average, water balance must always be equal to 0.

130. Why is water balance important for normal homeostasis?

When water balance does not equal 0, the organism is in a relative state of either dehydration (net water loss) or overhydration (water gain). Because the body is approximately 65% water, this delicate balance is critical for the overall regulation of cellular function. The control of C_{H_2O} is the body's feedback mechanism used to maintain normal water balance from the standpoint of water loss.

131. Is water balance also affected by water intake?

Thirst and drinking are the other factors used to maintain the balance between intake and excretion of fluids. When water loss exceeds water intake, the P_{osm} increases, and this rise in P_{osm} is sensed by the osmoreceptors, which signal the preoptic and paraventricular nuclei of the hypothalamus. The rise in P_{osm} triggers the release of ADH from the neurohypophysis, which serves to help restore water balance to 0 by decreasing water excretion. At the same time, the hypothalamus maintains neural projections to the anterior regions, which signal the desire and drive for thirst and drinking. Thus, the organism seeks the available water for resolving negative water balance both by increasing water intake and by reducing water excretion.

132. Does excess ADH release ever occur?

The **syndrome of inappropriate ADH secretion (SIADH)** is sometimes observed in patients for various reasons, including malignant (ectopic) neoplasms (e.g., bronchogenic carcinoma), CNS disorders (e.g., trauma), and pulmonary disorders (e.g., tuberculosis).

133. What effect does SIADH have on fluid and electrolyte homeostasis?

In this syndrome, excess ADH is released into the systemic circulation, and the hypothalamus no longer responds to normal changes in plasma osmolality. The elevated plasma concentrations of ADH maintain the kidneys in a constant state of water reabsorption leading to excess retention of water. A number of electrolyte disturbances result from this syndrome, including hypokalemia, hyponatremia, and decreased plasma oncotic pressure.

134. What are the functional consequences of a lack of ADH release?

The lack of circulating ADH is the form of diabetes termed **diabetes insipidus**. In the absence of ADH, the organism tends to have excess urine flow and water excretion, because without ADH, the collecting ducts are relatively impermeable to water. Thus, individuals with diabetes insipidus are in a **permanent** state of water loss because of excess renal excretion of water. Under these circumstances, P_{osm} increases, causing continual thirst and drinking. These individuals seek water on a continual basis and maintain their normal water balance primarily through the thirst mechanism.

Diabetes insipidus may be caused by deficiencies in either **hypothalamic** or **renal** mechanisms. **Hypothalamic** diabetes insipidus is the lack of ADH secretion and release from the neurohypophysis. This form of diabetes insipidus can be treated easily with administration of ADH on a regular basis. In **nephrogenic** diabetes insipidus, the hypothalamopituitary axis secretes ADH normally, but the distal tubules and collecting ducts do not respond appropriately to the presence of the hormone. Effective treatment for nephrogenic diabetes insipidus has not yet been developed.

REGULATION OF SODIUM EXCRETION AND PLASMA VOLUME

135. Why is the regulation of sodium intake and excretion important in plasma volume regulation?

The regulation of sodium intake and output is extremely important in the regulation and maintenance of a normal plasma volume. The major cation found in the ECF is sodium with its accompanying anions (primarily chloride and bicarbonate). Together, these ions comprise greater than 90% of the osmolytes in the ECF. Because plasma osmolarity is tightly controlled by ADH, which regulates renal water handling, any changes in extracellular sodium lead to changes in ADH and the accompanying changes in plasma volume.

136. Explain what is meant by sodium balance.

The term *balance* refers to the requirement that the intake and output of sodium (or any other substance) must be equal if an individual is in a steady state. For the body, dietary sodium intake must equal the excretion of sodium plus any insensible losses, sweating, and fecal losses. Because sodium intake is largely dependent on behavior, and insensible losses generally are quite small and usually not under tight physiologic control, the renal handling of sodium is the critical link to ensure that the body remains in a steady state. If the normal adult human consumes 8–10 g of NaCl per day, to remain in balance, 8–10 g of NaCl must be excreted per day.

137. How do the kidneys normally handle sodium?

Kidneys handle sodium through two basic mechanisms: **filtration** and **reabsorption**. Changes in neural, hormonal, and physical factors alter both filtration and reabsorption to decrease or increase sodium excretion to maintain sodium balance.

138. How much of the filtered sodium is normally reabsorbed in each tubular segment?

Proximal tubule	60–70%
Loop of Henle	20–25%
Distal convoluted tubule	3–5%
Collecting duct	2–4%

139. Why does reabsorption of filtered sodium vary from normal values?

Values vary depending on the volume status of the individual. When excess sodium must be excreted, reabsorption decreases to increase excretion. In contrast, in cases of volume depletion in which sodium must be conserved, sodium reabsorption is increased in the individually regulated nephron segments.

140. Summarize how changes in sodium intake and plasma volume can be sensed by the body.

Changes in plasma volume are sensed by the body at three main sites:

1. Low-pressure baroreceptors on the venous side of the systemic circulation
2. High-pressure baroreceptors on the arterial side of the systemic circulation
3. Intrarenal mechanisms (intrarenal baroreceptor and macula densa)

141. Where are the low-pressure baroreceptors?

Low-pressure baroreceptors are located within the **great veins,** the **atria,** and the **pulmonary vasculature**.

142. How do the low-pressure baroreceptors affect renal function?

Because they are located on the low-pressure side of the circulation, low-pressure baroreceptors respond to changes in fullness or central filling pressure by stretching and sending afferent signals via the vagus nerve to the cardiovascular control center in the hypothalamus and brain stem. In this region of the brain, the signals from the low-pressure and high-pressure baroreceptors are integrated, and reflex changes in renal nerve activity and arginine vasopressin release are mediated. In general, a change in venous volume of 5–10% is usually required before the low-pressure baroreceptors are activated.

143. Where are the high-pressure baroreceptors?

High-pressure baroreceptors are found in the **aortic arch** and **carotid artery**.

144. How do the high-pressure baroreceptors affect renal function?

These baroreceptors respond to changes in arterial pressure with afferent signals sent to the cardiovascular control center, where changes in renal sympathetic activity and arginine vasopressin release are regulated. These baroreceptors are fast acting and respond to a 5–10% change in arterial pressure. Despite the sensitivity of the arterial baroreceptors, much larger changes in volume occur in the highly compliant venous circulation before systemic arterial pressure is elevated 5–10%. The high-pressure baroreceptors therefore are not as sensitive to changes in plasma volume as the low-pressure baroreceptors.

145. What are the intrarenal mechanisms that sense changes in plasma volume?

Intrarenal baroreceptor
Macula densa

146. How do they function?

The **intrarenal baroreceptor** is a mechanism by which alterations in stretch of the afferent arteriole lead to changes in renin release. If increased intrarenal arterial pressure is sensed, renin release is inhibited. Conversely, renin release is stimulated when there is decreased stretch of the afferent arteriole.

The **macula densa** also alters renin release after changes in NaCl delivery. In response to increased NaCl delivery to this nephron segment, the macula densa signals the juxtaglomerular cells to release renin. When sodium chloride delivery to this segment is increased, the signal to the juxtaglomerular cells is to decrease renin release.

147. Explain how the signals from the high-pressure and low-pressure baroreceptors, the intrarenal baroreceptors, and the macula densa are integrated to regulate renal sodium handling.

The intrarenal and extrarenal mechanisms that sense the **fullness** of the extracellular space act in concert to regulate the renal handling of sodium. When volume is sensed to be high and increased sodium is delivered to the macula densa, the systems involved in the conservation of sodium and water are suppressed or inactivated, depending on the degree of fullness of the system. In contrast, when the volume (pressure) is judged to be low and macula densa sodium delivery is decreased, the systems that favor the conservation of sodium and water are activated.

148. List the systems primarily involved in sodium and plasma volume regulation.

Renin-angiotensin
Aldosterone
Renal sympathetic nerves
Atrial natriuretic peptide
ADH
Physical factors

149. What is the renin-angiotensin system?

The renin-angiotensin system is a cascade of biochemical reactions that leads to increased levels of the biologically active octapeptide angiotensin II. Renin is an enzyme found in the juxtaglomerular cells of the renal afferent arteriole; when this enzyme is released into the circulation, it cleaves angiotensinogen, a circulating polypeptide produced by the liver, into the decapeptide angiotensin I. Angiotensin I is then cleaved to angiotensin II by angiotensin-converting enzyme, which is found in endothelial cells in the lung and the kidney. By themselves, renin, angiotensinogen, angiotensin I, and angiotensin-converting enzyme have little to no biologic activity. The active peptide is angiotensin II, which is a potent vasoconstrictor, stimulator of aldosterone release, and stimulator of tubular sodium reabsorption.

150. Name the stimuli that activate the renin-angiotensin system.

1. **Reductions in renal perfusion pressure** are sensed by intrarenal baroreceptors in the afferent arteriole, which leads to renin release.
2. **Decreased delivery of NaCl to the macula densa** also stimulates renin release from the juxtaglomerular cells.
3. **Stimulation of renal sympathetic nerves** directly increases renin release.

Each of these stimuli is activated when the body needs to conserve or retain sodium.

151. What are the principal effects of the renin-angiotensin system on renal function?

The overall effect of the renin-angiotensin system is to **decrease sodium and water excretion** by decreasing filtered load and increasing tubular sodium reabsorption. Angiotensin II is a potent systemic vasoconstrictor, and stimulation of the renin-angiotensin system also leads to **increased total peripheral resistance,** which tends to increase blood pressure by direct effects. The renin angiotensin system is activated in conditions when sodium needs to be conserved.

152. How does the renin-angiotensin system alter renal vascular function?

Angiotensin II increases renal vascular resistance. In the human kidney, this peptide appears to constrict the efferent arteriole preferentially at normal circulating levels. After hemorrhage or other insults that lead to hypovolemia or lowering of renal perfusion pressure, elevated levels of angiotensin II constrict the preglomerular vasculature as well as the postglomerular efferent arteriole, leading to a decrease in GFR and RBF.

153. Does the renin-angiotensin system influence tubular sodium transport?

Angiotensin II directly stimulates proximal tubule sodium reabsorption. Angiotensin II also acts at the level of the adrenal gland to increase aldosterone secretion; aldosterone then has potent effects to stimulate sodium reabsorption and potassium secretion in the distal portions of the nephron.

154. What is aldosterone?

A mineralocorticoid produced in the zona glomerulosa of the adrenal gland. In response to increased angiotensin II or increased extracellular potassium levels, the synthesis of aldosterone and its release into the blood are increased. Of the two stimuli for aldosterone release, changes in extracellular potassium are the most potent.

155. How does aldosterone affect renal function?

The net effect of aldosterone on renal function is to **decrease sodium excretion** and **increase potassium excretion** without affecting renal hemodynamics (GFR and RBF). The mechanism of aldosterone action occurs at the level of the connecting tubule and collecting duct, where this steroid hormone binds to cytoplasmic receptors. This binding leads to increased synthesis and insertion of sodium channels into the tubular membranes to increase sodium reabsorption in exchange for potassium, which is secreted into the tubular lumen.

156. What is meant by *physical factors*, and how do physical factors affect renal sodium handling?

This a term used to describe collectively changes in hydrostatic and oncotic forces in the capillaries and renal interstitial space.

1. In the case of an expansion of ECF volume, plasma protein is diluted (plasma oncotic pressure decreases), and glomerular and peritubular capillary hydrostatic pressure increases. Increased glomerular capillary pressure increases the driving force for ultrafiltration, whereas dilution of plasma protein decreases the forces opposing filtration; for these reasons, the filtered load of sodium increases under volume-expanded conditions.
2. The increase in capillary hydrostatic pressure and decrease in plasma protein lead to less favorable conditions (elevated hydrostatic and reduced oncotic pressure) for reabsorption in the peritubular and vasa recta capillaries and tend to reduce the reabsorption of fluid from the tubules.

157. Explain how renal sympathetic nerves affect sodium handling.

In response to decreased volume and stretch from the low-pressure and high-pressure baroreceptors, renal sympathetic nerves are stimulated. The renal sympathetic nerves are activated in conditions of hypovolemia and serve to retain sodium. Renal sympathetic stimulation leads to sodium retention by three mechanisms:

- Decreasing filtered load
- Increasing tubular reabsorption
- Increasing renin release

158. What is atrial natriuretic factor?

A peptide found in the atria and great veins that is released in response to increased atrial stretch (increased ECF volume); also known as atrial natriuretic peptide.

159. What does atrial natriuretic factor do to affect renal function?

When atrial natriuretic factor is released, it increases sodium and water excretion by increasing GFR and decreasing collecting duct sodium reabsorption. Atrial natriuretic peptide is released in conditions of hypervolemia and acts to increase sodium excretion.

160. What is the pressure-natriuretic-diuretic mechanism?

The phenomenon by which increased renal perfusion pressure leads to an increase in sodium and water excretion owing to an intrinsic property of the kidney. The increased sodium and water excretion serves to decrease ECF volume and leads to a normalization of arterial pressure. Conversely, when arterial pressure is decreased, the pressure-natriuretic mechanism is shifted to a lower operating point, and the kidney tends to decrease sodium and water excretion to increase extracellular volume and return arterial pressure to control levels.

161. What is the importance of the pressure-natriuretic-diuretic mechanism?

This intrinsic feedback mechanism of the kidney is hypothesized by some scientists as one of the primary regulators of ECF volume and arterial blood pressure.

162. List other paracrine or autocrine systems or mechanisms that can alter renal sodium handling.

Natriuretic or Diuretic	*Antinatriuretic or Antidiuretic*
Prostaglandins	Thromboxane
Nitric oxide	Endothelin
Urodilatin	
Kinins	

163. How do all these systems act to regulate plasma volume?

The different neural, hormonal, and intrinsic mechanisms that regulate sodium and water excretion act in an integrated fashion in response to changes in sodium and water intake to maintain homeostasis. When dietary sodium is increased, output lags behind intake, and ECF space is expanded. The ECF expansion triggers a number of events:

- Activation of low-pressure baroreceptors, which inhibits sympathetic activity and vasopressin release
- Stretch of the atria, which leads to release of atrial natriuretic peptide
- A slight elevation of systemic arterial blood pressure, which shifts the pressure-natriuretic relationship to a higher level of pressure
- Inhibition of the renin-angiotensin-aldosterone axis by intrarenal mechanisms

These mechanisms operate in concert to maintain a constancy of the body's internal environment by excreting the excess sodium. In contrast to the changes that occur when sodium intake is elevated, these systems (sympathetic nerves, renin-angiotensin, vasopressin, aldosterone, pressure natriuresis-diuresis) are activated to conserve sodium in conditions of decreased dietary sodium intake or in other conditions in which the ECF is decreased.

164. How are these systems affected in disease states?

1. **Pathologic conditions:** In response to **hemorrhage, shock, severe vomiting,** or **severe diarrhea,** the mechanisms to conserve sodium and water are activated in the normal physiologic response to decreased ECF volume or decreased arterial pressure.

2. **Pathophysiologic conditions:** In **heart failure,** the inability of the heart to function adequately as a pump leads to a fall in cardiac output and mean arterial pressure. The fall in blood pressure leads to activation of sympathetic nerves, the renin-angiotensin system, vasopressin release, and aldosterone synthesis. These combined conditions lead to retention of fluid and water, which can actually exacerbate the heart condition by increasing the preload on the diseased heart.

3. It is also not uncommon to observe patients in which an **abnormality in one of the controlling systems** leads to alterations in renal sodium (and water) handling and the consequential effects on body fluids. In **hypoaldosteronism,** in which insufficient aldosterone is produced by the adrenal gland and large amounts of sodium are excreted, leading to decreased ECF volume, hypotension, and, if left untreated, circulatory shock and death.

ACID-BASE BALANCE AND EXCRETION OF POTASSIUM

165. Why is regulation of plasma K^+ concentration important?

The regulation of plasma K^+ concentration is critical to the overall function of the body because the K^+ concentration difference across cell membranes can dramatically influence the resting membrane potential of all cells. This resting membrane potential is particularly important for normal contraction of skeletal and cardiac muscle and function of nerve cells.

166. What is the normal range for plasma K^+ concentration?

3.0–5.0 mM/L.

167. How does the kidney participate in the control of K^+ balance?

The kidney and adrenal cortex work in concert as the primary organs that regulate plasma K^+

through the control of renal K^+ excretion. This regulation is accomplished by the release of aldosterone from the adrenal cortex, which regulates renal tubular K^+ handling.

168. Does aldosterone provide short-term or long-term control over Na^+ reabsorption and K^+ excretion?

Aldosterone should be considered a relatively **long-term** controller of Na^+ reabsorption and K^+ excretion. Aldosterone acts in the principal cells of the distal tubule and cortical collecting duct. It is a relatively long-term controller of Na^+ and K^+ balance because it is a steroid hormone, which activates transcription and translation of new protein.

169. How does aldosterone affect K^+ excretion and K^+ balance?

One mechanism by which aldosterone functions is to activate the tubular cell Na^+, K^+-ATPase. Stimulation of this basolateral cell enzyme not only increases Na^+ reabsorption into the interstitium, but also increases intracellular K^+ concentration. The increased intracellular K^+ promotes secretion of K^+ from inside the cell into the tubular lumen through apical channels and thereby promotes overall K^+ excretion. This gradient is under the complete influence of aldosterone, and for this reason aldosterone is often referred to as the **plasma K^+ controller**.

170. Does plasma K^+ concentration affect the secretion of aldosterone?

The concentration of K^+ in the plasma may be the most potent controller of aldosterone secretion from the adrenal zona glomerulosa cells. These cells are highly influenced by the circulating K^+ concentration. An elevation of plasma K^+ from 4.5 to 5.5 mEq/L provides near-maximum elevation of circulating aldosterone concentrations. Reduction of plasma K^+ below 3.0 mEq/L decreases aldosterone secretion and reduces plasma aldosterone to low values.

171. Do any other ions in the plasma affect plasma K^+?

The level of acidosis and plasma acidification can have a pronounced influence on the excretion of K^+ by the kidney. During chronic acidosis, elevation of extracellular H^+ ion greatly influences the plasma K^+ concentration. Both H^+ and K^+ are relatively permeable to movement into and out of cells. Thus, in the presence of excess H^+, the tendency is for H^+ to diffuse into cells and K^+ to diffuse out of cells to maintain electroneutrality.

172. How does acidosis affect plasma K^+?

Acute acidosis tends to decrease Na^+, K^+-ATPase and decrease the K^+ permeability of the apical membrane and thereby decrease potassium secretion and excretion. Chronic metabolic acidosis, however, induces **hyperkalemia,** which stimulates aldosterone release and has a net effect to increase potassium secretion and excretion.

173. What are the major mechanisms by which the kidney regulates acid-base balance?

Renal regulation of acid-base occurs via H^+ excretion and HCO_3^- reabsorption. Control of either H^+ excretion or the buffering capacity for H^+ with HCO_3^- has the net effect of controlling the overall state of extracellular fluid H^+ concentration.

174. What are the nephron segments responsible for regulating H^+ excretion?

Excretion of fixed acid (H^+) occurs in the proximal tubule, thick ascending limb, and intercalated cells of the distal tubule and collecting duct. In the proximal tubule and thick ascending limb, H^+ ion secretion occurs on the lumenal membrane in exchange for Na^+ ion. The intercalated cells contain specific proton pumps in the lumenal membrane that directly utilize ATP to secrete H^+. These proton pumps secrete H^+ into the tubular lumen of the distal tubule and collecting duct and assist in acidifying the urine.

175. How does HCO_3^- reabsorption contribute to the urine acidification process?

The removal of HCO_3^- from the tubular fluid is extremely important under normal conditions in which excess acid must be excreted from the body. The near complete reabsorption of filtered HCO_3^- is necessary to maintain the body's acid-base status since the CO_2/HCO_3^- buffer system is extremely important in acid-base regulation. The reabsorption of HCO_3^- from the tubular fluid is highly effective in the proximal tubule, thick ascending limb of Henle, and intercalated cells of the collecting duct and under normal circumstances 99.9% of the filtered load is reabsorbed.

176. How is HCO_3^- reabsorbed in the PCT?

The lumenal membrane of the PCT is relatively impermeable to HCO_3^- ions. Therefore, all HCO_3- must be reabsorbed in the form of CO_2. H^+ ion, which is secreted in exchange for Na^+, combines with HCO_3^- to form CO_2 and water, and this reaction is catalyzed by the presence of carbonic anhydrase on the PCT brush border membranes. CO_2 diffuses down its concentration gradient into the PCT cell because the lumenal membrane is permeable to this molecule (similar to all cells). Inside the cell, the CO_2 combines with water, again catalyzed by the presence of intracellular carbonic anhydrase, forming H^+ and HCO_3^-. From the inside of the cell, the HCO_3^- is able to diffuse down its concentration gradient into the blood and effectively complete the reabsorptive process.

177. How does acidosis increase the secretion of H^+ from the interstitial spaces into the tubular lumen?

Acidosis or increased plasma H^+ concentration is removed from the blood in a substrate-specific manner. As plasma H^+ concentration increases, the supply of substrate to the various transport processes in the kidneys also is increased. Therefore, H^+ secretion in the PCT and collecting duct is increased because of elevated substrate availability to the specific transporters in those sites.

178. What are the other mechanisms that the kidney uses to excrete H^+ ions and acidify the urine?

Other mechanisms include the excretion of PO_4^-, SO_4^-, and NH_3/NH_4^+. In the case of NH_3, acidosis increases ammoniagenesis through the deamination and metabolism of glutamine and glutamate. This deamination process in the PCT creates excess NH_3, which diffuses into the tubular lumen and combines with filtered H^+ ion to form NH_4^+. The NH_4^+ is then trapped in the tubular lumen and cannot diffuse back into the cell. Thus, the ammonia becomes an excellent carrier of excess H^+ into the excreted urine.

BIBLIOGRAPHY

1. Brenner BM: The Kidney, 5th ed. Philadelphia, W.B. Saunders, 1996.
2. Guyton AC, Hall JE: Textbook of Medical Physiology, 9th ed. Philadelphia, W.B. Saunders, 1996.
3. Koeppen, BW, Stanton BA: Renal Physiology, 2nd ed. St. Louis, Mosby, 1997.
4. Navar LG, Inscho EW, Majid SA, et al: Paracrine regulation of the renal microcirculation. Physiol Rev 76:425–536, 1996.
5. Windhager EE: Handbook of Physiology: Section 8. Renal Physiology, vol 1. Oxford, Oxford University Press, 1992.

7. GASTROINTESTINAL PHYSIOLOGY

Lenard M. Lichtenberger, Ph.D.

GASTROINTESTINAL SECRETION AND ITS REGULATION

1. Describe the different pathways by which gastrointestinal (GI) peptides can affect the metabolic or functional activity of a target cell and give examples of each.

1. **Endocrine:** Endocrine peptides are released by endocrine cells of the GI tract in response to a meal and travel by way of the circulation to the target cell to exert their respective actions. Examples include:

Gastrin
Cholecystokinin (CCK)
Secretin
Glucose-dependent insulinotropic peptide (GIP)

2. **Neurocrine:** Neurocrine peptides are released at nerve endings and affect a target cell by diffusing short distances through the interstitial fluid separating the two cell types. Examples are:

Vasoactive intestinal peptide (VIP)
Somatostatin
Substance P
Neurokinin A
Neurokinin B
Gastrin-releasing peptide (GRP)
Calcitonin gene-related peptide (CGRP)
Enkephalin
Nitric oxide (NO)

3. **Paracrine:** Paracrine factors are released by endocrine or endocrine-like cells and diffuse short distances through interstitial fluid to affect a neighboring target cell. In some cases, cytoplasmic processes have been identified that appear to extend from the cell releasing the paracrine factor to the target cell. Examples include:

- Histamine—released from enterochromaffin-like (ECL) cells and affecting parietal cell secretory activity
- Somatostatin—released from D cells and locally affecting the activity of both parietal cells of the oxyntic mucosa and gastrin-containing G cells of the antral mucosa

2. Which of the GI peptides are structurally related?

GI Family of Peptides

Secretin	*Tachykinins*
Secretin	Substance P
GIP	Neurokinin A (NKA)
VIP	Neurokinin B (NKB)
Glucagon-like peptide (GLP)	*Epidermal Growth Factor (EGF)*
Gastrin	EGF
Gastrin	Transforming growth factors (TGF-α, TGF-β)
CCK	Fibroblast growth factors (FGF-β)
Pancreatic Polypeptide (PP)	*Other GI Peptides*
PP	Somatostatin
Neuropeptide Y (NPY)	Motilin
Peptide YY (PYY)	GRP
	CGRP

3. What are the major characteristics of salivary secretion?

Salivary secretion generally is a hypotonic fluid of high volume, relative to tissue weight, that contains mucus, α-amylase (ptyalin), lipase (lingual lipase), and a number of factors to limit the growth of bacteria in the oropharyngeal cavity. These **antibacterial factors** include lysozyme, immunoglobulin A, and lactoferrin. Salivary secretion also **protects the oropharyngeal mucosa** against the injurious actions of either ingested substances (e.g., hot or acidic drinks, spicy foods) or regurgitated GI secretions (gastric juice, bile) by diluting or neutralizing these factors. If the salivary glands are destroyed (e.g., radiation therapy), a condition of **xerostomia** develops, which results in a decrease or abolition of salivary secretion associated with severe ulceration of the oropharyngeal epithelium, bacterial overgrowth, and an increased incidence of dental caries. In contrast to other GI secretions, salivary secretion is primarily under the regulation of the autonomic nervous system.

4. What are the major physiologic functions of salivary secretion?

- To lubricate the ingested food to facilitate its movement down the GI tract
- To initiate the hydrolysis of dietary carbohydrates and fat
- To limit the colonization of bacteria in the oropharyngeal cavity

5. What is the functional role of ptyalin or salivary amylase?

This enzyme catalyzes the hydrolysis of internal α-1,4-glycosidic bonds present in dietary starch molecules. This results in the generation of maltose, maltotriose, and α-limit dextrins, which contain the 1,6-branch points of the starch molecule. The salivary gland enzyme is identical to pancreatic amylase and has a pH optimum near neutrality. The products of salivary and pancreatic amylase catalyzed hydrolysis, in turn, are broken down to glucose by maltase and isomaltase (1,6-dextrinase) in the small intestine, where the monosaccharide is rapidly absorbed by an active transport mechanism.

6. Are any dietary nutrients other than carbohydrate broken down by saliva?

Yes. It appears that saliva contains a nonspecific lipase enzyme, called lingual lipase, that catalyzes the hydrolysis of triglycerides to fatty acids and monoglycerides acylated in the 2-position. Lingual lipase, which has a broad pH optimum, promotes the breakdown of dietary fat during both the cephalic and the gastric phase of digestion. As its name implies, the enzyme is primarily localized to the epithelial cells of the tongue and secreted into the saliva.

7. Are the salivary enzymes active only in the oropharyngeal cavity?

No. Lingual lipase has activity even at moderately acidic pH and thereby promotes the hydrolysis of dietary lipid at low pH found in the stomach between meals. Because of the buffering capacity of many foods, the pH of the stomach can rise to between 5 and 6 during the first few postprandial hours. This fact together with the observation that incomplete mixing and layering of foods can occur in the orad stomach (shielding midlayers from the pH of the luminal fluid) strongly suggests that the digestion of dietary starch by α-amylase may also proceed during the gastric phase of digestion.

8. What are the major salivary glands in humans?

- Parotid gland, located between the angle of the jaw and the ear
- Submaxillary gland, located below the jaw
- Sublingual gland, located below the tongue

9. Which of the three major salivary glands secretes a nonmucoid watery fluid?

The parotid gland, which is entirely made up of serous cells. In contrast, the submaxillary and sublingual glands contain mucous cells as well as serous cells and have a mixed secretion.

10. Name the basic functional components of the secretory unit of a salivary gland.

This unit is referred to as the **salivon** and includes the acinus, the blinded tube composed of acinar cells that empty into the intercalated duct region, which, in turn, empties into the striated duct. The **acinar cells** secrete both protein and electrolytes, and the latter inorganic components are modified by the ductule cells lining the striated duct. **Myoepithelial cells** are located along the basement membrane of both the intercalated and the striated ducts and on contraction promote the movement of salivary gland fluid distally into ducts of increasingly larger diameter, which empty into the oropharyngeal cavity (see figure).

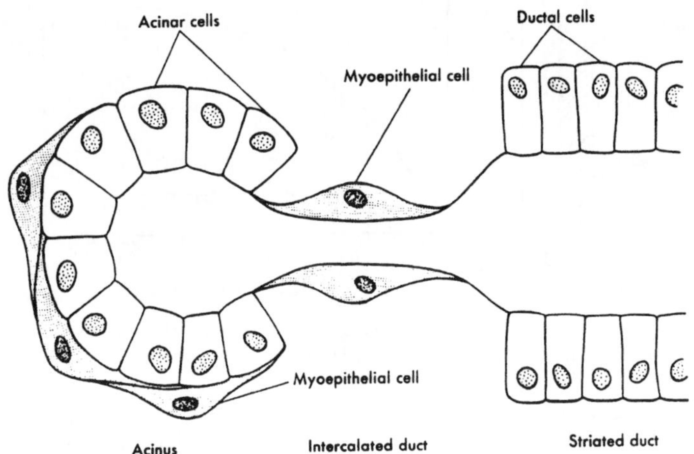

Cells lining the various portions of the salivon. (From Johnson LR: Gastrointestinal Physiology, 4th ed. St. Louis, Mosby, 1991, with permission.)

11. What are the notable blood flow characteristics of the salivary gland?

The direction of the arterial blood flow runs opposite to that of salivary fluid moving through the salivon. It appears that separate capillary beds serve the acinus and ductular region of the salivary gland unit, both of which are characterized by having a high capillary filtration coefficient to facilitate fluid and gas exchange. The blood flow to the salivary glands is high, approximately 20 times greater than most tissues when calculated per gram wet weight, which appears to be responsible for the high rate of salivary secretion that can be generated by these small excretory glands.

12. How do the inorganic constituents of saliva change as the secretory rate increases?

At high secretory rates, the ionic constituents of saliva approach, but in all cases (except K^+) are less than, their respective concentrations in plasma. As the rate of salivary secretion decreases, the Na^+ and Cl^- concentrations of salivary gland fluid decrease proportionally, whereas the K^+ and HCO_3^- remain fairly constant (see figure, top of next page). At low flow rates (< 10 mL/min), the major inorganic components of saliva are KCl and $KHCO_3$.

13. What is the effect of secretory rate on the tonicity of saliva?

Saliva becomes clearly hypotonic at low flow rates and approaches isotonicity as the flow rate increases to a maximal value. The explanation for these changes is that the ions are initially secreted into the lumen of the acinus at isotonic concentrations (with Cl^- being actively secreted and the remainder entering the lumen passively to maintain electroneutrality) and that as the saliva travels through the ducts, Na^+ and Cl^- are actively reabsorbed, whereas K^+ and HCO_3^- are actively secreted into the lumen of the ducts. In some cases, there is evidence for the presence of Cl^-/HCO_3^- exchanger at the luminal membrane of the ductule cells. It is clear that if the rate of fluid movement is slow, a greater number of ions are reabsorbed into the ductal epithelium than are secreted into the lumen, accounting for the decrease in tonicity of saliva. The ability of the salivary gland ducts to secrete HCO_3^- and to reabsorb H^+ in exchange for K^+ accounts for the fact that saliva is slightly alkaline (pH = 8).

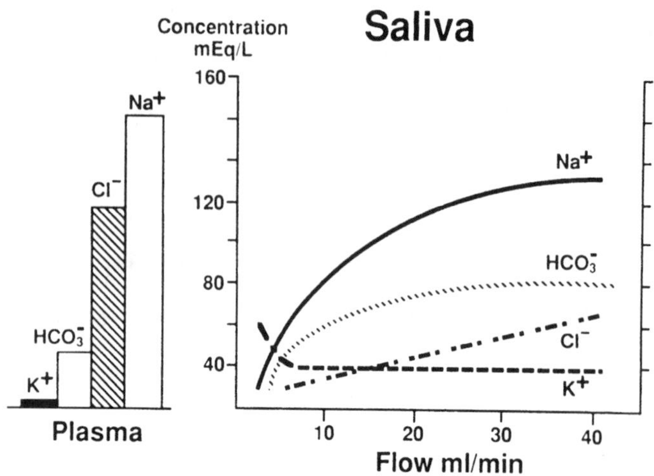

Concentrations of major ions in the saliva as a function of the rate of salivary secretion. Values in plasma are shown for comparison. (From Johnson LR: Gastrointestinal Physiology, 4th ed. St. Louis, Mosby, 1991, with permission.)

14. Is there a difference in the permeability characteristic of the luminal membrane of the acinar and ductal epithelium to water?

Yes. In contrast to the acinus, which is freely permeable to water, the ductal epithelial membrane appears to be relatively impermeable to water. This accounts for the fact that salivary gland fluid is isotonic when it leaves the acinus, whereas it becomes hypotonic at the level of the striated duct and thereafter.

15. How is salivary secretion regulated physiologically?

In contrast with other GI excretory organs, whose secretions are regulated by both hormones and nerves, salivary secretion is primarily regulated by the autonomic nervous system. Stimulation of both parasympathetic and sympathetic nerve trunks elicits an increase in salivary secretion, with the former playing the dominant role.

Stimulation of **parasympathetic** fibers induces the release of acetylcholine at the nerve terminals, which then interact with muscarinic receptors on both salivary gland epithelial and vascular tissue. This causes an activation of phosphatidylinositol-specific phospholipase C, resulting in the generation of inositol 1,4,5-triphosphate (IP_3), diacylglycerol, and a subsequent increase in cytosolic calcium and an activation of protein kinase C to promote protein phosphorylation. In response to the signal transduction cascade, transporters in both the acinar and the ductal cells become activated, and myoepithelial cells contract to expel salivary fluid distally. Furthermore, parasympathetic stimulation induces an increase in local blood flow to the salivary glands as a result of a direct vasodilator action and an increase in metabolism resulting in the generation of vasodilator metabolites and bradykinin (which is generated by the release of the enzyme, kallikrein).

Sympathetic stimulation results in the release of norepinephrine from nerve terminals, which activate adrenergic receptors on both acinar and ductal epithelial cells, resulting in the activation of adenylate cyclase and protein kinase A, to promote protein phosphorylation. In general, cyclic adenosine monophosphate (cAMP) is believed to activate the secretion of the organic constituents of salivary secretion (mucus and enzymes), whereas the IP_3-Ca^{++} system mediates the secretion of fluid and electrolytes. Additionally, sympathetic stimulation induces myoepithelial cells to contract and a vasoconstrictor response followed by a secondary and prolonged vasodilation as vasodilator substances are generated because of the increase in metabolic activity. Sympathetic stimulation thus results in a biphasic change in blood flow, with an initial decrease followed by a prolonged period of increased perfusion. Sympathetic stimulation is required for salivary gland growth because section of sympathetic neural connections results in rapid atrophy of the glands.

16. Is salivary secretion affected by central nervous system activity and emotions?

Yes. The act of chewing or even thinking of an appetizing meal **stimulates** salivary secretion, as does nausea and the ingestion of sour or spicy foods, whereas salivary secretion is **inhibited** during sleep, dehydration, and the emotional states of anxiety and fear. The CNS centers for parasympathetic and sympathetic outflow are still being identified but appear to converge in secretory centers in the medulla.

17. What are the major components of gastric juice?

Hydrochloric acid
Pepsin
Mucus
Intrinsic factor

18. Discuss the physiologic role of the major components of gastric juice.

Hydrochloric acid and **pepsin** initiate the hydrolysis of dietary protein, to be completed by pancreatic and brush border proteases when the food bolus enters the small intestine. The acidic environment of the stomach, which can approach a pH of 1.0 between meals, plays an important role in limiting the growth of aerobic bacteria and thus keeping the stomach in a semisterile state. **Intrinsic factor** plays an essential role in binding to and promoting the transport of vitamin B_{12} across the mucosa of the distal small intestine.

19. Why is intrinsic factor the only gastric factor that is required for life?

In the past, patients who suffered from atrophic gastritis frequently died, not from a GI or nutritional disturbance, but from **pernicious anemia.** This condition can now simply be corrected by giving patients parenteral injections of vitamin B_{12}. Similarly, patients who have their stomachs surgically removed (gastrectomy) also require injections of vitamin B_{12} to prevent them from developing pernicious anemia.

20. Describe the functional anatomy of the stomach.

The gastric mucosa can be functionally subdivided into the **oxyntic mucosa,** which occupies the proximal fundus and central body regions of the stomach, and the **antral mucosa,** present in the distal pyloric region of the stomach.

The major cell types present in the **oxyntic mucosa** are the **mucous cells,** present on the mucosal surface, the pit region, and the neck regions of the gastric gland; the **parietal cells,** which line the midregions of the gland; and the **chief cells,** which are present in the distal glandular regions (see figure, next page). The **surface mucous cells** secrete a viscous neutral mucous glycoprotein that is primarily responsible for the mucus gel lining that coats the luminal surface of the stomach, whereas the **mucous neck cells** secrete a soluble acidic and sulfated mucous glycoprotein. In addition, there is evidence that both classes of mucous cells of the oxyntic mucosa synthesize group I pepsinogen isozymes. The chief cell is the major source of pepsin in the body and synthesizes and secretes pepsinogen I. The parietal cell in humans is the source of hydrochloric acid and intrinsic factor. **Endocrine cells** are scattered throughout the oxyntic mucosa, with the most numerous being the **enterochromaffin-like (ECL) cells,** which secrete histamine, and the **delta (D) cells,** which synthesize and release somatostatin. Both cell types are localized in close proximity to the parietal cell and appear to have a paracrine regulatory influence on its activity.

The **antral mucosa,** which is structured in a glandular arrangement, primarily consists of mucous and endocrine cells. The mucous cells are similar to the glandular mucous cells of the oxyntic mucosa and synthesize and secrete pepsinogen group II isozymes. The major endocrine cells of the antral mucosa are the **gastrin-containing G cells** and the **somatostatin-containing D cells,** which are localized in the middistal regions of the pyloric glands, with the G-to-D cell ratio being approximately 4:1. Similar to the case of the parietal cell, the D cell is thought to have a paracrine influence on gastrin release from the G cell.

The progenitor regions of the oxyntic mucosa are the neck regions of the oxyntic gland, and immature cells migrate both upward to the surface and distally down the glands, where they differentiate into mucous, parietal, chief, and endocrine cells. In contrast, the proliferative cells of the antral mucosa are localized to the distal regions of the pyloric glands, and the daughter cells migrate upward to differentiate into mucous and endocrine cells.

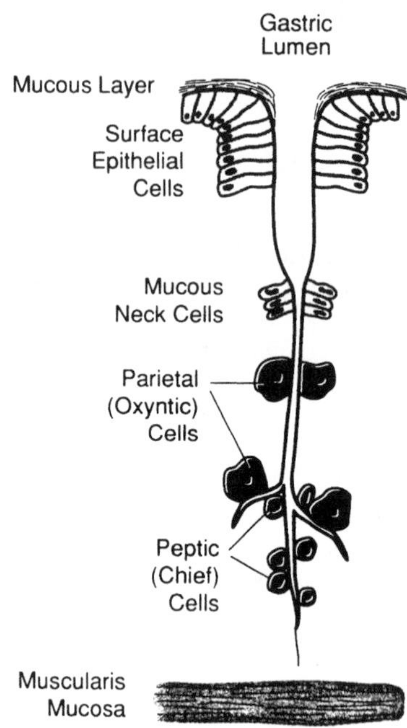

Oxyntic gland and pit, showing the positions of the various cell types. (From Johnson LR: Essential Medical Physiology, 2nd ed. Philadelphia, Lippincott-Raven, 1997, with permission.)

21. Describe the morphologic transformation of the parietal cell.

Parietal cells are rather large pyramidal-shaped cells that possess a large number of mitochondria (to generate adenosine triphosphate [ATP] required for hydrochloric acid secretion) and an intricate canalicular membrane that is contiguous with the surface membrane. In the quiescent state, multiple small vesicles, called **tubulovesicles,** are present in close proximity to the canalicular membrane. When the parietal cell is activated by the administration of a secretory stimulant (e.g., gastrin or histamine), the tubulovesicles fuse with the canalicular membrane, forming an intricate **secretory canaliculus**. This results in a morphologic transformation of the cell, markedly increasing the surface area of the canaliculus and inducing the formation of microvilli within the canalicular network.

22. What is the significance of this transformation to hydrochloric acid secretion?

This transformation brings two important transport elements together (from the tubulovesicle and canalicular membranes) that are required for hydrochloric acid secretion.

23. How does the proton pump work and what is its relationship to the morphologic transformation of the parietal cell?

The key enzyme involved in the ability of the parietal cell to transport H^+ actively against a millionfold chemical gradient is the **H^+, K^+-ATPase,** also called **the proton pump,** which resides in the membrane of the tubulovesicles. For this enzyme to be active and to pump protons unidirectionally, a K^+ gradient needs to be established in the opposite direction to that of the desired movement of protons. Because the tubulovesicle membrane is impermeable to K^+, such a gradient is not established until the tubulovesicles fuse with the canalicular membrane, which is permeable to the cation. Thus, the **morphologic transformation of the parietal cell** results in the translocation of the H^+, K^+-ATPase to the canalicular membrane in close proximity to K^+ channels, and it is the presence of this cation on the luminal face of the ATPase that both activates and provides the driving force to pump protons into the lumen. The initiating event in HCl secretion appears to be the cAMP-dependent opening of Cl^- channels, allowing K^+ (and its counter ion Cl^-) to diffuse out of the parietal cell and concentrate in the canalicular space where it can activate the proton pump (see figure).

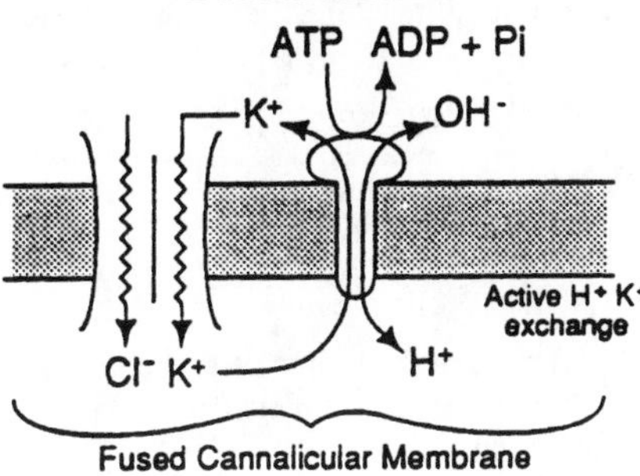

Molecular mechanism of proton secretion by the parietal cell.

24. Can the proton pump be blocked pharmacologically?

Yes. A family of compounds in the benzimidazole class can effectively, irreversibly bind to and inhibit the proton pump. Omeprazole (Prilosec) was the first of these drugs to be developed. It was determined that omeprazole enters the systemic circulation and, as a basic compound, will accumulate in high concentrations in acidic compartments. As a consequence, omeprazole becomes trapped in the canalicular space, becomes activated (to a sulfonamide), and forms a disulfide bond with the H^+, K^+-ATPase, irreversibly inhibiting the enzyme (see figure, top of next page). Other members of this class of **proton pump inhibitors (PPIs)** are lansoprazole (Prevacid), rabeprazole (Aciphex), and esomeprazole (Nexium).

25. What is the alkaline tide?

For every proton molecule that is pumped into the lumen, an OH^- remains in the cytoplasm of the parietal cell. To prevent intracellular alkalization and cell death, the enzyme carbonic an-

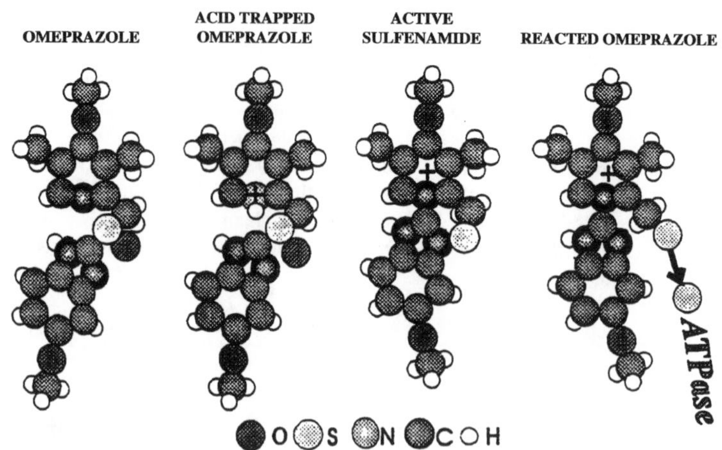

Acid-catalyzed activation of omeprazole resulting in its covalent binding to an available cysteine in H^+, K^+-ATPase.

hydrase catalyzes the formation of HCO_3^- from CO_2 and the remaining OH^-. The HCO_3^-, in turn, is transported across the basolateral membrane in exchange for Cl^-. Thus, for every proton molecule secreted, a HCO_3^- molecule enters the capillaries, accounting for the **alkaline tide.** This ability of the activated parietal cell to increase locally the concentration of this buffer in its own immediate microenvironment may also serve to protect the cell from the damaging effects of protons that back-diffuse into the tissue from the lumen.

26. What is the range that hydrochloric acid is secreted into the gastric juice?

- At low secretory rates: 10–20 mM
- At high secretory rates: 130–150 mM

27. What is the range of concentrations of remaining ions in the gastric juice?

- At low secretory rates: NaCl, 130–140 mM
- At high secretory rates: NaCl, 10–20 mM

28. What are the major physiologic regulators of gastric acid secretion?

The three major stimulants of gastric acid secretion are **gastrin, histamine,** and **acetylcholine.** The parietal cells are known to be innervated by both intrinsic and extrinsic nerves of the parasympathetic nervous system. **Acetylcholine** released from the nerve terminals binds to muscarinic (M_3) receptors and activates the cell through the IP_3-Ca^{++} pathway. **Histamine** has been demonstrated to act on specific H_2 receptors of the parietal cell, which then activate adenylate cyclase through a G-protein linking mechanism. The resultant increase in cytoplasmic cAMP results in the activation of protein kinase A and the phosphorylation of proteins that regulate the opening of Cl^- ion channels in the canalicular membrane. The two major cells that have been demonstrated to synthesize and release histamine are the mast cells and the **ECL cells** of the oxyntic mucosa. **Gastrin** is the major endocrine stimulant of the parietal cell. Gastrin is synthesized, stored, and secreted by the G cells of the antral mucosa. The activity of this endocrine cell is regulated by luminal/dietary nutrients, nerves, and paracrine factors. The major luminal stimulatory factors are peptides, amino acids, and amines, with luminal acid being a potent physiologic inhibitor of hormone release. The threshold for this inhibitory effect of acid on gastrin release is a pH of 3.0, and it becomes maximal at pH values between 2.0 and 2.5. The G cell is also activated by cholinergic and noncholinergic fibers of the parasympathetic nervous system. The mediator of the noncholinergic fibers is **GRP,** which is structurally similar to the frog peptide bombesin. Finally, gastrin release from the G cell can be inhibited by somatostatin released from neighboring D cells. This paracrine form of regulation may play a role in both the ability of luminal acid to inhibit gastrin release, as somatostatin release is stimulated by luminal acid, and the ability of the parasympathetic nervous system to stimulate gastrin release, because cholinergic agonists inhibit somatostatin release from the D cell.

29. In what way is gastrin unique as a stimulant of gastric acid secretion?

Gastrin appears to stimulate the parietal cell by both a **direct** and an **indirect pathway.** Directly, gastrin has been demonstrated to bind to a receptor on the parietal cell, called the **CCK-B receptor,** inducing a G-protein mediated increase in IP_3 and cytosolic calcium and the phosphorylation of key proteins involved in the morphologic transformation of the parietal cell. (Acetylcholine is also thought to activate the cell in a similar manner.) Indirectly, gastrin and acetylcholine stimulate the local release of histamine from neighboring ECL cells, which act in a paracrine manner to stimulate the parietal cell by a process mediated by cAMP.

30. In what way is histamine of clinical importance as a physiologic stimulant of gastric acid secretion?

H_2-receptor antagonists (cimetidine [Tagamet], ranitidine [Zantac], nizatidine [Axid], and famotidine [Pepcid]) are highly effective in reducing gastric acid secretion and promoting ulcer healing in humans.

31. What are the major phases of gastric secretion?

- Cephalic: 20–30% of the acid secretory response to a meal
- Gastric: 60–70% of the acid secretory response to a meal
- Intestinal: approximately 10% of the acid secretory response to a meal

32. How are the phases of gastric secretion regulated?

The **cephalic phase** is activated by the ingestion of a meal (before its entry into the stomach) or even merely the contemplation of an appetizing meal. It is primarily regulated by long vagal fibers traveling from the central nervous system, which, in turn, innervate either the parietal cell or the G cell. The second phase is initiated when the food bolus enters the stomach.

The **gastric phase** is dependent on neural, chemical, and endocrine regulation of parietal cell activity. Both long (vagovagal) and short (intrinsic) neural pathways have been identified that either act directly on the parietal cell or affect its activity by altering the release of gastrin or somatostatin. In addition, noncholinergic fibers have been demonstrated to stimulate the release of GRP. Evidence exists that distention of the body or antrum can activate a number of these neural pathways to stimulate both gastrin release and gastric acid secretion. Dietary factors (peptides, amino acids, and amines) also stimulate gastrin release from the G cell during the gastric phase of secretion. Gastrin release as a result of chemical nutrients or parasympathetic stimulation can be abruptly inhibited by acidification of the antrum to $pH < 3.0$, by a mechanism that is mediated, in part, by the paracrine inhibitory actions of somatostatin. The third phase of gastric acid secretion occurs when the food empties into the small intestine.

The **intestinal phase** is partly due to the release of gastrin from the proximal duodenum as approximately 30% of the gastrin is present in the proximal small intestine. There is also some evidence that distention of the proximal duodenum can stimulate gastric acid secretion by an undefined mechanism and that amino acids that are absorbed by the small intestinal mucosa travel by way of the systemic circulation to stimulate the parietal cells directly by interacting with receptors on the cell's basolateral membrane. Gastric acid secretion is inhibited as the food bolus continues to move into the small intestine; this may be attributable to the withdrawal of gastric stimulants and the release of intestinal hormones into the circulation (secretin, CCK, enteroglucagon, GIP, PYY, and neurotensin), also called enterogastrones, that have documented ability to inhibit gastric acid secretion.

33. What are the unique chemical characteristics of gastrin?

The molecule is processed as it moves through the endoplasmic reticulum–Golgi network; processing continues as it is stored in the secretory granule. The major biologically active forms of the hormone are a 17-amino acid peptide (G-17) and a 34-amino acid peptide (G-34) that can either be sulfated (G-17II, G-34II) or not (G-171, G-341). These molecules share an active site of four amino acids on the C-terminus of the molecule that possesses all the activity of the larger molecules (see figure). It is critical, however, that the phenylalanine molecule at the C-terminus be amidated to prevent exopeptidases from degrading the molecule.

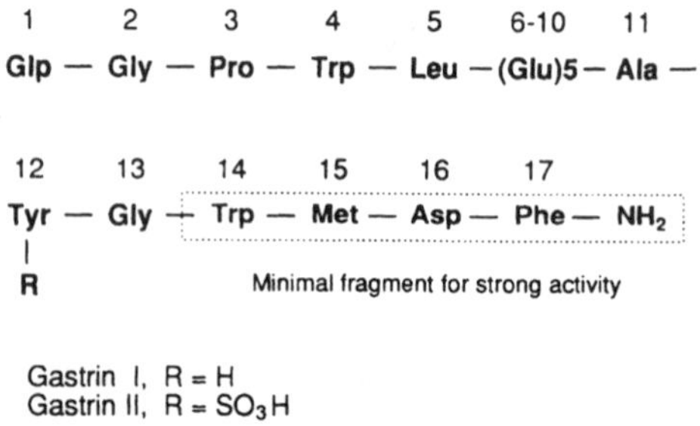

1 2 3 4 5 6-10 11
Glp — Gly — Pro — Trp — Leu —(Glu)5— Ala —

12 13 14 15 16 17
Tyr — Gly — Trp — Met — Asp — Phe — NH_2
|
R

Minimal fragment for strong activity

Gastrin I, R = H
Gastrin II, R = SO_3H

Structure of human "little" gastrin (HG-17). (From Johnson LR: Essential Medical Physiology, 2nd ed. Philadelphia, Lippincott-Raven, 1997, with permission.)

34. Does gastrin share properties with other GI peptides?

Similar to many peptide hormones, gastrin constitutes a family of related peptides that are formed from a preprohormone. The same active site is also shared by the CCK family of peptides.

35. Describe the unique features of pepsin.

Pepsin is stored intracellularly as an inactive precursor molecule, **pepsinogen.** Pepsinogen represents a family of closely related isozymes that have been divided into two classes. Group I pepsinogens are found in the chief cell and in the mucous cell of the oxyntic mucosa, whereas group II pepsinogens are present in the antral mucosa and the submucosal Brunner's glands of the proximal duodenum. The pepsin isozymes are unique in that their pH optima fall within the acidic range, and depending on the isozyme, the pH optimum occurs between pH values of 1.5 and 5.0. Pepsin is an endopeptidase that cleaves peptide bonds between two hydrophobic amino acids. Although not essential for life, pepsin plays a fundamentally important role in initiating the breakdown of dietary proteins in the stomach.

36. How are the activity and secretion of pepsin regulated?

Pepsinogen is secreted into the gastric lumen in response to vagal stimulation and the presence of acid in the gastric lumen. At acidic pH, pepsinogen is converted to the active molecule, pepsin. At neutral pH, pepsin is denatured and devoid of activity.

37. Is the secretion of intrinsic factor physiologically regulated?

Yes. In humans, intrinsic factor is synthesized by parietal cells, and its release into the gastric lumen is under the same control as is gastric acid secretion, being stimulated by cholinergic agonists, histamine, and gastrin.

38. What are the major chemical constituents of gastric mucus?

The major chemical constituent of gastric mucus is mucus glycoprotein. Phospholipids, sphingolipids, and glyceroglucolipids are synthesized and secreted by gastric mucous cells and contribute to both the structure and the properties of mucus.

39. How are the chemical constituents organized?

Mucus glycoprotein is a heavily glycosylated polymeric protein having a molecular weight of approximately $2–10 \times 10^6$. It is composed of glycosylated subunits of smaller size (molecular weight $= 0.07–0.5 \times 10^6$) that polymerize to form the parent molecule. Glycoproteins, phospholipids, sphingolipids, and glyceroglucolipids interact with each other and luminal acid to promote the formation of a hydrophobic and viscous mucus gel that coats the surface of the gastric mucosa.

40. What are the major physiologic functions of gastric mucus?

1. Mucus plays a fundamentally important role as a boundary lubricant for both the GI mucosa and the food bolus traveling down the GI tract, to minimize frictional forces and tissue injury.

2. Mucus appears to play a fundamentally important role in protecting the gastric mucosa against the corrosive actions of the acidic and proteolytic properties of gastric juice by

- Trapping HCO_3^- ions released into the luminal space and thereby generating a pH gradient between the luminal bulk solution and the gastric epithelium
- Creating a hydrophobic interfacial layer to repel the movement of acidic gastric fluid from back-diffusing into the tissue

41. How is gastric mucus secretion physiologically regulated?

Mucus secretion is stimulated by both **parasympathetic stimulation** and by **chemical/mechanical irritation.** The former mechanism primarily stimulates soluble mucus secretion from mucus neck cells, whereas the latter stimulates the gel-forming mucus from surface mucous cells. Chemical and mechanical–induced mucus secretion may, in part, be mediated by the generation of **prostaglandins,** which are known both to stimulate mucus secretion and to protect the tissue from injurious factors in the lumen. Prostaglandin biosynthesis is regulated by two major enzymes: **phospholipase A_2 (PLA_2),** which generates arachidonic acid from the breakdown of membrane phospholipids, **cyclooxygenase (COX),** which subsequently converts arachidonic acid to the active prostaglandins. The ability of **nonsteroidal anti-inflammatory drugs (NSAIDs)** to inhibit the COX enzymes of the gastroduodenal mucosa, and in turn the generation of prostaglandins, is thought to be in part responsible for these drugs' ulcerogenic activity. Mucus can be released as a consequence of **exocytosis** (individual mucus granules being discharged), **compound exocytosis** (multiple mucus granules being discharged), **apical expulsion** (the entire mucus granule package being discharged), or the **exfoliation** of the mucus cell into the gastric lumen.

42. What are the major causative factors in duodenal ulcer disease?

- Infection with the gram-negative bacteria ***Helicobacter pylori***
- Consumption of **NSAIDs**

43. Explain the pathophysiologic mechanisms involved in duodenal ulcer disease.

Evidence suggests that greater than 90% of duodenal ulcer patients are infected with ***H. pylori.*** The bacteria most often colonize the mucus gel layer of the gastric antrum and induce a chronic active gastritis associated with increased gastric acid secretion and circulating gastrin levels. In addition to an increase in gastric aggressive factors and inflammatory cells and mediators, there also appears to be a weakening of the barrier properties of the gastroduodenal mucosa, with an attenuation in the thickness and hydrophobic properties of the mucus gel layer and a decrease in bicarbonate secretion. As a consequence of our understanding of the etiologic role of the bacteria, duodenal ulcer patients are presently effectively treated with a combination of antibiotics. **NSAID consumption** has been linked to approximately 60% of gastric ulcer patients. These drugs are being consumed at ever-increasing rates by our populace not only to treat chronic inflammatory diseases (e.g., arthritis), fever, pain, and inflammation, but also to prevent heart disease, stroke, and colon cancer. NSAIDs are thought to induce gastric injury by a direct topical injurious action and by inhibiting COX, the rate-limiting enzyme in the biosynthesis of gastroprotective prostaglandins.

44. How is *H. pylori*–induced duodenal ulcer treated?

With a combination of antibiotics together with either a proton pump inhibitor (e.g. omeprazole [Prilosec]) or a bismuth compound (e.g., bismuth subsalicylate [Pepto-Bismol], ranitidine bismuth citrate [Tritec]).

45. What are the physiologic functions of pancreatic juice?

Pancreatic juice contains essential enzymes to catalyze the breakdown of dietary carbohydrates, lipids, and proteins to basic molecular units (monosaccharides and disaccharides, monoglycerides, fatty acids, amino acids, and dipeptides and tripeptides) that can be readily absorbed by the small intestine by either active or passive transport mechanisms. Without these enzymes, proper nutrition would not be maintained, and malnutrition and death would ensue. For this reason, patients with pancreatic insufficiency are prescribed pancreatic enzyme supplements to be taken with their meals. Pancreatic HCO_3^- also plays an essential role in humans to neutralize acidic gastric fluid that empties into the proximal duodenum. This is important, first to promote the digestion of the dietary nutrients by pancreatic and intestinal enzymes whose pH optima range between pH 7 and 8, and second to prevent the formation of intestinal ulcers because the intestinal mucosa, in contrast with the gastric mucosa, is not provided with a strong barrier to luminal acid. The role of pancreatic HCO_3^- in these physiologic processes can be appreciated in individuals who secrete an abnormally high concentration of gastric hydrochloric acid, owing to the presence of a gastrin-producing tumor, referred to as **Zollinger-Ellison syndrome.** In this pathologic state, pancreatic HCO_3^- no longer can neutralize all the gastric acid being emptied into the small intestine, and these patients suffer from steatorrhea (lipid malabsorption) and intestinal ulceration that can extend down to the jejunum.

46. Describe the functional anatomy of the pancreatic exocrine secretory unit.

The functional exocrine secretory unit is composed of an acinus lined by **zymogen-containing acinar cells** that drain into a pancreatic ductule. These cells, which represent approximately 80% of pancreatic tissue, synthesize and secrete the full complement of pancreatic enzymes (which are packaged within zymogen granules) along with electrolytes, which are thought to be primarily NaCl and some $NaHCO_3$. The cells localized at the mouth to the duct are called the **centroacinar cells,** and those lining the ductules are called the **duct cells** (see figure). The major function of these two cell types (centroacinar and duct cells), which represent approximately 5% of the pancreatic tissue, is to secrete $NaHCO_3$. In addition, the pancreas contains a small amount of endocrine tissue (approximately 2% of the pancreatic mass), referred to as the islets of Langerhans, that is made up of insulin-, glucagon-, and somatostatin-containing endocrine cells. The pancreatic **islets of Langerhans** play a vital role in the regulation of carbohydrate metabolism. If this tissue becomes compromised due to disease or surgery, **diabetes mellitus** will ensue.

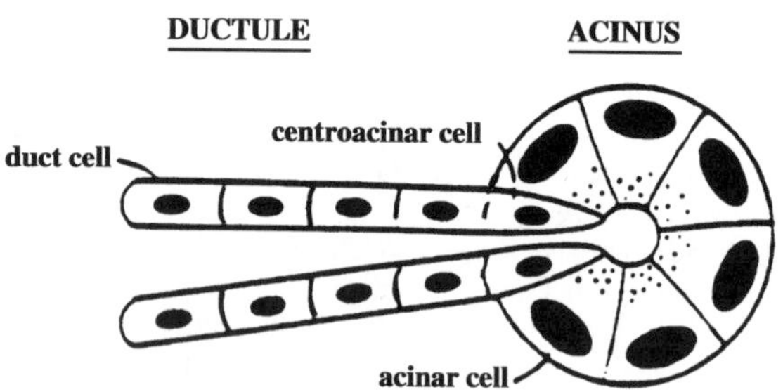

47. Describe the mechanism by which the pancreatic exocrine tissue secretes $NaHCO_3$.

The major cellular elements present in the duct and centroacinar cells that are required for pancreatic HCO_3^- secretion are depicted in the accompanying figure. These cells possess the ubiquitous Na^+, K^+-ATPase at their basolateral membrane, which drives the pumping of three Na^+ molecules out of the cell in exchange for two K^+ molecules. This creates an electrochemical driving force that promotes the diffusion of Na^+ into the cell. The presence of a Na^+-H^+ exchanger, also along the basolateral membrane, results in the pumping of intracellular protons into the interstitium by a secondary active transport process, as Na^+ molecules enter the cell. The remaining OH^- ions are then condensed with CO_2 by a reaction catalyzed by **carbonic anhydrase** to produce HCO_3^-, which is then actively transported (secondary active transport) across the luminal membrane in exchange for Cl^-. There is evidence for the presence of **Cl^- channels** in the luminal membrane that can be activated by cAMP, a second messenger that can be generated by peptides in the secretin family. This initial flux of the anion out of the cell sets up the driving force required for the exchange pump and the movement of HCO_3^- into the lumen of the pancreatic duct. Na^+ molecules enter the ductule lumen (primarily across the paracellular space) to associate with HCO_3^- to maintain electroneutrality. Water molecules also enter the pancreatic lumen as a result of osmotic forces generated by the secreted $NaHCO_3$.

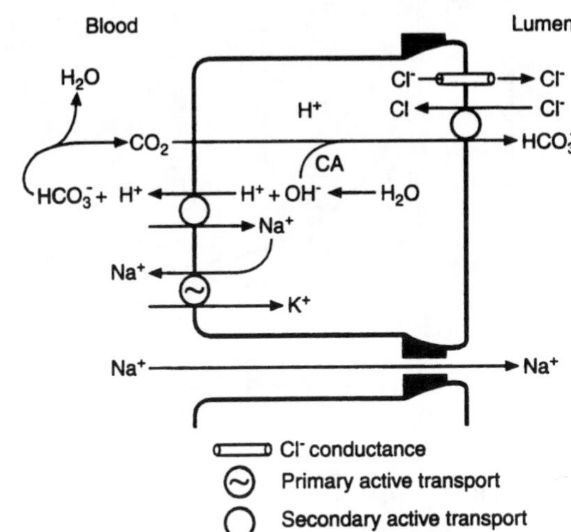

Cellular processes that best account for the secretion of HCO_3^- by the pancreatic ductule cells.

48. How does the electrolyte concentration of pancreatic juice vary with secretory rate?

The $NaHCO_3$ concentration increases toward isotonicity (reaching a maximal value at approximately 120 mEq) at high secretory rates (see figure, top of next page). As the secretory rate decreases, the NaCl concentration increases at the expenses of the buffer. The reciprocal relationship between the two anions can best be explained by the presence of Cl^--HCO_3^- exchanger in the luminal membrane of centroacinar and duct cells, which remodels pancreatic juice as it moves down the duct system. Thus, at slow secretory rates, luminal HCO_3^- is exchanged for Cl^-. This exchange process would be limited at more rapid secretory rates.

49. What is the two-component hypothesis?

Another possible explanation for the reciprocal relationship between these two ions comes from the two-component hypothesis, which postulates that at low secretory rates, NaCl is predominantly secreted by one cell type (e.g., acinar cells), whereas during stimulation with an agent, such as the peptide hormone secretin, the duct and centroacinar cells secrete a fluid enriched in $NaHCO_3$.

50. How does pancreatic juice compare in tonicity with salivary secretion and gastric secretion?

In contrast with salivary secretion and similar to gastric secretion, pancreatic juice is isotonic at all rates of secretion.

51. What are the major phases of pancreatic secretion?

- Cephalic—approximately 20% of the pancreatic secretory response to a meal
- Gastric—5–10% of the pancreatic secretory response to a meal
- Intestinal—approximately 80% of the pancreatic secretory response to a meal

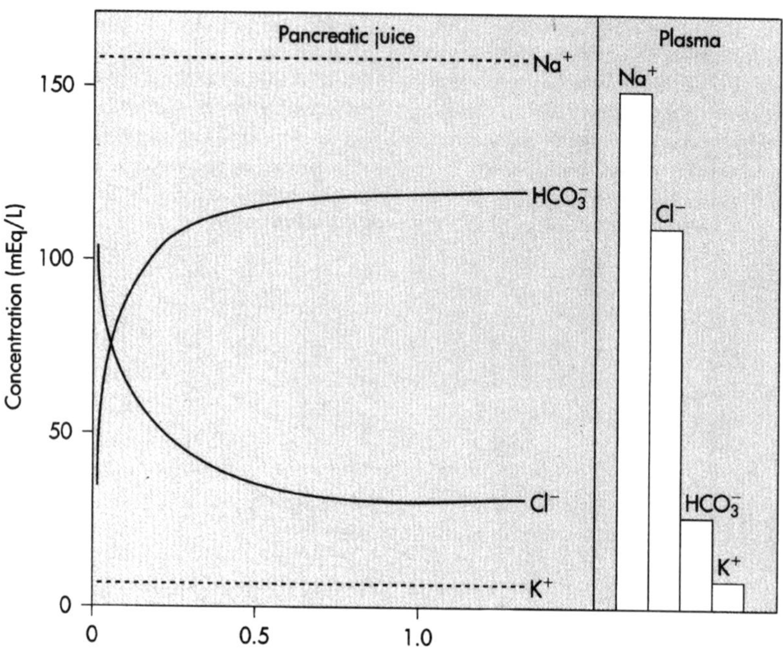

Relationship between the rate of secretion of pancreatic juice and the concentrations of its major ions. (From Johnson LR: Gastrointestinal Physiology, 4th ed. St. Louis, Mosby, 1991, with permission.)

52. How is pancreatic exocrine secretion regulated during the cephalic, gastric, and intestinal phases of digestion?

Similar to gastric secretion, pancreatic secretion is under the dual regulation of nerves from the autonomic nervous system and GI hormones, whose contribution to the response varies with the location of the ingested food and timing of the meal. The pancreas secretes an enzyme-rich, low-volume fluid during the **cephalic phase** of a meal. This is primarily due to the central activation of vagal efferents that innervate and stimulate the pancreatic acinar cells. The neuromediator is acetylcholine, which binds to and activates muscarinic receptors of the acinar cells and through the IP_3-Ca^{++} signal transduction system induces the exocytosis of zymogen granules. In addition to enzyme output, there is a small increase in pancreatic juice volume and $NaHCO_3$ concentration. Because gastrin and CCK share the same active site, there is a possibility that some of the enzyme secretory response may be attributable to the release of gastrin into circulation during the cephalic phase.

Pancreatic secretion continues as the food bolus enters the stomach during the **gastric phase** of digestion. This again is primarily a low-volume, enzyme-rich fluid that is thought to be mediated by cholinergic fibers, which are activated by a gastropancreatic reflex arc that is stimulated by gastric distention. The role of gastrin as a humoral mediator of pancreatic secretion has not been proven in humans.

The **intestinal phase** represents the major component of the pancreatic secretory response. During this phase, $NaHCO_3$, protein (pancreatic enzymes), and volume are all markedly increased. The major mediators of this response are the GI hormones, secretin and CCK, with cholinergic nerves playing an important permissive role. The exocrine pancreas is innervated by vagal fibers, and it is known that both pancreatic enzyme and bicarbonate output are markedly diminished by the administration of muscarinic antagonists (atropine) or after section of the vagus nerve.

53. Discuss the role of the hormone secretin in the intestinal phase of pancreatic secretion.

Secretin is secreted into the blood by the S cell of the duodenum. The major stimulant of secretin release is an acidic pH in the duodenum, with a pH of 4.5 being the threshold for S cell activation and maximal secretin release being achieved at pH ≤ 3.0 (see figure). It is thought that as the pH decreases below the threshold value, increasingly longer lengths of duodenum become acidified, resulting in the activation of increasing numbers of secretin-containing S cells. Secretin has been reported to bind to a specific class of receptors on duct, centroacinar, and acinar cells to activate adenylate cyclase through a G-protein heterodimer complex. The resultant increase in cAMP then activates the cell, by a mechanism yet to be defined but that appears to be related to the phosphorylation of a number of proteins, one of which affects the open probability of Cl^- channels on the luminal membrane of these target cells. It has been demonstrated that the postprandial increase in pancreatic bicarbonate secretion and the rise in secretin levels in the blood can be effectively blocked if animals or humans are pretreated with an H_2-receptor antagonist to inhibit gastric acid secretion.

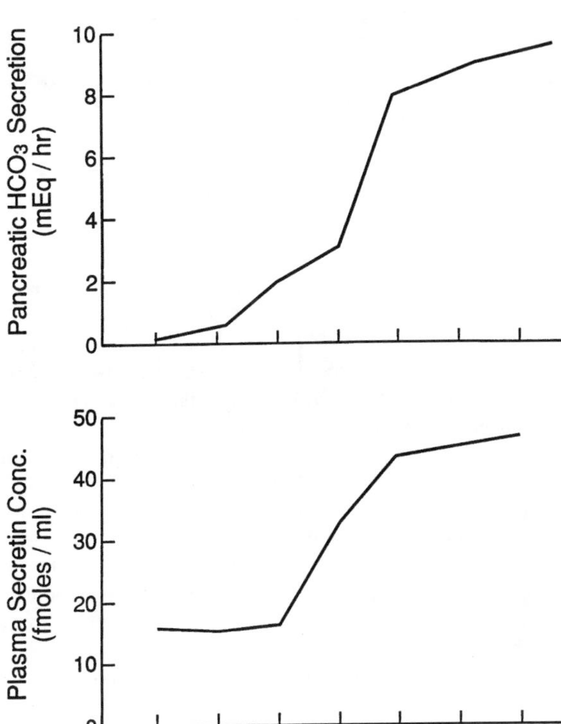

pH dependence of secretin-induced pancreatic bicarbonate secretion.

54. Discuss the role of CCK in the intestinal phase of pancreatic secretion.

The presence of proteins, lipids, or their breakdown products in the duodenum stimulates pancreatic enzyme secretion by a mechanism mediated by the peptide hormone CCK. This hormone, which is synthesized and released from the I cells of duodenum, has chemical homology to gastrin, sharing the active site at the C-terminus of the molecule. As depicted in the figure, the major difference in the two molecules resides in the fact that the tyrosyl group in CCK is located in the seventh position from the C-terminus (as compared with being in the sixth position from the C-terminus in gastrin) and that for the molecule to possess CCK-like activity, it is imperative for this amino acid to be sulfated. On stimulation with hydrolytic products of the digestion of dietary proteins (certain amino acids and dipeptides) and fats (fatty acids having > 8 carbons in length), CCK is released into the blood and travels to the exocrine pancreas, where it binds to CCK-A receptors on acinar, centroacinar, and duct cells to activate secretion through an IP_3-Ca^{++} signal transduction system. The major secretory response to CCK is the secretion of pancreatic enzymes, and its interaction with receptors on duct and centroacinar cells is primarily to potentiate the action of secretin to stimulate bicarbonate secretion.

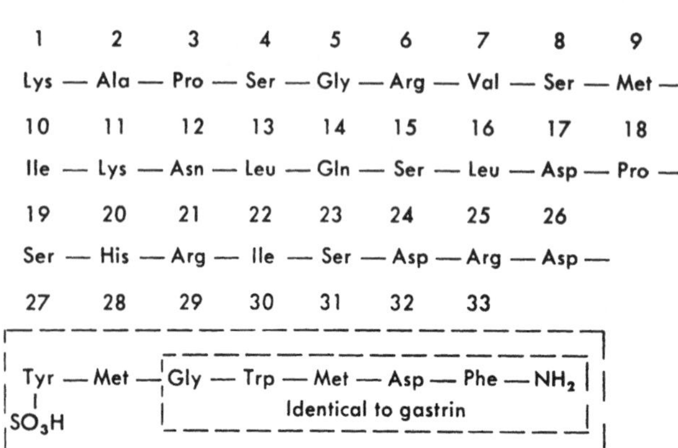

Porcine cholecystokinin. (From Johnson LR: Gastrointestinal Physiology, 4th ed. St. Louis, Mosby, 1991, with permission.)

55. Describe the physiologic importance of potentiative interaction of secretin, CCK, and acetylcholine on pancreatic secretion.

The evidence is clear that the secretory response of the exocrine pancreas to a specific stimulant is significantly increased if the two other secretagogues are also present. The physiologic importance of this potentiative interaction becomes particularly significant in the pancreatic bicarbonate response to intestinal acidification that is mediated by secretin. Because the pH of the proximal duodenum in humans reaches the threshold value for secretin release (pH approximately 4.5) only for short periods of time after a meal, resulting in the release of small quantities of secretin into the blood, it is important for the duct and centroacinar cells to be sensitized for activation by being simultaneously stimulated by CCK and acetylcholine. If the effects of either agent are blocked (by the administration of a CCK-A receptor antagonist or the muscarinic antagonist, atropine), the postprandial secretory response is markedly reduced. Similarly, it is possible that secretin and acetylcholine may sensitize the acinar cells to respond to CCK. The molecular basis for the potentiative interaction is that different stimulants (e.g., secretin and CCK or acetylcholine) act through different intracellular mediators, resulting in the phosphorylation of different proteins that are required for an optimal secretory response. Thus, if two agents act through different intracellular mediators, the response of administering the two simultaneously generally exceeds the additive response of the two agents alone. In contrast, if the two agents are acting through the same intracellular mediator (acetylcholine and CCK), the response is expected to be additive if the two agents are simultaneously administered at a submaximal concentration.

56. What are the physiologic inhibitors of pancreatic secretion?

Both **pancreatic bicarbonate** and **enzyme secretion** are self-limited because the stimulants for CCK release (amino acids, peptides, fatty acids) or secretin release (duodenal acidity) are removed by the end organ response (e.g., secretion of proteolytic and lipolytic enzymes and bicarbonate). In addition, the pancreatic enzyme **trypsin** appears to be a potent inhibitor of CCK release, perhaps by breaking down a GRP-like peptide in the GI lumen that serves as a paracrine (local) stimulant of CCK secretion.

57. What GI hormones affect insulin release from the endocrine tissue of the pancreas?

- Glucose-dependent insulinotropic peptide (GIP)
- Glucagonlike peptide (GLP)

It has been postulated that glucose stimulates the release of an intestinal hormone called an **incretin** that enters the blood and activates the insulin-containing β-cells of the pancreas. Present evidence strongly indicates that GIP and GLP have this property because the release of both peptides is stimulated by glucose in the intestinal lumen, and both have the capacity to stimulate insulin release. Because the evidence is somewhat stronger for GIP, it is considered a physiologically important hormone by many investigators.

58. Describe the major physiologic functions of bile.

Bile plays an essential role in the digestion and absorption of **dietary lipids.** It accomplishes this by initially emulsifying dietary lipids into colloidal particles that can be readily acted on by pancreatic lipase/colipase. Second, bile salts form colloidal aggregates called **micelles** and **mixed micelles,** which serve to facilitate the intestinal absorption of the products of lipid digestion (**free fatty acids** and **2β-monoglycerides**) and lipid-soluble vitamins. Bile also plays an important role in the excretion of **cholesterol** and its derivatives, **bile pigments (bilirubin),** and other toxic chemicals present in the circulation that are not readily filtered by the kidney.

59. Describe the features of the hepatic exocrine tissue that serve in its function to synthesize, secrete, and remodel bile.

Similar to the situation in the salivary gland and pancreas, the **hepatic parenchymal cells** (also called **hepatocytes**) are situated along a blinded end of a tube, called a **canaliculus,** which drains into a ductule, then into ducts of increasing larger diameter, and finally out into the common bile duct, which empties into the proximal duodenum. The hepatic parenchymal cells secrete both electrolytes and organic material (bile salts and pigments) into the canaliculus, either across the canalicular membrane or by paracellular route. **Ductule cells** (also called **cholangiocytes**) also secrete electrolytes (primarily $NaHCO_3$) and remodel its composition. Between meals, the sphincter of Oddi, a cuff of smooth muscle positioned where the common bile duct drains into the duodenum, is closed, and bile flows in a retrograde direction up the cystic duct and into the gall bladder, where it is stored and concentrated (see figure). During meals, the gallbladder forcefully contracts and the sphincter of Oddi relaxes, propelling bile into the duodenum.

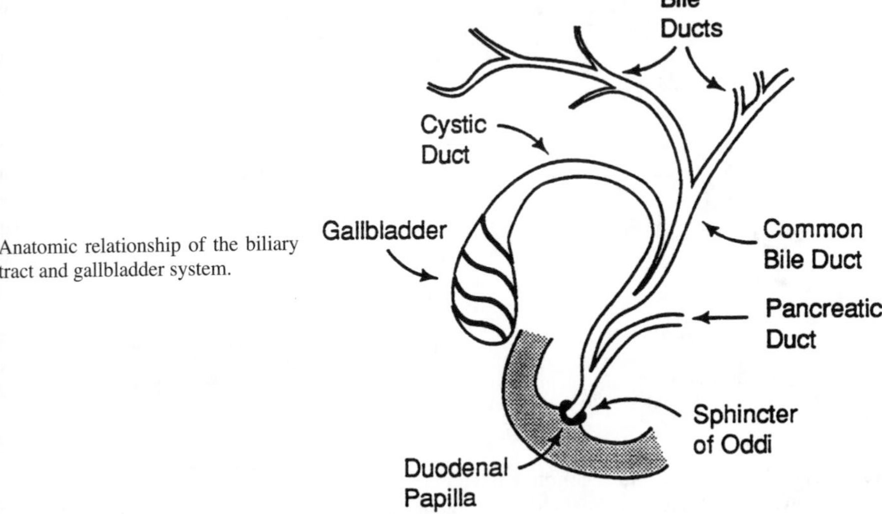

Anatomic relationship of the biliary tract and gallbladder system.

60. What two major blood vessels bring blood to the hepatic exocrine tissue?

The **portal vein** and the **hepatic artery.** Blood leaves these major vessels and perfuses the exocrine tissue through hepatic sinusoids, highly permeable channels that are in direct contact with the basolateral membrane of hepatic parenchymal cells (see figure). The blood flow through the sinusoidal space runs in the opposite direction (counterflow) to that of the canalicular fluid which drains into the hepatic duct system. This organization promotes the uptake of bile salts returning to the liver via the portal blood by the hepatic exocrine tissue and its resecretion across the canalicular membrane into the bile.

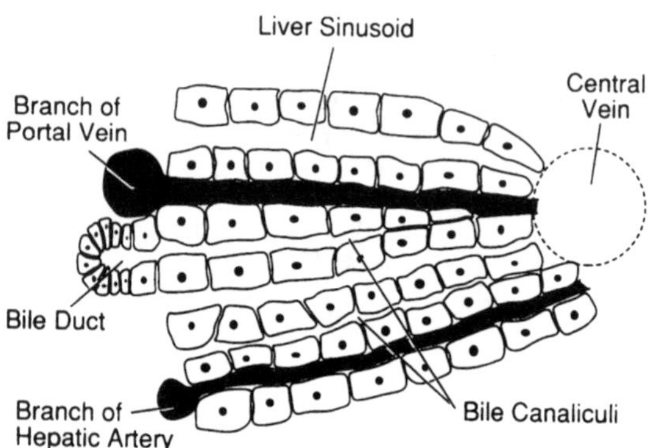

Schematic diagram of the relationship between blood vessels, hepatocytes, and bile canaliculi in the liver. Each hepatocyte is exposed to blood at one membrane surface and a bile canaliculus at the other. (From Johnson LR: Essential Medical Physiology, 2nd ed. Philadelphia, Lippincott-Raven, 1997, with permission.)

61. What are bile acids?

Bile acids constitute approximately 50% of the organic material of bile. Bile acids are formed as a consequence of the breakdown of cholesterol, with the rate-limiting enzyme being **7α-hydroxylase,** also called **cholesterol 7α-hydroxylase (CYP7A)** (see figure).

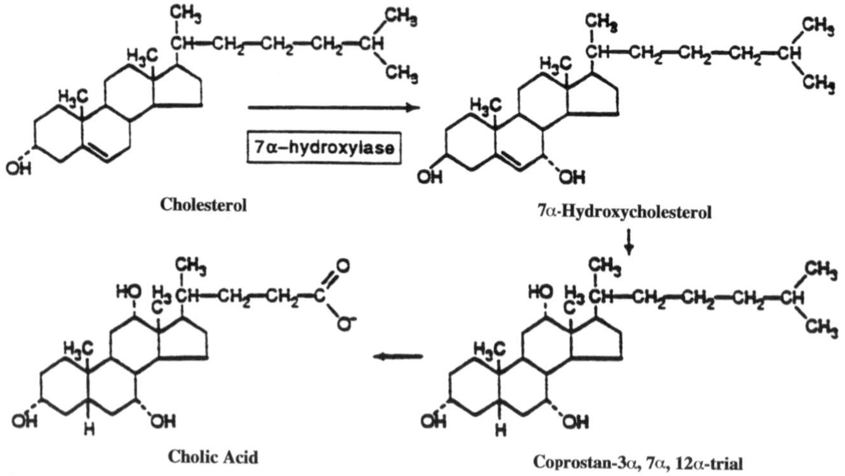

7α–hydroxylase

Cholesterol

7α-Hydroxycholesterol

Cholic Acid

Coprostan-3α, 7α, 12α-trial

Formation of bile acids from cholesterol in the liver. The 7α-hydroxylation step, which appears to be rate limiting, is inhibited by bile acids that have been taken up by the hepatocyte from the portal blood.

62. Define the primary and secondary bile acids.

The two major bile acids synthesized in humans by hepatic exocrine tissue are **cholic** and **chenodeoxycholic acid** (see figure). These are the **primary bile acids.** Both molecules possess a sterol nucleus, which is hydroxylated in the 3 and 7 position (dihydroxylated = **chenodeoxycholic acid**) or 3, 7, and 12 positions (trihydroxylated = **cholic acid**). When the primary bile acids enter the small intestine, they may be dehydroxylated in the 7 position to either **deoxycholic acid** or **lithocholic acid,** by intestinal flora. These molecules, which are the **secondary bile acids,** along with the primary bile acids, can be reabsorbed by the enterohepatic circulatory system and resecreted back into the bile. At any one time, bile contains a mixture of primary and secondary bile acids and trace amounts of chemical modifications of the four molecules.

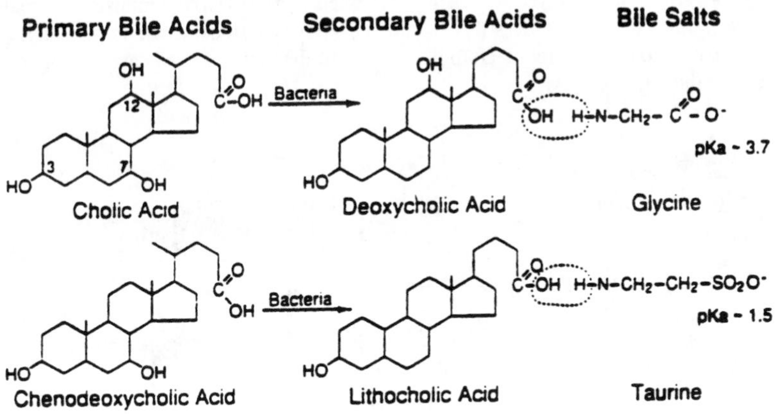

Principal organic constituents of bile. The two primary bile acids may be converted to secondary bile acids in the intestine. Each of the four bile acids may be conjugated to either glycine or taurine to form bile salts. (From Johnson LR: Essential Medical Physiology, 2nd ed. Philadelphia, Lippincott-Raven, 1997, with permission.)

63. What are the ratios of these four molecules in human bile?

4 cholic acid:2 chenodeoxycholic acid:1 deoxycholic acid:trace amounts of lithocholic acid.

64. What are the solubility characteristics of bile acids?

The aqueous solubility of bile acids depends, in part, on their state of hydroxylation, with the trihydroxylated bile acid, **cholic acid,** having the greatest solubility, and the monohydroxylated secondary bile acid, **lithocholic acid,** having the lowest solubility in water. All bile acids, as the name implies, possess a branched side-chain ending in a carboxyl group. The pKa of this carboxyl group can vary between 5 and 7, depending on the bile acid, meaning that, unless modified, greater than 50% of the molecules would be in the undissociated, lipid-soluble state under the mildly acidic pH of the proximal duodenum. This would result in their precipitation.

65. How does the body modify the bile acids to enhance their solubility in the biliary tract and prevent precipitation?

To prevent precipitation from occurring, the hepatic parenchymal cell conjugates the primary and secondary bile acids to either **glycine** or **taurine,** which results in a decrease of the pKa to 3.7 (glycodeoxycholic acid) and 1.5 (taurodeoxycholic acid). This **conjugation step** thus ensures that these molecules are ionized at all the pHs encountered within the biliary tract and intestinal lumen. Because these molecules are negatively charged and ionically associated with cations, mostly Na^+, they are accurately called **bile salts.**

66. What is the difference between bile acids and bile salts?

A **bile acid** represents the undissociated molecule, which has a low water solubility. Conjugation of the molecule with glycine or taurine molecules ensures that the molecule is in an ionized water-soluble state within the biliary and GI tract system, which electrostatically associates, mostly with Na^+, as a **bile salt.** Conjugated bile salts are the predominant molecular species within the biliary and GI tract.

67. How does the chemical structure of bile salts contribute to their amphipathic properties?

Three-dimensional analysis of bile salts reveals that the OH^-, SO_2O^-, and COO^- groups are oriented along one plane of the molecule and the hydrocarbon chain on another (see figure). This allows the molecule to orient at oil–water interfaces (with the charged groups facing the water) lowering the interfacial surface tension forces. When this occurs in the GI tract, the presence of bile salts converts dietary triglycerides from oil droplets to a stable microemulsion of smaller particles, possessing a diameter of less than 1 mm. This physical transformation also facilitates the ability of lipase and colipase to attach to the surface of the emulsion and catalyze the hydrolysis of dietary triglycerides.

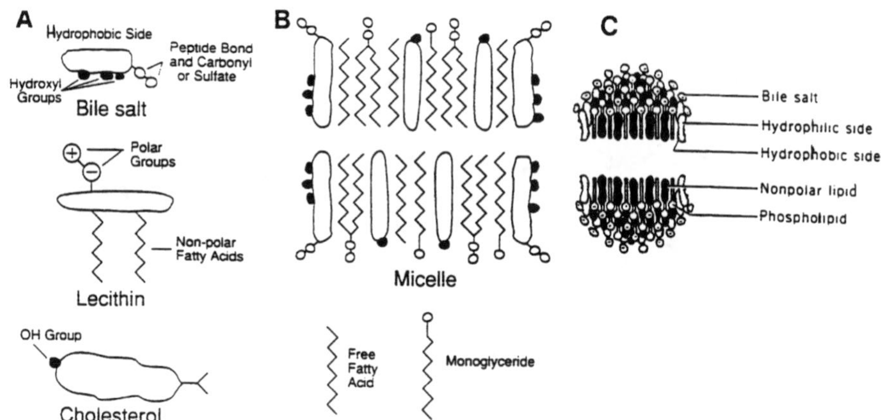

Structures of components of micelles and micelles themselves. *A,* Representations of bile salt, lecithin, and cholesterol molecules, illustrating the separation of polar and nonpolar surfaces. *B,* Cross-section of a micelle, showing the arrangement of these molecules plus the principal products of fat digestion. *C,* Micelles are cylindrical disks whose outer curved surfaces are composed of bile salts. (From Johnson LR: Essential Medical Physiology, 2nd ed. Philadelphia, Lippincott-Raven, 1997, with permission.)

68. What are the other organic constituents of bile?

1. **Phosphatidylcholine** is present in bile in high concentration and represents approximately 40% of the organic constituents of bile. Similar to bile salts, phosphatidylcholine has clear amphipathic properties, with the phosphorylcholine head group orienting into the water phase and diacyl glycerol having clear hydrophobic properties. The physiologic function of biliary phosphatidylcholine has yet to be resolved but may be to increase the aqueous solubility or dispersibility of bile salts and the other organic constituent, cholesterol, within the biliary tract system and to detoxify the detergent actions of bile salts, which can otherwise readily solubilize or disrupt cellular membranes.

2. Another constituent of bile is **cholesterol,** which represents approximately 4% of its organic material. Increasing the sterol concentration much beyond this value may result in the crystallization and precipitation of cholesterol as gallstones. Bile represents the principal fluid by which the body disposes this atherogenic sterol either as free cholesterol or as a bile acid derivative. Bile pigments, which are tetrapyrrolic products of the breakdown of hemoglobin by the reticuloendothelial system, are excreted into the bile.

3. **Bilirubin** is the major bile pigment, formed by the reticuloendothelial system. It travels in the blood in association with albumen, taken up by the hepatic parenchymal cells by special anion transporters on the basolateral membrane, conjugated intracellularly to glucuronic acid, and secreted into the bile as **bilirubin glucuronide** (see figure, top of next page).

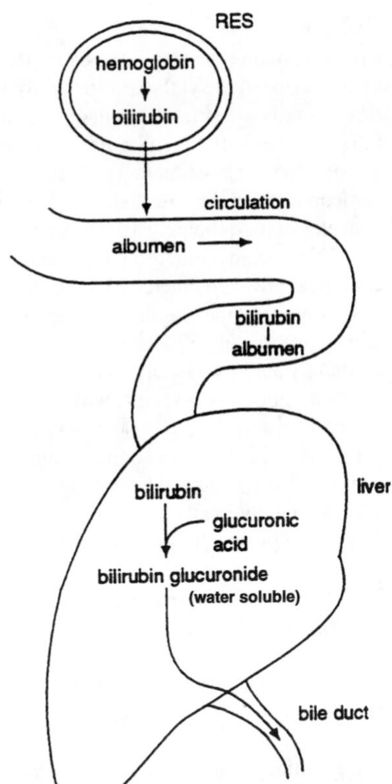

Transport of bilirubin from the reticuloendothelial system (RES) into bile.

69. What are micelles?

Bile salts have the capacity to self-aggregate to form macromolecular structures, called **micelles.** These macromolecules, which are schematically depicted in the figure in question 67, orient in such a fashion that the hydrophilic plane of the molecule faces the outside aqueous solution, whereas the hydrophobic molecular regions are inwardly directed toward the core of the macromolecule. These macromolecules, which generally possess a diameter of less than 100 Å, often take the shape of cylinders or spheres and do not contain an aqueous lumen (in contrast with vesicles).

70. How are micelles formed?

Bile salts form micelles only when they are present at or above a certain concentration, referred to as the **critical micellar concentration** (CMC), which, depending on the bile salt, can vary from 0.5 to 5 mM. Biliary phosphatidylcholine and cholesterol are readily incorporated into micelles to form **mixed micelles,** and these amphipathic molecules orient accordingly so that their hydrophilic groups are on the surface of the mixed micelles and their hydrophobic groups are facing inward.

71. What is the physiologic function of micelles?

To serve as a vehicle to take up the products of triglyceride metabolism (long-chain fatty acids and 2β-monoglycerides, plus lipid-soluble vitamins) and promote their uptake across into the jejunal epithelium.

72. Describe the enterohepatic circulation of bile salts.

The small intestine has developed an efficient mechanism to reabsorb secreted bile salts, return them to the liver via the portal vein, and resecrete them back into the bile. It has been estimated that 95–98% of the 20–30 g of bile salts secreted daily enter the enterohepatic circulatory system and are returned to the liver. The returning bile salts, in turn, inhibit the rate-limiting enzyme in bile acid synthesis, 7α-hydroxylase (CYP7A), so that the hepatic exocrine tissue synthesizes only the small amount of bile salts that are excreted into the feces, which range between 0.6 and 1.2 g daily. Even so, this is not an insignificant amount of the total bile acid pool of 2–2.5 g. The apparent discrepancy between this figure and the 20–30 g of bile salts that are secreted per day comes from the fact that each bile salt may be secreted and reabsorbed several times during a meal, or approximately 10 times per day.

The intestinal mucosa has several mechanisms to reabsorb bile salts. Intestinal flora can deconjugate bile salts, thereby increasing their lipid solubility. These molecules are then absorbed passively along the length of the small bowel. The remaining conjugated bile salts, which constitute approximately 50% of the available molecules, are actively transported by a sodium coupled secondary active transport system present on the brush border membrane of the ileal mucosa. The returning bile salts associate with plasma albumen and return to the liver via the portal blood. A mechanism similar to that present in the ileal mucosa then transports the bile salts into the hepatic parenchymal cells (by a sodium–taurocholate cotransporter polypeptide [ntcp]) across the cell's sinusoidal membrane. The conjugated bile salt molecules returning from the intestine together with the newly synthesized and conjugated molecules are then secreted across the canalicular membrane by an ATP-dependent bile salt export pump (BSEP).

73. Do bile salts secreted into the canalicular lumen influence bile secretion?

Yes. Approximately 50% of bile flow is considered to be dependent on the biliary output of bile salts. This dependence is partly due to the ability of bile salts to draw water osmotically into the biliary tract system and their ability to activate ionic pumps/exchangers to promote the secretion of electrolytes and water.

74. Is biliary electrolyte secretion regulated by hormones?

Yes. The GI hormone secretin stimulates biliary HCO_3^- secretion by the hepatic ductule cells (cholangiocytes). This is considered to be a component of bile flow that is independent of bile acid output.

75. What is the function of the gallbladder epithelium?

The gallbladder epithelium actively transports Na^+, Cl^-, and HCO_3^- from the lumen into the tissue, which osmotically pulls water into the tissue. Although other species appear to possess a neutral carrier mechanism to transport these salts, in humans the process may be driven solely by an active transport of Na^+.

76. List the concentrations of the constituents of bile.

Approximate Values for Major Components of Liver and Gallbladder Bile

COMPONENT	LIVER BILE	GALLBLADDER BILE
Na^+ (mEq/L)	150	300
K^+ (mEq/L)	4.5	10
Ca^{++} (mEq/L)	4	20
Cl^- (mEq/L)	80	5
HCO_3^- (mEq/L)	25	12
Bile salts (mEq/L)	30	315
pH	7.4	6.5
Cholesterol (mg/100 mL)	110	600
Bilirubin (mg/100 mL)	100	1000

77. Explain how even though the concentration of electrolytes in liver or gallbladder bile exceeds isotonicity, both bile solutions are iso-osmolar to plasma.

This apparent paradox is explained by the fact that the cations that accumulate in gallbladder and liver bile at concentrations that exceed their levels in plasma are electrostatically associated with negatively charged (dissociated) bile acids, which are present as a micellar suspension. Because this colloidal suspension is not in true solution, it does not have osmotic activity.

78. Describe how bile acid output is physiologically regulated.

CCK is released from the I cells of the intestine in response to fatty acids having more than eight carbons as well as products of protein metabolism. CCK then travels in the blood to the gallbladder, where it stimulates the contractile activity of gallbladder smooth muscle. CCK also induces a relaxation of the sphincter of Oddi, promoting the movement of gallbladder bile into the small intestine. Vagal fibers innervating gallbladder smooth muscle are also important in this response, as the postprandial increase in gallbladder activity can be attenuated or blocked if these nerve fibers are severed or in the presence of cholinergic antagonists. Certain presynaptic vagal fibers that innervate gallbladder smooth muscle have been reported to have CCK-A receptors. These may activate an intramural cholinergic reflex due to elevations in circulating CCK levels that contributes to the gallbladder contractile response. (See figure.)

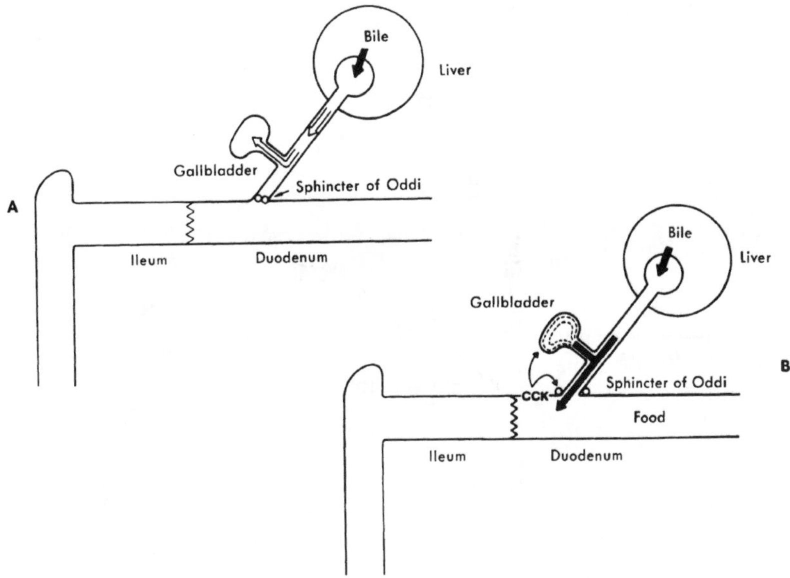

A, Bile flow between periods of digestion. Bile is secreted continuously by the liver and flows toward the duodenum. In the interdigestive period, the gallbladder is readily distensible, and the sphincter of Oddi is contracted. Therefore, bile flows into the gallbladder rather than into the duodenum. *B,* On eating, both hormonal (CCK) and neural stimuli cause contraction of the gallbladder and relaxation of the sphincter of Oddi. Thus, bile flows into the bowel. Bile secretion by the liver increases as bile acids are returned via the enterohepatic circulation. (From Johnson LR: Gastrointestinal Physiology, 4th ed. St. Louis, Mosby, 1991, with permission.)

79. What normally protects the hepatocyte from the injurious effects of bile salts, and when this fails, what are the signs of liver failure or cholestasis?

Increases in the intracellular concentration of bile salts will activate a number of feedback mechanisms to reduce the levels of this detergent-like molecule within the hepatocyte, including decreasing the activity and expression of CYP7A, the rate-limiting enzyme in bile acid biosynthesis, and decreasing the mRNA expression of ntcp and increasing the mRNA expression of the bsep, the principal influx and efflux transporters for bile salts, respectively. The accumulation of bile pigments in the blood is frequently associated with **cholestasis** or **liver failure.** The clearance from blood of bile pigments, like bilirubin, is normally very efficient, but during cholestasis, the resultant increase in circulating levels of bilirubin imparts a yellow pigmentation to the skin and eyeballs. This condition is referred to as **jaundice.** Another sign of cholestasis is an elevation of the hepatocyte enzymes lactic dehydrogenase (LDH), aspartate transaminase (AST or SGOT), alanine transaminase (ALT), and alkaline phosphatase in plasma. These are also diagnostic of alcoholic-induced liver disease or hepatitis that is most frequently of viral origin (e.g., **hepatitis A, B, or C**).

80. What are the metabolic products of bilirubin glucuronide?

Bilirubin is secreted into the bile as a glucuronide. In the intestinal lumen, bacterial flora deconjugate some of the bilirubin and reduce it to urobilinogen. This latter molecule can be excreted into the feces, where it is oxidized to stercobilin (accounting for the brown pigment of stool); the remainder is reabsorbed into the portal blood. Any bilirubin not taken up by liver and secreted into the bile enters the systemic circulation, where the urobilinogen is readily filtered by the kidney and excreted into the urine where it is oxidized to urobilin. Urobilin has a yellow-brownish color, accounting for the color of urine (see figure).

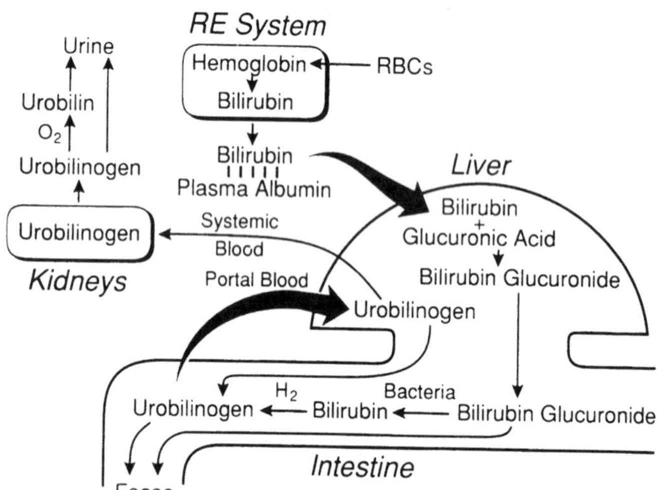

Bilirubin excretory pathways. Heavy arrows represent active processes. (From Johnson LR: Essential Medical Physiology, 2nd ed. Philadelphia, Lippincott-Raven, 1997, with permission.)

81. What are the two major forms of gallstones?

1. Cholesterol stones
2. Pigment stones

82. How does gallstone formation occur?

- **Cholesterol stones** are caused by the precipitation of the sterol from supersaturated bile.
- **Pigment stones** are caused by deconjugation of bilirubin glucuronide to the less soluble free bilirubin, as a consequence of gallbladder infection or inflammation (**cholecystitis**).

DIGESTION AND ABSORPTION

83. Describe the architecture of the small intestinal mucosa.

The epithelial cells of the small intestine or enterocytes are derived from a stem cell population in the crypts of Lieberkühn. This is the region where proliferation occurs, and the daughter cells then migrate to cover the fingerlike villi of the small intestine. During this migration, which takes 3–6 days to complete, the epithelial cells differentiate to form columnar-shaped enterocytes, mucus-secreting goblet cells, or endocrine cells.

84. Discuss the role of the small intestinal mucosa in digestion and absorption of dietary nutrients.

The **enterocyte** possesses a **brush border membrane,** which, in addition to increasing markedly the surface area of the tissue, plays a seminal role in the digestion and absorption of nutrients via brush border enzymes (involved in contact digestion) and carrier mechanisms. Intestinal secretion of electrolytes primarily occurs in the **crypts,** whereas the **goblet cells** play a central role in the secretion of mucus glycoprotein, which coats the apical surface of the mucosa. Once the mature enterocytes migrate to the apex of the villi, they are exfoliated into the lumen and are replaced by neighboring cells. Thus, small intestinal epithelial cells represent a dynamic population of cells that are turning over at a rapid rate to meet changing environmental and dietary conditions.

85. Describe the two mechanisms by which nutrients are digested in the GI tract.

1. The first major mechanism by which nutrients are digested is by **luminal** or **cavital** digestion. This form of digestion is catalyzed by enzymes that are secreted by exocrine tissue (e.g., salivary, pancreatic enzymes, pepsin) into the lumen of the GI tract.

2. The second form of digestion is called either **membrane** or **contact** digestion, as occurs when the substrate molecules come in direct contact with enzymes present on the **brush border membrane** of the small intestine. The products of membrane or contact digestion are then rapidly absorbed across the small intestinal mucosa by both active and passive transport pathways.

86. List the digestive enzymes of the GI tract and indicate if they are involved in luminal or membrane digestion.

In the accompanying table, the enzymes involved in contact digestion are marked with an asterisk; all others act by luminal digestion.

Digestive Enzymes of the GI Tract

SOURCE	ENZYME	SOURCE	ENZYME
Salivary glands	Amylase	Intestinal mucosa	Enterokinase
	Lingual lipase		Disaccharidases
Stomach	Pepsin		Sucrase*
Pancreas	Amylase		Maltase*
	Trypsin		Lactase*
	Chymotrypsin		Trehalase*
	Carboxypeptidase		α-Dextrinase
	Elastase		(isomaltase)*
	Lipase/colipase		Peptidases
	Phospholipase A_2		Amino-oligopeptidase*
	Cholesterol esterase		Dipeptidase*
	(nonspecific)		

*Acts by contact/membrane digestion.

87. Explain how diet can affect the activity of digestive enzymes secreted by the GI tract.

There currently is ample evidence that the pancreatic enzymes synthesized and packaged in zymogen granules are influenced by diet. This process is called **adaptation.** It has been demonstrated, for example, that pancreatic amylase activity increases in response to a carbohydrate-rich diet, whereas pancreatic lipase is increased if fat-rich diets are consumed. It is also known that placing animals on soy-enriched diets results in an increase in the output of pancreatic enzymes, most probably as a result of the presence of a trypsin inhibitor. The activity of the brush border enzymes sucrase, isomaltase, and maltase also appear to be increased in humans who are switched to a starch-rich diet.

88. Give an example of a digestive enzyme that is not directly altered by diet.

The activity of **lactase,** another brush border enzyme, undergoes a developmental decrease in activity in children after 6 years of age, which coincides with a similar decrease in the consumption of milk. This age-dependent decrease in lactase activity, which is "hard-wired" in our genetic makeup, does not appear to occur in individuals in Scandinavian countries, where milk consumption continues into adulthood.

89. How much of the human diet is composed of carbohydrate?

Approximately 50%, in the form of starch.

90. Describe how dietary carbohydrate is digested within the GI tract.

Starch derived from plants is in the form of amylopectin, which consists of a highly branched D-glucose polymer. The glucose molecules of the backbone of amylopectin are bound in α-1,4-linkages, whereas at the branch points they are bound in α-1,6-linkages (see figure). Amylose represents the major form of animal starch. In this polymer, the D-glucose molecules are bound in straight 1,4-linkages. Both of these starch molecules can serve as the substrate for luminal digestion by salivary gland and pancreatic α-amylase. These enzymes are essentially identical in structure with a pH optimum near neutrality and hydrolyze interior α-1,4-linkages of starch to produce the disaccharide, **maltose;** the trisaccharide, **maltotriose;** and the branched-chain saccharides, **α-limit dextrins.** The last-mentioned compounds are formed from the hydrolysis of amylopectin and are short polymers containing the 1,6-branch points with short 1,4-linked groups at one or both ends of the molecule. The products of α-amylase catalyzed hydrolysis are then acted on by brush border enzymes. Maltase-glucoamylase cleaves the α-1,4-linkages of maltose, maltotriose, and limit dextrins. Isomaltase, also called **α-dextrinase,** cleaves the short polymers at the α-1,6-bond. There is some crossover activity because isomaltase can cleave the 1,4-bonds of maltose and maltotriose as well.

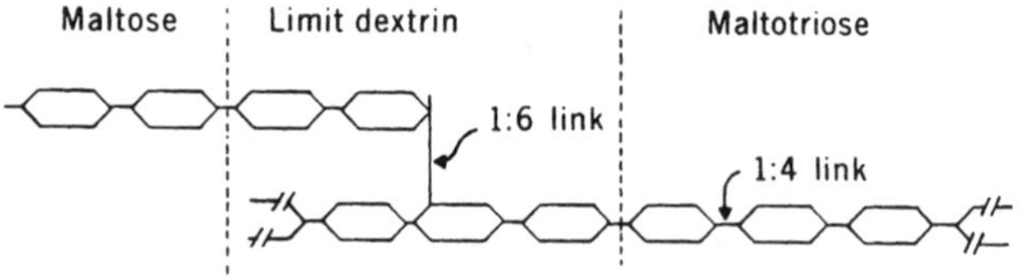

Maltose
Limit dextrin
Maltotriose
1:6 link
1:4 link

Products of starch hydrolysis by α-amylase. (From Johnson LR: Gastrointestinal Physiology, 4th ed. St. Louis, Mosby, 1991, with permission.)

91. What is the final product of starch digestion?

Free **glucose,** which is readily taken up across the brush border membrane and into the enterocyte by a sodium-coupled secondary active transport system (see Na^+-S carrier in the figure, top of next page).

92. What are two other major carbohydrates in the diet?

1. **Sucrose,** a disaccharide, is particularly abundant in the plant world and is the predominant constituent in cane sugar. Sucrose is a disaccharide of glucose and fructose and is readily cleaved by contact digestion by the brush border enzyme, sucrase. Although glucose is actively transported, fructose is taken up into the enterocyte by facilitated diffusion. It appears that one gene synthesizes a larger precursor protein called **sucrase-isomaltase,** which is then cleaved by pancreatic proteases to sucrase and isomaltase on the surface of the brush border.

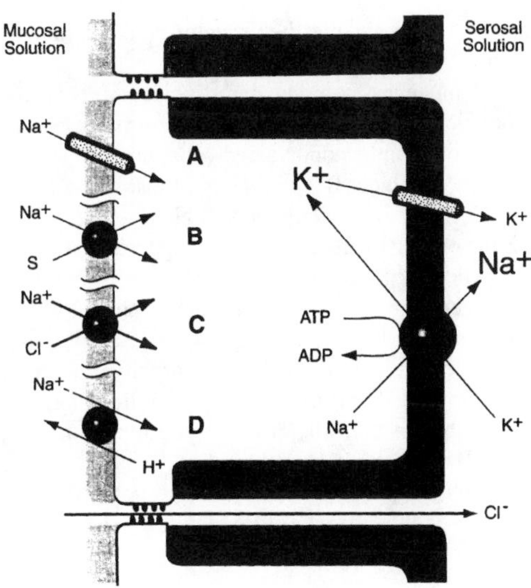

A composite model illustrating the four different mechanisms responsible for the movement of Na^+ from the luminal solution across the apical membranes of small and large intestinal cells. *S*, organic solute. (From Johnson LR: Essential Medical Physiology, 2nd ed. Philadelphia, Lippincott-Raven, 1997, with permission.)

2. **Lactose,** abundant in dairy products, is a disaccharide of glucose and galactose. The brush border enzyme, lactase, cleaves the 1,4-bond to produce glucose and galactose, both of which are actively transported into the tissue. All the brush border enzymes have a pH optimum at or near 6.0.

93. Which of the monosaccharide products are actively transported across the small intestine?

D-Glucose and D-galactose.

94. Describe the mechanisms involved in active transport of D-glucose and D-galactose.

D-Glucose and D-galactose are actively transported from the lumen into the tissue by a **sodium-coupled carrier mechanism** that is driven by the sodium concentration gradient established by the Na^+, K^+-ATPase (sodium pump) localized at the basolateral membrane of the enterocyte (see figure in question 91). Because the same carrier protein is used for both sugars, luminal galactose can competitively inhibit glucose transport and vice versa. The active transport of both sugars can be blocked by inhibitors of oxidative phosphorylation, ouabain (which blocks the sodium pump), or the absence of Na^+ salts in the luminal bathing solution (if Na^+ is replaced with choline). Because this carrier mechanism has sites for both Na^+ and glucose and plays an important role in the intestinal absorption of both substances, the presence of increasing concentrations of glucose in the lumen, which increase Na^+ flux into the tissue, can be monitored electrophysiologically (lumen becoming negative to tissue). Once the sugars are actively transported into the enterocytes, they are transported across the basolateral membrane and into the blood by a facilitated diffusion process, which according to the definition of **facilitated diffusion,** demonstrates saturation kinetics but does not require ATP or oxygen. Facilitated diffusion also plays a central role in the transport of fructose from the lumen into the blood.

95. What are some of the pathophysiologic mechanisms accounting for abnormal carbohydrate digestion and absorption?

Much of the adult population of the world (except people from Northern Europe or who have Scandinavian ancestry) have problems digesting milk, owing to an adult-onset deficiency in the brush border enzyme **lactase.** Although the enzyme is quite high during the neonatal period and through infancy, it begins to decline rather sharply in children older than 6 years of age. In certain cases, lactase activity is deficient from birth. These lactase-deficient children suffer from bouts of (osmotic) diarrhea after the consumption of milk and need to be placed on strict nondairy diets.

A much less common digestive/absorptive problem occurs in individuals who have inherited a deficiency of the enzyme **sucrase-isomaltase** or lack the glucose-galactose carrier. All of these conditions can be noninvasively diagnosed by an oral tolerance test, in which the sugar (lactose, sucrose, or glucose) is dissolved in a solution (10–15%) and ingested, and blood is drawn at 5, 10, 15, 30, 45, and 60 minutes. If glucose levels fail to increase in the blood at least 25 mg/dL after the oral challenge, it strongly suggests that the enzyme or carrier protein is lacking.

The diagnosis for lactase or sucrase-isomaltase deficiency can be further established by taking an endoscopic biopsy specimen of the intestinal mucosa and performing the appropriate enzyme assay. Other diseases (celiac disease, Whipple's disease) associated with blunting of the villus can result in abnormalities in carbohydrate digestion and absorption. All the aforementioned conditions result in an excess concentration of monosaccharides or disaccharides in the GI lumen, which then osmotically draw water into the lumen, resulting in osmotic diarrhea.

96. List the pancreatic enzymes responsible for the digestion of dietary protein, indicating the bonds they attack and which are exopeptidases and which are endopeptidases.

Principal Pancreatic Proteases

ENZYME	PRIMARY ACTION
Endopeptidases	Hydrolyze interior peptide bonds of polypeptides and proteins
Trypsin	Attacks peptide bonds involving basic amino acids; yields products with basic amino acids at C-terminal end
Chymotrypsin	Attacks peptide bonds involving aromatic amino acids, leucine, glutamine, and methionine; yields peptide products with these amino acids at C-terminal end
Elastase	Attacks peptide bonds involving neutral aliphatic amino acids; yields products with neutral amino acids at C-terminal end
Exopeptidases	Hydrolyze external peptide bonds of polypeptides and protein
Carboxypeptidase-A	Attacks peptides with aromatic and neutral aliphatic amino acids at C-terminal end
Carboxypeptidase-B	Attacks peptides with basic amino acids at C-terminal end

97. What prevents these proteolytic enzymes from attacking and breaking down the exocrine GI tissue where they are synthesized and stored?

All of the protease enzymes are stored in their cell of origin as inactive **proenzymes** and become active only when they are secreted into the lumen. The pancreatic proenzyme trypsinogen is activated by an enzyme released from the intestinal mucosa called **enterokinase.** The trypsin molecule formed in this reaction then converts other trypsinogen molecules and the remaining pancreatic proenzymes (chymotrypsinogen, proelastase procarboxypeptidase-A, and procarboxypeptidase-B) to the activated state (see figure, top of next page).

98. Do pancreatic and gastric proteases account for all GI protein digestion?

No. It has been estimated that approximately 60% of protein digestion occurs when protein or its peptide products are acted on by a family of peptidases localized on the brush border membrane of enterocytes.

99. How are the products of digestion of dietary proteins absorbed across the small intestinal mucosa?

Similar to the situation for glucose transport, a sodium-coupled secondary active transport mechanism is responsible for intestinal absorption of most free L-amino acids. There appear to be separate but related carriers for neutral, dibasic, imino, and dicarboxylic amino acids. As in the

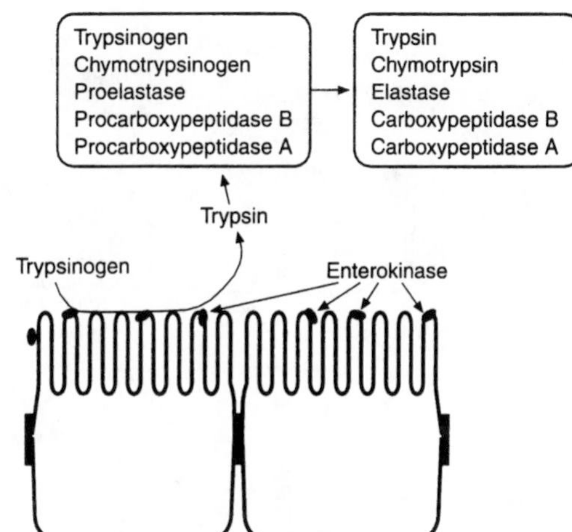

Means of activating the pancreatic proteases that are secreted as proenzymes. Trypsinogen is activated by enterokinase. The resulting trypsin converts the other proenzymes plus additional trypsinogen. (From Johnson LR: Essential Medical Physiology, 2nd ed. Philadelphia, Lippincott-Raven, 1997, with permission.)

case of active glucose transport, the active transport of the L-amino acids is dependent on Na^+, oxygen, and ATP, and amino acids transported by the same carrier system can competitively inhibit one another (e.g., phenylalanine inhibiting the uptake of methionine; aspartate inhibiting the uptake of glutamate). There is also compelling evidence that certain dipeptides and tripeptides are actively transported across the small intestinal mucosa. Some of the carrier systems appear to require luminal sodium to actively transport peptides into the tissue. Carrier mechanisms are presently being identified in the transport of cytoplasmic amino acids and peptides across the basolateral membrane and into the blood.

100. List the lipid constituents of the human diet.

Triglycerides
Phospholipids
Free and esterified sterols

101. Describe how dietary triglyceride is digested in the GI tract.

Digestion is initiated in the stomach by lingual lipase. This enzyme plays a rather minor role in humans and is responsible for breaking down less than 10% of dietary triglyceride. In preparation of the intestinal handling of dietary lipid, the stomach through its churning and mixing action initiates the emulsification of the lipid into smaller fat droplets, a process that continues as the food bolus is exposed to amphipathic chemicals in bile (bile salts and phospholipids) that are potent emulsifying agents. This results in the generation of a disperse microemulsion, which facilitates the binding and action of pancreatic lipase to the surface of the lipidic particle (which now has a diameter < 1 mm). Although bile salts are known to activate this enzyme and adjust its pH optimum to 6.0 (to match that of the lumen of the proximal intestine), they also rapidly remove the lipase from the surface of the lipidic particles as a result of their detergent-like properties. To prevent this from happening, pancreatic exocrine tissue also secretes a factor called **procolipase.** When activated by trypsin to colipase, the protein binds to the surface of the lipid droplet and stabilizes the lipase at the oil–liquid interface. The lipase, which is also called **glycerol ester hydrolase,** catalyzes the hydrolysis of ester linkages at the 1 and 3 positions of glycerol, resulting in the formation of **free fatty acid** and **2-monoglycerides** (see figure, top of next page). Pancreatic lipase, in contrast with pancreatic protease, is stored by pancreatic exocrine tissue in active form and is secreted in excess of need, even with the triglycerol-rich diet of Western countries.

Cholesterol ester hydrolase, also called **nonspecific esterase,** is stored and secreted by the pancreas in active form and, as the name implies, catalyzes the hydrolysis of cholesterol esters to

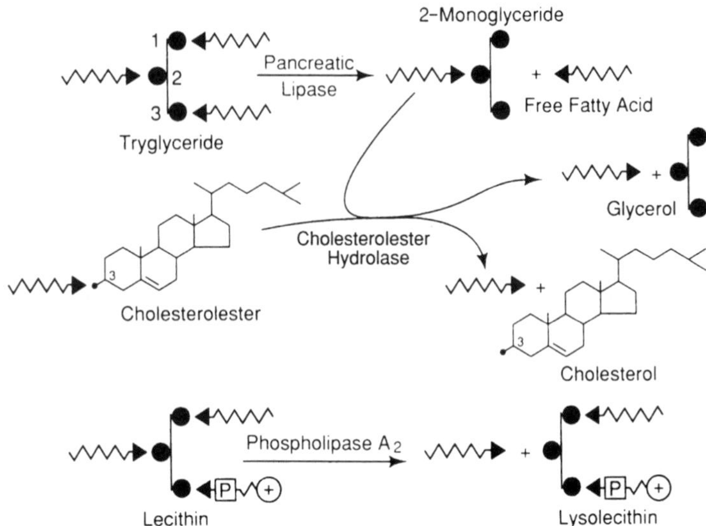

Three major classes of dietary fat and their digestion products. The primary enzymes involved in digestion are also illustrated. (From Johnson LR: Essential Medical Physiology, 2nd ed. Philadelphia, Lippincott-Raven, 1997, with permission.)

cholesterol and free fatty acid. Being a nonspecific esterase, it also attacks the 1, 2, and 3 positions of triglycerides, forming free fatty acids and glycerol. **Phospholipase A_2** is a third pancreatic enzyme involved in dietary lipid digestion. It is biosynthesized and secreted by pancreatic exocrine tissue as a proenzyme and activated in the intestinal lumen by trypsin. Phospholipase A_2 catalyzes the hydrolysis of phosphatidylcholine or lecithin at the 2-position forming free fatty acid and lysolecithin. This enzyme is activated by bile salts and plays a fundamental role in the digestion of not only dietary lecithin (approximately 2 g/day), but also phospholipids that enter the GI tract from the bile and GI epithelial cells that are sloughed into the lumen.

102. Describe the mechanism by which the products of lipid digestion are absorbed by the GI tract.

The major mechanism by which fatty acids (having a chain length of > 8 carbons), 2-monoglycerides, phospholipids, cholesterol, and lipid-soluble vitamins (vitamins A, D, E, and K) are absorbed is in association with **bile salt micelles.** This generally takes place in the jejunum and proximal ileum. Evidence suggests that the micelles primarily act to deliver the lipids to the brush border membrane, where they passively diffuse into the tissue. The bile salts are then absorbed independently, either passively by passive diffusion (primarily deconjugated bile salts) or actively (conjugated bile salts) by a secondary sodium-dependent, active-transport mechanism in operation across mucosa of the distal ileum. Short-chain fatty acids, having fewer than 8 carbons, are mostly water soluble, and are absorbed primarily by diffusion between cells (paracellular).

103. How are the products of lipid digestion handled intracellularly?

The long-chain fatty acids and 2-monoglycerides bind to specific fatty acid binding proteins. The protein-lipid complex then traffics to the smooth endoplasmic reticulum, which contains the full complement of enzymes and cofactors required to resynthesize them back into triglycerides either by the **monoglyceride acylation pathway** (where acyl coenzyme A [CoA] derivatives of fatty acids react with either monoglycerides or diglycerides to form triglycerides), which is predominant, or the less frequently used **phosphatidic acid pathway** (where the acyl CoA derivatives of fatty acids are reacted with α-glycerophosphate to form phosphatidic acid, which, in turn, is dephosphorylated to a diglyceride). The absorbed cholesterol is primarily reesterified with fatty acids. The newly synthesized triglyceride and cholesterol esters are then packaged by the Golgi apparatus into lipidic particles called **chylomicrons,** whose diameters range between 750 and 6000 Å. The surface of the chylomicrons is coated with a mixture of phospholipids, cholesterol, and specific **apoproteins** (Apo AI, Apo AIV, Apo B, and Apo CII). A number of these apoproteins are critical in the transport of the chylomicron out of the enterocyte and into intestinal lacteals, which empty into larger lymphatic vessels that drain the splanchnic beds and finally empty into circulation via the thoracic duct. In contrast with the lymphatic route taken by chylomicrons, short-chain and medium-chain fatty acids can enter the capillary system directly by diffusing across the basolateral membrane of the enterocyte.

104. How are salts and water absorbed across the intestinal mucosa?

Electrolytes can be absorbed across the mucosa of the small and large intestine either paracellularly or transcellularly. To be transported by the **paracellular** route, an ion needs to traverse the tight junctional structures, or **zona occludens,** between neighboring enterocytes. In the small intestine, this appears to be a low-resistance pathway for the diffusion of ions and water, and for this reason it is referred to as a **leaky epithelium.** Because of this property, ions and water are primarily absorbed across the small intestinal mucosa, and the osmotic activity of the intraluminal fluid is close to that of plasma. Of the 7–10 L of water that enter the small intestine, only 0.6 L reach the colon. In contrast, the tight junctions of the large intestine are relatively impermeable to ions and water, and for this reason this tissue is said to be a **tight or high-resistance epithelium.** Because of this property, only a small fraction of ion and water transport occurs across the large bowel mucosa, and it is not uncommon for the fluid contained within the lumen of the colon to be hyperosmolar to that of plasma.

The mucosa of both the small and large intestine transport ions and water **transcellularly.** This takes place through specific channels or by carrier proteins. In many cases, the transport of one ion is linked to the cotransport or countertransport of another ion or nonelectrolyte (glucose or amino acids). Multiple transport pathways exist for Na^+ to cross the apical and basolateral membrane of the enterocyte or colonocyte. Because of these transcellular and paracellular pathways for the absorption of sodium, the concentration of this cation decreases from approximately 140 mEq in the duodenum to approximately 40 mEq in the colon. Water molecules are osmotically drawn across the apical membrane (through water channels) in response to the absorption of both electrolytes and nonelectrolytes. Further, water also moves into the intercellular space, as these osmotically active molecules concentrate there. The net result is buildup in the hydrostatic forces in this microenvironment, causing the bulk flow of water and solutes through the basement membrane and into the capillaries draining the intestine. This is referred to as the **osmotic gradient hypothesis** of solute and water absorption.

105. Describe the mechanisms regulating chloride absorption in the GI tract.

Chloride is absorbed across the small intestinal epithelia by two secondary active transport mechanisms. The first is mediated by a **cotransport carrier protein** that has sites for both Cl^- and a cation (which in most cases is Na^+ but can also be K^+). Thus, Cl^- is actively transported into the tissue as Na^+ moves down its concentration gradient from the lumen into the enterocyte, a process dependent on the activity of the sodium pump at the basolateral membrane. The Na^+-Cl^- cotransport mechanism can be blocked by the so-called loop diuretics such as furosemide.

The second mechanism by which Cl^- is actively transported into the epithelium is in **exchange for HCO_3^-**. This mechanism depends on carbonic anhydrase to generate a HCO_3^- concentration gradient from the tissue to the lumen to provide the driving force for this countertransport mechanism. It has been determined that in contrast with the enterocyte that uses both transport mechanisms, the colonocyte absorbs Cl^- primarily by the latter, Cl^--HCO_3^- exchanger.

106. Describe the mechanisms regulating chloride secretion in the GI tract.

Cl^- is the major anion secreted by the small and large intestine. In contrast with the absorptive pathways that occur in enterocytes present on the villus, secretion takes place in the intestinal and colonic crypts. As depicted in the accompanying figure, these cells have a Na^+ (or K^+)-Cl^- cotransport pathway on the basolateral membrane that drives the secondary active transport of Cl^- into the tissue. This, in turn, generates a Cl^- concentration gradient, driving the diffusion of the anion out of the tissue. The apical membrane of the cell, which has a low basal permeability to Cl^-, possesses two types of Cl^- channels, which are normally closed. One channel is activated by elevations in cytosolic calcium, and the second, which is identical to the **cystic fibrosis transmembrane conductance regulator (CFTR)** of the upper airways, is activated by the cAMP–protein kinase A mechanism. When one of these two channels is activated, Cl^- is rapidly secreted into the lumen, with Na^+ following by the paracellular route, to maintain electroneutrality. Intestinal and colonic secretion of NaCl can be physiologically regulated by cholinergic nerves (by increasing intracellular Ca^+) and certain GI hormones that are members of the secretin family of peptides (secretin, VIP, and glucagon).

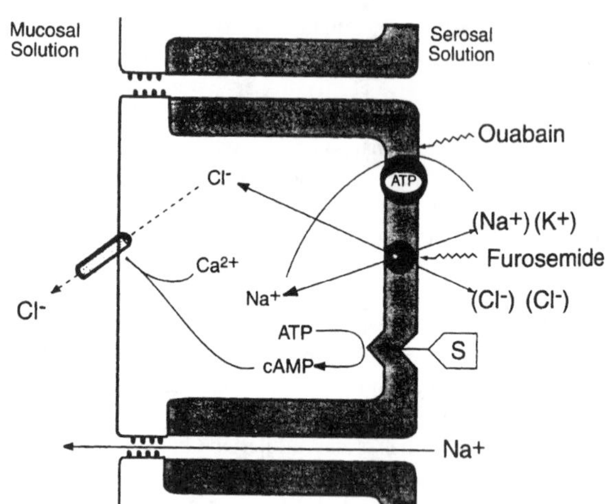

Cellular model of secondary active Cl^- secretion accompanied by passive Na^+ secretion by secretory cells in the crypts of the small and large intestines. *S,* secretagogue. (From Johnson LR: Essential Medical Physiology, 2nd ed. Philadelphia, Lippincott-Raven, 1997, with permission.)

107. What are some pathologic consequences of elevated chloride secretion?

Intestinal secretion can be elevated by certain pathogenic bacteria and viruses (rotavirus), resulting in acute episodes of diarrhea that may be life-threatening. For example, ***Vibrio cholerae*** and certain strains of *Escherichia coli* secrete **enterotoxins** that stimulate the adenylate cyclase activity of intestinal crypt cells, causing the CFTR-regulated Cl^- channels to open. The marked secretion of NaCl that follows osmotically draws large volumes of water into the lumen, resulting in secretory diarrhea that can bring about the loss of several liters of fluid per day. A much rarer condition is a pancreatic tumor that produces an abnormally high concentration of the GI peptide VIP. This condition, called **pancreatic cholera** or **watery diarrhea syndrome,** also results in secretory diarrhea, which is mediated by sustained increases in cytoplasmic calcium.

108. How can cholera-induced secretory diarrhea be managed?

The severe secretory diarrhea caused by microorganisms can be controlled to some extent by **oral rehydration therapy.** This form of therapy was developed from knowledge of physiologic transport mechanisms: certain sugars and amino acids are actively absorbed by the small and large intestine by sodium-coupled secondary active transport mechanisms. Thus, administering a drink containing high concentrations of glucose, an amino acid, and NaCl promotes the intestinal uptake of both the nonelectrolytes and electrolytes, which, in turn, osmotically drives luminal water into the tissue. This net absorption of water counterbalances (all or in part) the secretion of electrolytes and water caused by the microorganism, serving to maintain homeostasis and preventing life-threatening episodes of dehydration.

GASTROINTESTINAL MOTILITY AND ITS REGULATION

109. What is the enteric nervous system?

A network of intrinsic nerves of the GI tract from the midesophagus to the colon. The enteric nervous system is grouped into two major networks:

- **Myenteric plexus,** located between the outer longitudinal and inner, circular muscle layer
- **Submucosal plexus,** localized between the circular muscle layer and the muscularis mucosa (see figure)

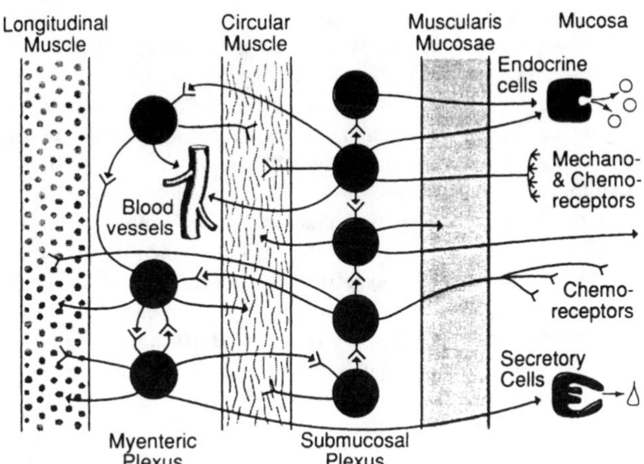

The enteric nervous system. Some reflexes may occur entirely within the wall of the GI tract. (From Johnson LR: Gastrointestinal Physiology, 4th ed. St. Louis, Mosby, 1991, with permission.)

110. What does the enteric nervous system regulate?

The myenteric plexus and the submucosal plexus are extrinsically innervated by afferent and efferent fibers of the parasympathetic and sympathetic nervous system, providing anatomic evidence for cross-talk and regulation between both nervous systems. The myenteric and submucosal plexuses constitute cell bodies, axons, dendrites, and nerve endings, which innervate a number of targets:

- Other ganglia
- Smooth muscle
- Endocrine cells
- Secretory cells

Numerous neurotransmitters or neurocrines are synthesized and released by these enteric fibers:

- Acetylcholine
- CCK
- Serotonin
- Nitric oxide
- Somatostatin
- Enkephalins
- VIP
- Dopamine
- Members of the substance P family of peptides (neurokinins)

111. Is functioning of the enteric nervous system dependent on the extrinsic nervous system?

No. Although it is clear that extrinsic nerves modulate the activity of the enteric nervous system, the enteric nervous system would function if all connections with the extrinsic nervous system were severed, as indicated by the maintenance of coordinated waves of contractions from the midesophagus to the colon in animals subjected to a truncal vagotomy.

112. Describe the physiologic events that coordinate the swallowing of ingested food to its movement into and down the esophagus.

The act of swallowing is initiated with the upward movement of the tongue against the hard palate. As the tongue sweeps backward, the food bolus is propelled into the oropharynx, and the nasopharynx is closed by the downward movement of the soft palate. Simultaneously a wave of contraction sweeps down the constrictor muscles of the pharynx, which results in the upward movement of the glottis and the downward movement of the epiglottis, sealing off the trachea, which is immediately preceded by the opening of the **upper esophageal sphincter** as a result of a relaxation of the cricopharyngeal muscle. Although the initial act of swallowing is voluntary in nature, once the food bolus enters the pharynx, a series of receptors become activated that send afferent impulses via the vagus and glossopharyngeal nerves to the swallowing center in the medulla. This evokes a sequential series of signals down efferent fibers to the muscles of the pharynx and the esophagus to coordinate the swallowing reflex. The coordination of this reflex and the initiation of the peristaltic wave of contraction from the pharynx to the esophagus are modulated by afferent signals from receptors in these tissues to the swallowing center. The importance of this central control of the swallowing reflex can be appreciated in individuals who are incapable of swallowing ingested food because of a neurologic lesion in the medulla.

Once the food bolus enters the esophagus, the upper esophageal sphincter closes (to prevent the swallowing of air), and a peristaltic wave of contraction sweeps down the esophagus. This **primary peristaltic wave** of contraction (which is preceded by the pharyngeal phase) moves slowly down the esophagus at a rate of 2–6 cm/s until it reaches the **lower esophageal sphincter (LES).** The smooth muscles of the LES are tonically contracted, and relax immediately before the peristaltic wave of contraction reaches the sphincter. The presence of food particles in the esophagus that have not been completely removed by the above-mentioned primary peristaltic contractions can induce a **secondary peristalsis** that is elicited by distention. The physiologic coordination of esophageal peristalsis is initially regulated by efferent vagal fibers from the swallowing center that innervate striated muscles of the body of the esophagus. In addition, visceral motor nerves also innervate enteric neurons of the myenteric plexus. Interruption of these neural connections produces abnormalities in the initiation of peristalsis in the upper regions of the esophagus composed of striated muscles, whereas peristaltic contractions proceed normally in the mid-distal esophageal regions, which are composed of smooth muscle. It appears that the tonic contraction of LES smooth muscle is myogenic in origin, and the relaxation of the muscle as the food bolus approaches the sphincter is mediated neurally by vagal fibers. The neurotransmitter that induces LES relaxation is still under investigation, but evidence suggests that both **VIP** and **nitric oxide (NO)** may be involved.

113. What is receptive relaxation?

The ability of the smooth muscles of the proximal or orad region of the stomach to relax, as food enters the stomach during the gastric phase of digestion. This allows the stomach to accommodate rather large volumes while gastric pressure is only minimally increased.

114. How is receptive relaxation controlled?

Receptive relaxation is regulated by vagal innervation, is coordinated with relaxation of the LES, and is abolished after vagotomy.

115. How does the contractile activity of the orad and the caudad stomach differ during the fasting and fed state?

Fasting: The contractile activity of the orad stomach is weak and infrequent, consistent with its thin complement of smooth muscle and quiescent electrical activity. Although for the most part the stomach does not contract during the fasting state, every 90 minutes or so, periods of vigorous contractions are initiated at the midportion of the stomach (lasting 3–5 minutes) and move slowly distally along the GI tract. This event is called the **migrating myoelectric** (or **motor) complex (MMC)** and is thought to play an important role in clearing the GI tract of mucus, exfoliated cells, and bacteria.

Fed: During the gastric phase of digestion, the MMC is replaced by more frequent gastric contractions that are initiated in the gastric body and sweep distally, increasing in force and velocity as they approach the pylorus. When the peristaltic contractions overtake the food bolus and reach the pylorus, they serve to propel the gastric material back into the stomach in an orad direction. This event, known as **retropulsion,** plays an important role in both the mixing and the breaking down of the food bolus into small particles, because it has been determined that food particles need to be less than 2 mm^3 before they empty into the duodenum.

116. What are gastric slow waves?

The intrinsic electrical activity of gastric smooth muscle cells that triggers the contractions of the caudad stomach.

117. How are slow waves generated?

An unstable membrane potential rhythmically depolarizes and repolarizes (see figure). When the membrane potential depolarizes to a threshold value, contraction of the smooth muscle occurs. When the plateau potential of the slow wave has spike potentials superimposed on it, the gastric contractions become more forceful, as may occur in the presence of cholinergic agonists or specific GI hormones (e.g., gastrin). The velocity and amplitude of the slow waves increase as they approach the pylorus, accounting for the proportional increase in gastric contractile activity. Furthermore, the slow-wave frequency during a meal (between 3 and 5/min) is the same as the frequency of gastric contractions, and for this reason it is also referred to as the **pacemaker potential.** This type of slow-wave activity does not occur in the orad stomach and is initiated at the gastric body at the border of the orad and caudad stomach, a region that is also called the **pacemaker.** The molecular basis for the unstable membrane potential of gastric smooth muscle cells is unknown, with evidence that they may be triggered by oscillations in the sodium pump, cytosolic calcium levels, or intrinsic activity of nonmuscle pacemaker cells, called the **interstitial cells of Cajal,** which are electrically coupled to smooth muscle cells.

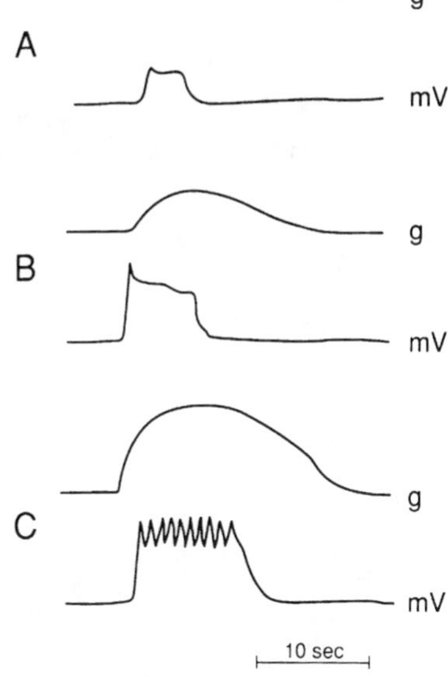

Three sets of mechanical (*g*) and electrical (*mV*) tracings from the caudad region of the stomach. *A,* Slow wave depolarization of insufficient magnitude to cause contraction. *B,* Increased depolarization results in contraction. *C,* Electrical slow wave with multiple spike potentials and extended plateau produces a vigorous and extended contraction.

118. How is gastric emptying regulated?

Liquids empty more rapidly than solids, and solid particles do not empty until they have been broken down to less than 2 mm^3 to ensure their rapid assimilation in the intestine. Both hyperosmotic and hypo-osmotic solutions have a delayed gastric emptying relative to saline, and receptors are present in the proximal duodenum that slow emptying in response to low pH, hyperosmolarity, and the presence of dietary lipid. The retardation in the rate of gastric emptying in response to dietary lipid in the intestine may, in part, be due to the release of CCK, which has been demonstrated to inhibit this gastric property.

119. What is the predominant form of contractile activity in the small intestine during the fasting state?

Although the smooth muscle of the small intestine contracts sporadically between meals, the most organized contractile activity is the **MMC.** This event, which occurs at approximately 90-minute intervals, is a continuation of the wave of intense contractile activity that is initiated in the gastric body and sweeps distally to clear the GI lumen of mucus, exfoliated cells, and other debris and limits the number of intestinal flora. It also takes approximately 90 minutes for the MCC to sweep the entire length of the small intestine, so that this activity is initiated in the proximal duodenum just when the wave of contractile activity reaches the ileocecal region.

120. What is segmentation?

During a meal, MMC activity disappears and is replaced by multiple contractions of variable frequency and amplitude up and down the small intestine (see figure). More frequently than not, this contractile event is local in nature and not coordinated with the contractile activity of adjacent proximal or distal intestinal tissue. This type of contraction, which results in the partial or complete occlusion of the intestinal lumen, thereby primarily serves to mix the food in this localized region and is called **segmentation.** The average frequency of these contractions is multiples of every 5 seconds, which is the frequency of slow-wave activity.

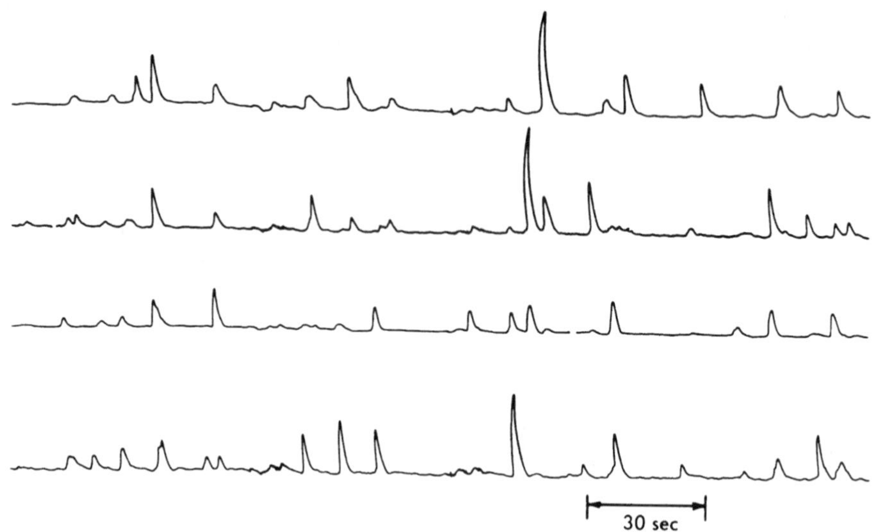

Intraluminal pressure changes recorded from the duodenum of a conscious man. Sensors placed 1 cm apart record changes in pressure that are phasic, lasting 4–5 seconds. Note that a rather large contraction can take place at one site, while nothing is recorded 1 cm away on either side. (From Johnson LR: Gastrointestinal Physiology, 4th ed. St. Louis, Mosby, 1991, with permission.)

121. Can contractile activity be coordinated in some instances?

Occasionally, contractile activity is coordinated after a short delay with contractions of an adjacent aboral region of the small bowel, resulting in a coordinated peristaltic wave that can propel the food bolus rapidly in an aboral direction (see figure, next page). It appears that in healthy individuals, **peristaltic contractions** move luminal material distally for only short distances of

1- to 4-cm lengths. This coordinated activity is followed by segmenting contractions, perhaps to expose the food bolus to the maximal digestive and absorptive capacity of a region of the small intestine before it is moved to the next intestinal region.

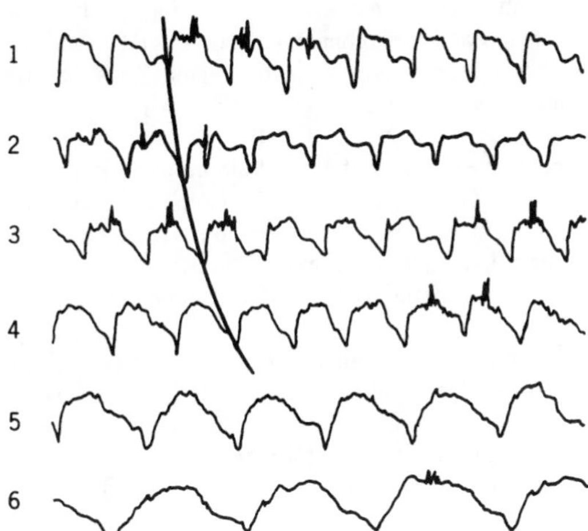

Slow waves and spike potentials from multiple sites in the small intestine. Tracings 1 to 6 illustrate activity from progressively distal areas. Solid line connecting the slow waves in tracings 1 to 4 denotes the apparent propagation in the region of a slow-wave frequency plateau. Tracings 5 to 6 show decreases in slow-wave frequency at more distal areas. The rapid transients that occur on the peaks of some of the slow waves represent spike potentials. (From Johnson LR: Gastrointestinal Physiology, 4th ed. St. Louis, Mosby, 1991, with permission.)

122. Does a small intestine contraction occur in association with every slow wave?

No. Although slow waves elicit a depolarization of the intestinal smooth muscle cells that approaches the threshold for muscle contraction, the latter contractile event is dependent on the presence of **spike potentials.** These rapid depolarizations of the membrane, which occur during the depolarization phase of the slow wave, cause the threshold for cell activation to be exceeded and are followed after several milliseconds by a smooth muscle contraction. Spike potentials do not occur with every slow wave. For this reason, the contractile activity of the small bowel occurs at intervals that are multiples of the slow-wave frequency of every 5 seconds, thereby occurring at intervals of 5, 10, 15, or 20 seconds.

123. How is small intestinal motility regulated?

Both GI hormones and neural activity regulate the contractile activity of the small intestine, primarily by affecting the frequency and intensity of spike potentials of intestinal smooth muscle cells. Parasympathetic activity stimulates, whereas sympathetic activity depresses, intestinal smooth muscle contractions. VIP and nitric oxide appear to play a mediatory role in neurally induced intestinal smooth muscle relaxation, whereas serotonin may play a role in mediating peristaltic events. A GI peptide called **motilin** also may play an important physiologic role in triggering or modulating the MMC that sweeps down the GI tract, as its circulating levels increase in the blood before such an event, and exogenous administration of the peptide can induce MMC activity. Although GI peptides and extrinsic nerves appear to affect small intestinal motility, the contractile activity is not solely dependent on these neurohormonal signals because both MMCs and peristaltic waves of contraction can be demonstrated in extrinsically denervated small intestine, underlying the importance of the enteric nervous system in controlling these events.

124. What are taeniae coli?

In contrast with the small intestine, in which the outer band of longitudinal muscle is continuous, the longitudinal muscle fibers of the large intestine are concentrated into three flat bands referred to as **taeniae coli,** running from the cecum to the rectum, at which point they fan out to form a more continuous muscle layer.

125. What are haustrations?

The large intestine appears to be subdivided into a chain of sacs that are called **haustra** or **haustrations.** The origin of these structures is not clear and may relate to points of concentration of smooth muscle coordinated with mucosal foldings. They appear to be more concentrated where the taeniae coli are located. Their location is not completely fixed because they disappear during and reappear after colonic contractions, and this form of segmental contraction of the intestinal wall may even reform at another region. Thus, haustra have both an anatomic and a functional origin.

126. Is the movement of the food bolus from the ileum into the cecum regulated?

Yes. Distention of the distal ileum induces a reflexive relaxation of the ileocecal sphincter, resulting in the movement of the food bolus into the cecum and colon. Also, distention of the walls of the colon induces a reflexive contraction of the sphincter, preventing the retrograde movement of luminal material back into the small bowel.

127. Describe the contractile activity of the large intestine.

Most of the contractile activity of the colonic smooth muscle is segmental in nature, thereby serving primarily to mix the luminal contents. These contractions last from 12 to 60 seconds and probably contribute to the formation of haustra. Approximately one to three times per day, a wave of peristaltic activity sweeps down the large intestine, called a **mass movement,** which serves to propel the luminal material toward the rectum. The haustrations and segmental activity of the large intestine temporarily disappear during a mass movement event. The electrophysiologic origin of segmental and peristaltic contractions of the large intestine is still under study but appears to be related to both slow-wave activity and the appearance of spike potentials.

128. What is the retrosphincteric reflex?

Normally the rectum is empty because of the segmental contractions of this most distal region of the large intestine, and the internal anal sphincter is tonically contracted. At the time of a mass movement, the walls of the rectum become distended and initiate a reflexive relaxation of the internal anal sphincter propelling the fecal material into the anal canal. Distention of the rectum to greater than 25% capacity initiates an afferent impulse centrally to provide an urge to defecate.

129. Describe how the act of defecation is controlled.

The act of defecation is controlled by the external anal sphincter. This sphincter is partially composed of striated muscle, in contrast with other GI sphincters, and is under voluntary control under the regulation of the pelvic nerve (parasympathetic) and the hypogastric plexus (sympathetic). In situations in which defecation is inappropriate, the external anal sphincter contracts; the receptors in the rectum accommodate, relieving the sensation to defecate; and the internal anal sphincter regains its tone. In situations in which defecation is appropriate, the external anal sphincter relaxes under voluntary control, and the longitudinal muscles of the colon and rectum contract as the musculature of the pelvic floor relaxes. The forces promoting defecation can also be increased with the contraction of thoracic and abdominal muscles.

130. How is large intestinal motility regulated?

Although it is clear that both segmental and peristaltic contractions occur in the large intestine tissue that has been surgically excised, presumably under the control of the enteric nervous system, it is also well documented that both parasympathetic and sympathetic nerves stimulate and inhibit the contractile activity of the colon. Extrinsically, the **parasympathetic** innervation of the cecum and ascending and transverse colon comes from the vagus nerve, whereas the pelvic nerve innervates the descending colon and rectum. **Sympathetic** innervation of the proximal regions of large intestine originates from the **superior mesenteric ganglion,** whereas more distal regions of the bowel receive their sympathetic innervation from fibers that originate in the **infe-**

rior mesenteric ganglion and the **hypogastric plexus.** GI peptides and other neurotransmitters also appear to play a role in the regulation of colonic motility with substance P and related tachykinins stimulating and VIP and nitric oxide inhibiting the contractile activity of GI smooth muscle.

131. What is the role of sensory afferent nerves which originate in the gastrointestinal tract?

Although extrinsic nerves are not absolutely required for many GI functions, many sensory afferent nerves project from the gut to the spinal cord and brain (via the sympathetic and parasympathetic pathways). These sensory nerves are known to be involved in certain reflexes in which distention of one region will affect (mostly inhibit) the activity of another (e.g., the intestinal inhibitory reflex). Sensory afferent pathways forming neural connections with the CNS and brain have been known to relay the sensation of pain and fullness and regulate the physiologic and behavioral functions affecting feeding behavior (satiety), gastric emptying, and local blood flow.

BIBLIOGRAPHY

1. Johnson LR (ed): Gastrointestinal Physiology, 6th ed. St. Louis, Mosby, 2000.
2. Johnson LR: Gastrointestinal physiology. In Johnson LR (ed): Essential Medical Physiology. Philadelphia, Lippincott-Raven, 1997.

8. ENDOCRINE PHYSIOLOGY

Hershel Raff, Ph.D.

PRINCIPLES OF ENDOCRINOLOGY

1. What is a hormone?

An **endocrine** hormone is classically considered a substance produced in small amounts, released into the blood where it is transported to a distant organ to exert its specific action on target tissue equipped with a **receptor** for the hormone. A hormone can also act on neighboring tissue within the same gland (**paracrine**) and can act on the tissue that produced it (**autocrine**). Hormones can also be synthesized and released into the bloodstream by nerves (**neurocrine**).

2. List general functions that hormones regulate.

- **Reproduction**—menstrual cycle, ovulation, spermatogenesis, pregnancy, lactation
- **Growth and development**—sexual differentiation, secondary sex characteristics, growth velocity
- **Maintenance of the internal environment**—extracellular fluid volume, blood pressure, electrolyte balance, and regulation of plasma ions such as calcium and sodium
- **Energy flux**—storage, distribution, and consumption of calories; heat production
- **Behavior**—food and water intake, sexual behavior, mood

3. What is the chemical nature of classic hormones, and where are they produced?

The chemical nature of hormones is determined by the site of synthesis and, in turn, determines the mode of transport in blood, the mechanism of action, and rate of metabolism.

	SITE OF RELEASE	HORMONE
Amines and tyrosine derivatives	Adrenal medulla	Catecholamines (epinephrine, norepinephrine, dopamine)
	Thyroid gland	Triiodothyronine (T_3), thyroxine (T_4)
Steroids	Gonads and placenta	Testosterone, estrogens, progesterone
	Adrenal cortex	Cortisol, aldosterone, adrenal androgens
	Diet/skin/liver/kidney	Secosteroids (vitamin D and its metabolites)
Polypeptides and proteins	Posterior pituitary	Oxytocin, vasopressin
	Hypothalamus	TRH, somatostatin, GnRH, CRH, GHRH
	Anterior pituitary	MSH, ACTH, prolactin, GH
	Gastrointestinal	Gastrin, somatostatin, cholecystokinin, secretin
	Endocrine pancreas	Insulin, glucagon, pancreatic polypeptide
	Placenta	Chorionic somatomammotropin
	Parathyroid/thyroid	PTH, calcitonin
	Many others	Examples: heart (atrial natriuretic peptide), liver (IGF-1)
Glycoproteins	Anterior pituitary	LH, FSH, TSH
	Placenta	hCG

TRH = thyrotropin-releasing hormone, GnRH = gonadotropin-releasing hormone, MSH = melanocyte-stimulating hormone, CRH = corticotropin-releasing hormone, GHRH = growth hormone–releasing hormone, ACTH = adrenocorticotropic hormone, GH= growth hormone, PTH = parathyroid hormone, LH = luteinizing hormone, FSH = follicle-stimulating hormone, TSH = thyroid-stimulating hormone, hCG = human chorionic gonadotropin

4. What are some examples of different categories of hormones?

Amines

OH
HO
HO
CH — CH_2 — NH_2
(Norepinephrine)

Thyroid Hormones

HO — O — CH_2 — CH — COOH, I, I, I, NH_2
(3,5,3'-triiodothyronine,T_3)

Polypeptides

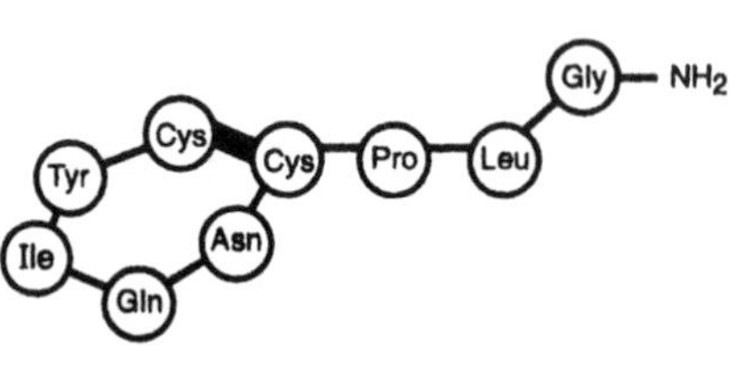

(Oxytocin)

Proteins

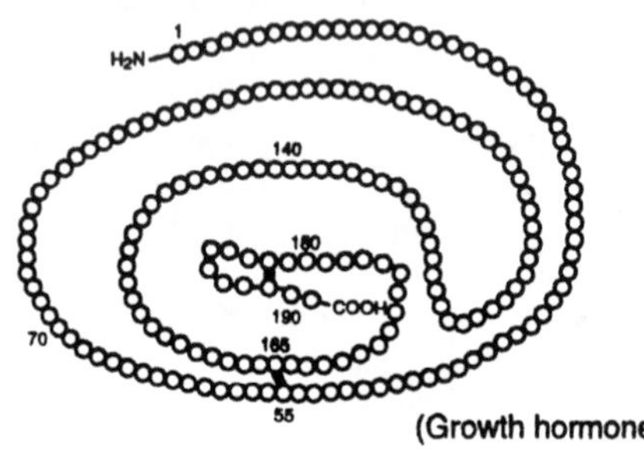

(Growth hormone)

Steroids

CH_2OH
C=O
HO
OH
O
(Cortisol)

OH
(Vitamin D3)

Examples of different categories of hormones. In the case of the protein hormone, each circle represents an amino acid, as shown for the polypeptide hormone. The structure of oxytocin is similar to arginine vasopressin. (From Griffin JE, Ojeda SR (eds): Textbook of Endocrine Physiology, 3rd ed. New York, Oxford University Press, 1996, p 7, with permission.)

5. Is there a pattern to the release of hormones?

Hormones are released with a variety of rhythms. Hormones can be released in **circadian rhythm,** such as cortisol, which peaks at 8 A.M. and reaches its nadir at midnight in diurnal animals. Hormones can be released in **ultradian rhythm,** with many regular pulses within a day (e.g., luteinizing hormone [LH]), and even have seasonal rhythms. Hormones can also be released primarily in response to specific stimuli (e.g., suckling-induced prolactin). Pulsatility appears to maintain receptor sensitivity to hormones.

6. What are the general principles of the control of hormone secretion?

The end-product (hormone, metabolite) inhibits the release of the hormone that stimulated the production of the end-product (feedback loop). Most hormones are under **negative feedback** (thermostatic) control. For example, glucagon stimulates glucose production; an increase in plasma glucose shuts off glucagon production.

7. Compare and contrast the general mechanism of action of each class of hormone.

Most hormones work via either a cell membrane receptor, which activates or inhibits a second messenger that alters the function (increases or decreases) of an existent cellular component (e.g., pump), or via an intracellular receptor, which activates specific gene transcription and translation of new protein (synthesis of a new cellular component [e.g., pump]). Some cell membrane hormone receptors also influence gene expression, and some intracellular hormone receptors may act via nongenomic mechanisms.

HORMONE	RECEPTOR LOCATION	SECOND MESSENGER	TIME TO EFFECT
Thyroid	Nuclear	Transcription	Slow
Steroid	Cytoplasmic	Transcription	Slow
Peptide	Cell membrane	cAMP/cGMP	Fast
Catecholamine	Cell membrane	cAMP/cGMP	Fast
Peptide	Cell membrane	IP_2/DAG	Fast

8. List some of the types of cell membrane receptors, and give an example of a hormone ligand.

Seven-transmembrane domain receptor: This classic cell membrane receptor is covered in detail in Chapter 2. The β-adrenergic receptor (catecholamine ligand) is the classic model. These receptors interact with another family of proteins (G-proteins) that mediate changes in adenylate cyclase activity and cyclic adenosine monophosphate (cAMP) production and turn on the classic phosphorylase cascade.

Protein tyrosine kinase activity: These receptors (e.g., epidermal growth factor [EGF] and insulin) catalyze the phosphorylation of tyrosine on intracellular proteins.

Guanylate cyclase-linked receptors: These receptors (e.g., for atrial natriuretic peptide) promote the production of the second messenger cyclic guanosine monophosphate (cGMP).

Cytokine receptor superfamily: Growth hormone (GH) and prolactin are examples of hormones that bind to these receptors, which activate tyrosine phosphorylation despite no apparent homology to known protein kinases.

9. Briefly describe the different second messengers that mediate the action of the cell surface hormone receptors.

Second messengers quickly transduce and amplify the signal generated by the binding of the hormone to the cell surface receptor. Among these second messengers are cAMP, cGMP, the calcium-calmodulin system, and the phosphatidylinositol-diacylglyceride-inositol 1,4,5 triphosphate (IP_3) system. The details of each of these can be found in Chapter 2. Briefly, although they are quite different in their biochemistry, the end result of each is the same in that they quickly act on an intracellular element either to inhibit or to activate some function (e.g., enzyme, pump, membrane potential, calcium release).

10. List and briefly describe some of the types of intracellular hormone receptors.

The intracellular receptors work mostly by altering gene expression. This is why they generally have a slower onset of action than cell membrane receptors, which quickly activate second messengers. **Steroid and thyroid hormones** bind either to a cytoplasmic receptor that is translocated to the nucleus or to nuclear receptors. The binding of steroid to the receptor either liberates the complex from heat-shock proteins (e.g., cortisol) or directly activates the receptor already bound to its respective hormone-responsive elements (HRE) on DNA (e.g., thyroid hormone, estrogen, $1,25(OH)_2D$). Either way, the activated receptor-ligand forms a complex (e.g., homodimer), binds to its HRE, and activates transcription of specific genes (mRNA production). This increase in specific mRNAs results in the synthesis (translation) of specific proteins (e.g., enzyme pumps).

11. List the general features of the metabolism (clearance) of hormones.

1. Some hormones are transported in plasma bound to carrier proteins. Hormones are metabolized from the plasma compartment; usually only the free (unbound) component of the circulating hormone is available for metabolism. It is the unbound hormone that is free to exert a biologic action.

2. Metabolic clearance is inversely proportional to the percent of total hormone circulating in the bound form. Thyroid hormone has a slow metabolic clearance (long half-life) because it circulates $>$ 99.6% bound. Protein binding of a hormone in the plasma compartment protects the hormone from metabolism because only the free hormone is biologically active and available for metabolism.

3. Within a class of hormones, metabolic clearance is also inversely proportional to protein binding in plasma. For example, the steroid cortisol circulates 95% bound and has a slower metabolic clearance than aldosterone, which circulates only 15% bound.

12. Discuss the general principles of endocrine disease.

In general, most disorders that are primarily attributable to hormones result from either their real or apparent underproduction or real or apparent overproduction.

Underproduction:

- **Primary underproduction** is due to loss of the function of the gland producing the active hormone. An example is destruction of both adrenal glands (primary adrenal insufficiency).
- **Secondary underproduction** is due to the loss of the hormone that normally stimulates the gland producing the active hormone. An example of this is hypopituitarism, in which the pituitary fails to produce trophic hormones (e.g., adrenocorticotropic hormone [ACTH]), which maintain normal function of a gland (e.g., adrenal cortex).
- **Apparent underproduction** (target cell insensitivity) is usually due to a receptor defect (mutation) such that, even if the hormone is present, the target cell cannot respond. An example of this is testicular feminization, in which a male genotype (XY) fetus has a mutation in the testosterone receptor and, as a result of loss of androgen activity, develops a female phenotype. Another example is pseudohypoparathyroidism, in which, despite normal or elevated parathyroid hormone (PTH) levels, the target cells for PTH cannot respond.

Overproduction:

- **Primary overproduction** is usually due to a neoplasm (tumor) arising from a cell population that normally produces the hormone such that the hormone is produced in excess regardless of any endogenous signal to stop its production. An example is an adrenocortical adenoma that produces cortisol even in the absence of ACTH.
- **Secondary overproduction** is due to excess input into the target gland. An example is a tumor arising from normal pituitary cells and producing too much trophic hormone (e.g., ACTH) such that an otherwise normal adrenal cortex is told to produce too much cortisol. Another example is secondary hyperparathyroidism, in which calcium, which inhibits PTH release, is not absorbed properly in the gastrointestinal tract, and PTH release is greatly increased to compensate for it.
- **Apparent overproduction** is due to activation of a receptor or cellular component owing to a mutation. Therefore, the function of the target gland is activated even in the absence of normal hormonal stimulation. An example of an activating mutation is Liddle's syndrome, in which the renal epithelial sodium channel is constitutively activated and mimics the effects of too much aldosterone, even though aldosterone is low.

PITUITARY PHYSIOLOGY

13. Describe the functional anatomy of the hypothalamic-pituitary interface.

The control of anterior and posterior pituitary hormone release is a classic example of **neuroendocrine** systems. The **anterior pituitary** (adenohypophysis, pars distalis) is controlled by hypothalamic releasing or inhibiting (hypophysiotropic) hormones synthesized in parvocellular neurons with cell bodies in nuclei in the hypothalamus (generally medial nuclei such as arcuate and medial paraventricular). Input to these cell bodies increases or decreases the release of stimulatory (releasing) or inhibitory hormones, which are released from terminals located on capillaries in the median eminence. They enter the long portal blood vessels and are transported to the anterior pituitary, where they stimulate or inhibit the release of hormones from the anterior pituitary. The **posterior pituitary** (neurohypophysis, pars nervosa) releases hormones directly into the blood from axons with magnocellular cell bodies located in the supraoptic and paraventricular (lateral) nuclei of the hypothalamus. Input into these cell bodies causes the increase or decrease in the release of posterior pituitary hormones (arginine vasopressin [AVP] or oxytocin) into capillaries in the posterior pituitary.

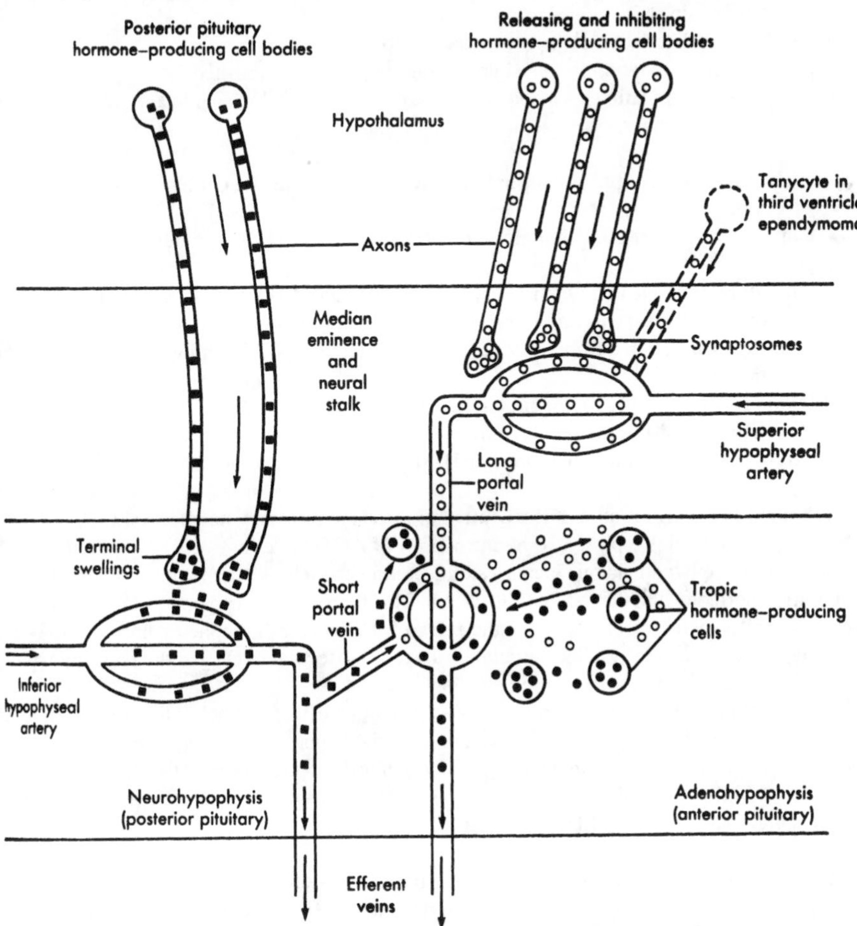

The functional anatomy of the hypothalamic-pituitary interface and its blood supply. Arrows indicate the direction of hormone movement. The posterior pituitary has direct arterial blood supply, whereas the anterior pituitary receives most of its blood (containing hypothalamic releasing and inhibiting factors) via portal blood. (From Genuth SM: The endocrine system. In Berne RM, Levy MN (eds): Physiology, 3rd ed. St. Louis, Mosby, 1993, with permission.)

ANTERIOR PITUITARY

14. What are the hormones of the anterior pituitary?

1. **Glycoproteins** (α-subunits identical; β-subunits confer specificity):

- Thyroid-stimulating hormone (TSH; thyrotropin): stimulates thyroid hormone synthesis and release

- Gonadotropins: LH and follicle-stimulating hormone (FSH)
  Female: stimulates ovarian function and steroidogenesis
  Male: stimulates testicular function and steroidogenesis

2. **Somatomammotropins** (single-peptide chain with disulfide bonds):

- GH (somatotropin): stimulates somatic growth (via insulin-like growth factor I [IGF-1]) and is counterregulatory to insulin
- Prolactin (mammotropin): promotes lactation in females

3. **Proopiomelanocortin (POMC) family** (precursor for small peptides produced by post-translational processing):

- ACTH: stimulates adrenal growth and steroidogenesis
- β-Lipotropin, β-endorphin: physiologic roles not firmly established
- Melanocyte-stimulating hormone (MSH): skin darkening in lower animals and at high concentration in humans; physiologic roles not established

15. List the factors (hypophysiotropic hormones) involved in the control of anterior pituitary secretion.

- **Corticotropin-releasing hormone** (CRH) stimulates POMC synthesis and ACTH secretion.
- **Gonadotropin-releasing hormone** (GnRH) stimulates LH and FSH secretion.
- **Growth hormone–releasing hormone** (GHRH) stimulates growth hormone release.
- **Somatostatin** (somatotropin release-inhibiting factor [SRIF]) inhibits growth hormone secretion.
- **Prolactin-stimulating factor** probably exists, but its exact nature has not been resolved.
- **Prolactin-inhibiting factor** (dopamine) inhibits the release of prolactin.
- **Thyrotropin-releasing hormone** (TRH) stimulates TSH and prolactin secretion.

16. What is the general model of the control of anterior pituitary hormone secretion?

The classic model is represented by the control of ACTH release (see figure on next page). Neural input to the hypothalamus increases or decreases the release of a hypothalamic releasing or inhibiting hormone into the long portal system. This hormone is transported to the anterior pituitary, where it increases or decreases the release of a trophic hormone or hormones. These trophic hormones enter the systemic circulation and exert effects at target glands. The target gland releases a hormone, which has systemic effects.

The target gland limits its own release by exerting **negative feedback** inhibition at the level of the pituitary gland, hypothalamus, or even input to the hypothalamus. Feedback actions mediated by target gland hormones are called long-loop. Short-loop feedback is the inhibition of hypothalamic function by pituitary trophic hormones. Ultra-short loop feedback is the inhibition of hypothalamic function by hypothalamic factors.

17. Is the control of all anterior pituitary hormones the same?

No, each is peculiar in its own way. Sometimes it is easier to remember the exceptions (in **bold**) to the general model:

CRH-ACTH-cortisol	Classic system
GHRH/somatostatin-GH-IGF-I	**Dual (stimulatory [GHRH] and inhibitory [somatostatin]) hypophysiotropic hormones**
TRH-TSH-T_3/T_4	**Majority of negative feedback of thyroid hormone exerted at pituitary (inhibition of TSH)**
GnRH-LH/FSH-testes	**Two pituitary hormones (parallel system) LH and FSH controlled by same hypothalamic factor**
GnRH-LH/FSH-ovaries	**Positive feedback of estrogen on LH during menstrual cycle**
Dopamine-prolactin	**Primarily inhibitory hypophysiotropic control (dopamine inhibition of prolactin release)**

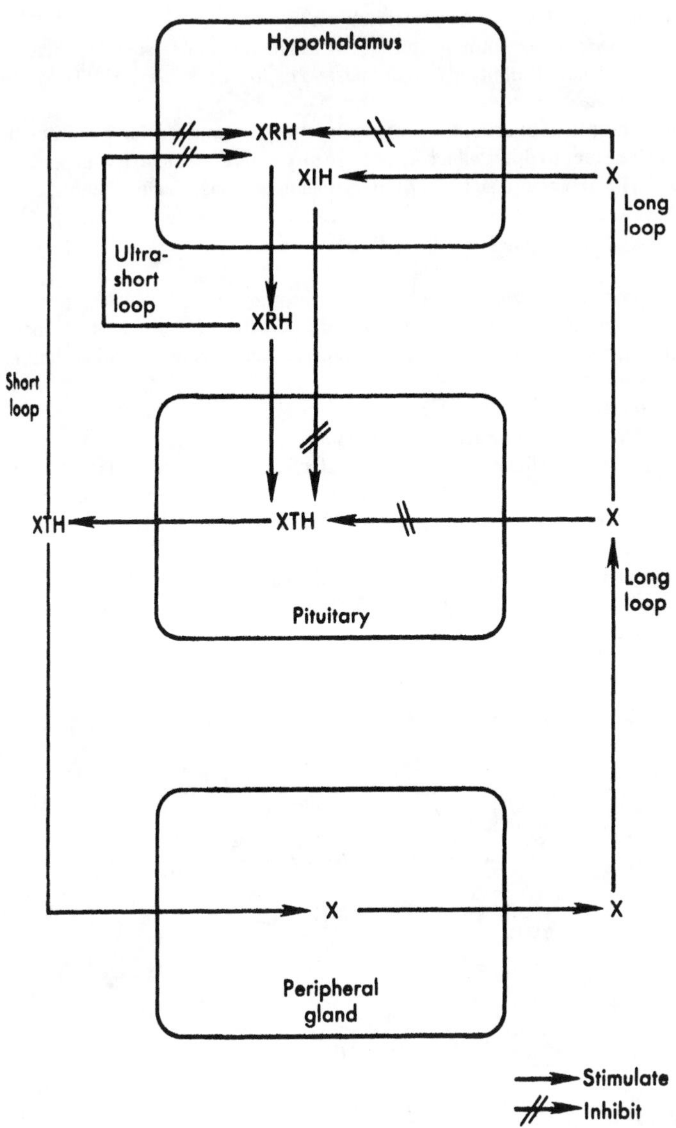

Classic feedforward and feedback regulation of anterior pituitary hormone secretion. Release (XRH) or inhibitory (XIH) hypothalamic hormones access the anterior pituitary via portal veins and either stimulate or inhibit the release of a pituitary tropic hormone (XTH). XTH then acts at target gland to stimulate peripheral gland hormone (X). X inhibits XTH either directly or by inhibiting XRH or stimulated XIH (long-loop negative feedback). XTH may inhibit XRH or stimulate XIH (short-loop negative feedback). It has even been suggested that XRH can inhibit itself (ultrashort-loop negative feedback). (From Genuth SM: The endocrine system. In Berne RM, Levy MN (eds): Physiology, 3rd ed. St. Louis, Mosby, 1993, with permission.)

18. Define hypopituitarism.

Hypopituitarism is a decrease in anterior pituitary function (although posterior pituitary function can be decreased).

19. What is meant by isolated hypopituitarism?

Only one or two anterior hormones are absent. Examples of these are GH deficiency (dwarfism) gonadotropin deficiency (Kallmann's syndrome, anorexia), and isolated ACTH deficiency.

20. Give an example of overactivity (hyperfunction) of an anterior pituitary hormone.

Tumors of the **lactotrophs,** which synthesize prolactin, can lead to **hyperprolactinemia.** This can suppress LH-FSH release and lead to hypogonadism in males and amenorrhea in females.

POSTERIOR PITUITARY—VASOPRESSIN

21. What is arginine vasopressin (AVP)?

AVP is a neurohormone synthesized and released from nerves. It is a nonapeptide with a disulfide bond between amino acids 1 and 6, which creates a ring and tail structure. Its structure is similar to oxytocin (see question 4).

22. Why is AVP also called antidiuretic hormone?

The two names describe both of its major effects. It is a potent vasoconstrictor, hence **vasopressin.** At even lower plasma concentrations, it increases passive water reabsorption in the renal collecting ducts, hence the name **antidiuretic** because its effect leads to a concentrated urine.

23. Are there any other prominent actions of AVP?

AVP appears to have effects within the central nervous system to improve memory, may be involved in blood clotting, and is well known to potentiate the effects of CRH on ACTH release (a hypophysiotropic effect).

24. Describe the control of AVP. (See figure.)

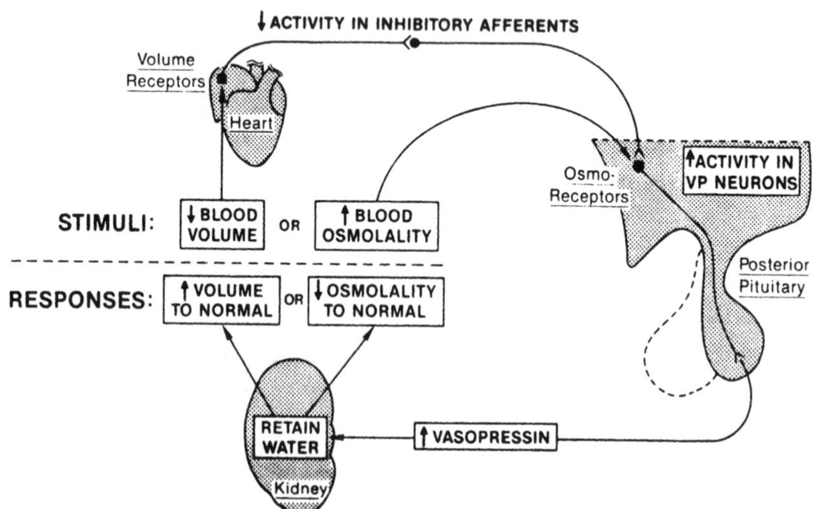

The two major vasopressin control loops. An increase in the osmolality of the blood stimulates vasopressin release, which increases renal passive water reabsorption (retaining the plasma solvent). A decrease in blood volume stimulates vasopressin release via low-pressure baroreceptors in the heart, which increase plasma volume by increasing renal water reabsorption. Although not shown, an increase in osmolality also increases thirst, thereby increasing solvent intake. (From Hedge GA, Colby HD, Goodman RL: Clinical Endocrine Physiology. Philadelphia, W.B. Saunders, 1987, with permission.)

Osmolar control loop: An increase in osmolality is sensed by **osmoreceptors** located in the portion of the anterior hypothalamus devoid of a blood-brain barrier. This allows these neural structures to sense small changes in plasma osmolality (usually plasma sodium). A signal from the osmoreceptor has input to the magnocellular vasopressin neurons located primarily in the supraoptic (SON) and lateral paraventricular nuclei (PVN) of the hypothalamus. These neurons have long axons that terminate on capillaries in the posterior pituitary, which, when depolarized, release AVP into the posterior pituitary capillaries, which drain into the systemic circulation. AVP increases passive water reabsorption in the kidney, helping to dilute the increase in plasma osmolality. AVP does *not* create new water; it just prevents the loss of water from the kidney. Hyperosmolality-induced increases in osmoreceptor activity also stimulate thirst.

Nonosmotic stimuli:

- **Blood volume control loop:** A small decrease in blood volume is sensed by low-pressure baroreceptors in the heart as a decrease in end-diastolic volume/pressure/wall stretch. Input from these afferent receptors to the hypothalamus (via a decrease in activity of inhibitory afferents), results in an increase in vasopressin, which increases water reabsorption, and a relative increase in plasma volume.
- **Others:** Arterial hypotension (via baroreceptors), hypercapnia (via central and peripheral chemoreceptors), hypoxia (via arterial chemoreceptors), pain (via nociception), and nausea all increase the release of vasopressin.

25. Define diabetes insipidus.

Diabetes (siphon/excess urine) insipidus (tasteless/hypo-osmotic) is a state of excess free water excretion (polyuria/hypo-osmotic urine) caused by either the lack of AVP or the inability of the kidney to respond to AVP. It is therefore a nonosmotic diuresis (as opposed to diabetes mellitus).

26. What are the types of diabetes insipidus?

Central (pituitary; neurogenic) diabetes insipidus is due to the total or partial loss of the ability to synthesize or release AVP. This results in an inability to concentrate the urine. The loss of free water leads to an increase in plasma osmolality. The hyperosmolality cannot increase AVP sufficiently but usually results in a large increase in thirst. In many patients with central diabetes insipidus, the patient has high water intake and output but can usually maintain a relatively normal plasma osmolality (normonatremia). It is only when water intake is restricted that the severe hyperosmolality becomes apparent.

Nephrogenic (renal) diabetes insipidus is due to the inability of the kidney to respond to vasopressin. Hyperosmolality (hypernatremia) also ensues, and vasopressin is elevated, but the kidney cannot respond appropriately.

27. Is there a disease of vasopressin excess?

The **syndrome of inappropriate antidiuretic hormone (SIADH)** is the overproduction of vasopressin not accounted for by hyperosmolality or nonosmotic stimuli to vasopressin (e.g., pain, nausea). The overproduction of vasopressin (usually from a pulmonary neoplasm) results in excess water reabsorption, an expansion of plasma volume (hypo-osmolality), and hyponatremia (low plasma sodium).

ADRENAL GLAND

28. Describe the functional zonation of the adrenal gland.

The adrenal gland is composed of layers:

- The outermost layer is the capsule.
- The next layer is the adrenal cortex, which constitutes approximately 90% of the mass of the adrenal gland and synthesizes steroid hormones.
- The innermost layer, the core of the adrenal gland, is the medulla, which is controlled primarily by the autonomic nervous system and secretes catecholamines.

ADRENAL CORTEX

29. Describe the histology of the adrenal cortex.

This is a classic example of functional zonation. The outermost zone is the **zona glomerulosa,** which synthesizes and releases the mineralocorticoid **aldosterone.** Next is the **zona fasciculata,** whose primary secretory product is the glucocorticoid **cortisol.** The innermost zone is the **zona reticularis,** whose primary secretory product is the adrenal androgen **dehydroepiandrosterone** (DHEA). The zonae fasciculata and reticularis are often considered together because they both secrete cortisol and DHEA to some degree.

30. Diagram the synthetic pathway for the adrenal steroids.

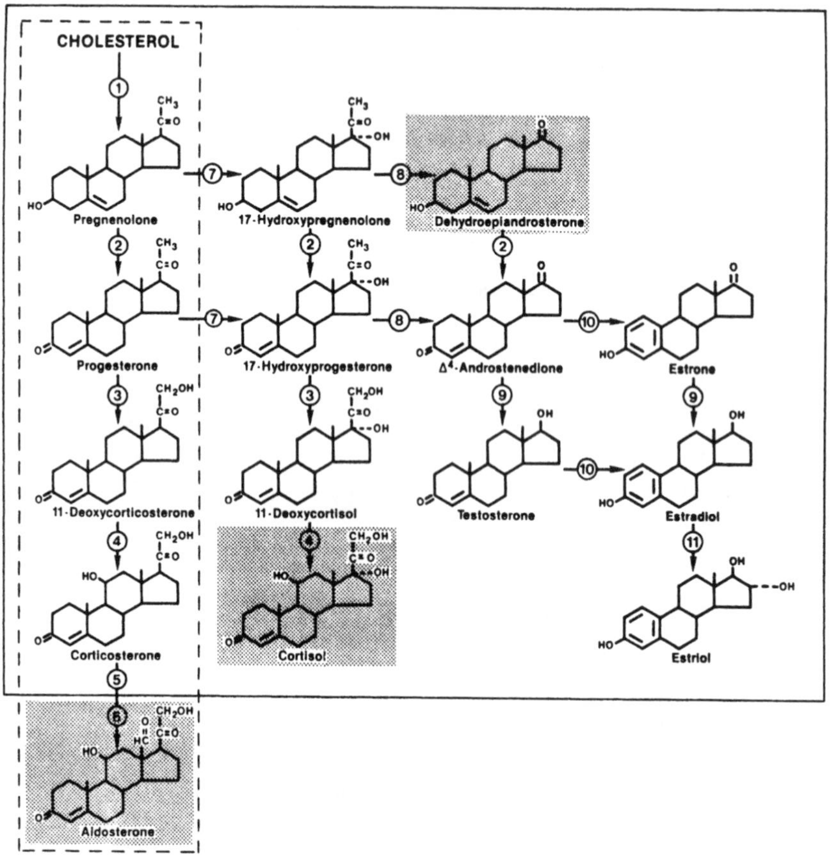

Steroidogenic pathways in the zona glomerulosa (dotted lines) that produce aldosterone and the zona fasciculata-reticularis (solid lines) that produce cortisol and adrenal androgens. Major secretory products are shaded. (From Hedge GA, Colby HD, Goodman RL: Clinical Endocrine Physiology. Philadelphia, W.B. Saunders, 1987, with permission.)

Enzymes (abbreviation/gene name) keyed by number to the figure above:

1. Side-chain cleavage (P450scc/*CYP11A1*). Rate-limiting step is cholesterol transport into the mitochondria
2. 3β-Hydroxysteroid dehydrogenase (3β-HSD/*HSD3B*)

3. 21-Hydroxylase (P450c21/*CYP21*)
4. 11β-Hydroxylase (P450c11β/*CYP11B1*) in zona fasciculata (*solid box*)

4–6. Aldosterone synthase (P450c11AS/*CYP11B2*) in the zona glomerulosa (*dotted box*). The zona fasciculata/reticularis does not produce aldosterone under normal conditions.

7. 17α-Hydroxylase (P450c17/*CYP17*) in the zona fasciculata and reticularis only (zona glomerulosa does not produce cortisol)
8. 17,20 Lyase (P450c17/*CYP17*). Steps 7 and 8 are catalyzed by same enzyme. Step 8 is required for steroid to enter the androgen and estrogen pathways.
9. 17-Hydroxysteroid dehydrogenase (17OHSD)
10. Aromatase (P450aro/*CYP19*)
11. 16α-Hydroxylase

31. What is the primary controller of cortisol synthesis?

ACTH from the pituitary gland increases the synthesis of cortisol acutely and maintains adrenocortical size and function chronically. ACTH binds to a specific cell surface receptor, which, via a guanine nucleotide-binding (G) protein, stimulates adenylate cyclase activity. This leads to an increase in cAMP, which stimulates protein kinase A. This leads to an increase in cholesterol transport from the cytosol into the mitochondria, where the first enzyme–side chain cleavage (P450scc) is located. Therefore, the rate-limiting step of steroidogenesis is cholesterol transport into the mitochondria.

32. What is the primary controller of aldosterone synthesis?

The control of aldosterone synthesis involves multiple stimulatory and inhibitory secretagogues. Classically, angiotensin II (Ang II) is used as a model secretagogue for aldosterone. Ang II binds to its receptor on the zona glomerulosa cell, which, via a G protein, activates phospholipase C. Phospholipase C catalyzes the production of the second messengers IP_3 and DAG, which directly (and indirectly by activating release of intracellular calcium) activates cholesterol transport into the mitochondria.

33. Are cortisol and aldosterone the most potent glucocorticoid and mineralocorticoid?

They are the most potent **endogenous** steroids of their class. There are several more potent synthetic steroids, such as the glucocorticoids dexamethasone, prednisone, and triamcinolone and the mineralocorticoid 9α-fluorocortisol. Furthermore, some intermediates of endogenous steroidogenesis have biologic activity, such as corticosterone (both glucocorticoid and mineralocorticoid activity) and deoxycorticosterone (mostly mineralocorticoid activity). The latter can cause hypertension in P450c11β deficiency.

34. How are adrenal steroids transported in the blood?

Steroids circulate in the free (dissolved) form and bind to carrier proteins. The free and bound plasma steroid compartments are in equilibrium. In the case of cortisol, about 95% circulates in the bound form primarily to corticosteroid-binding globulin (CBG), a high-affinity, low-capacity carrier, and albumin, a low-affinity, high-capacity carrier. The **free form** is biologically active and is available for metabolism.

35. List the physiologic effects of cortisol.

Central nervous system	Suppresses CRH and AVP Increases food intake
Cardiovascular system	Maintains ability to respond to vasoconstrictors
Liver	Increases gluconeogenesis (glucose synthesis)
Lungs	Necessary for lung maturation and surfactant production in the fetus
Pituitary	Inhibits ACTH synthesis and secretion
Kidney	Increases glomerular filtration rate

Bone	Increases resorption/decreases formation
Muscle	Increases protein catabolism (increase in gluconeogenic precursors)
	Decreases insulin sensitivity (decrease in glucose uptake)
Immune system	Immunosuppressive (pharmacologic?)
Connective tissue	Decreases fibroblast activity and collagen synthesis

It is well known that cortisol deficiency is a lethal disorder that must be treated promptly. The exact biologic reason for this is not known, although it is presumed that the ability to maintain blood pressure and volume is the main factor. Some of the effects above are probably relevant only when the hormone is used in pharmacologic doses.

36. Why is cortisol called a glucocorticoid?

One of the long-term effects of cortisol is to increase blood glucose (hyperglycemia). It does this in two general ways: First, cortisol leads to an increase in glucose production in the liver (gluconeogenesis). The liver uses amino acids from muscle and glycerol from fat as gluconeogenic precursors, so, in that sense, cortisol is catabolic. Second, cortisol prevents insulin-mediated glucose uptake in muscle and fat, which prevents glucose from leaving the plasma compartment. The combination of increased gluconeogenesis and decreased insulin-stimulated glucose uptake leads to hyperglycemia. This is thought to be an important mechanism in maintaining plasma glucose levels during a prolonged fast.

37. How is ACTH synthesized?

ACTH is synthesized in pituitary corticotrophs as part of a large precursor molecule, POMC. Posttranslational processing of POMC produces big (22 kilodaltons) ACTH, from which ACTH is produced. POMC is also the precursor for β-LPH, which is further cleaved to γ-LPH and β-endorphin. ACTH contains within it the MSH sequence; hence, when plasma ACTH levels are high (e.g., primary adrenal insufficiency, Nelson's syndrome), skin darkening can occur.

38. Draw the overall control of cortisol secretion.

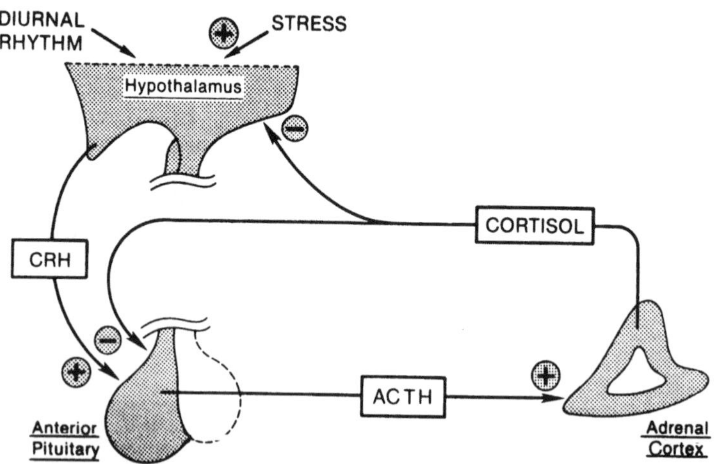

Regulation of the hypothalamic-pituitary-adrenal (HPA) axis. + indicates that stress stimulates CRH, that CRH stimulates ACTH, and that ACTH stimulates cortisol (feedforward control). − indicates that cortisol inhibits CRH and ACTH release (negative feedback). (From Hedge GA, Colby HD, Goodman RL: Clinical Endocrine Physiology. Philadelphia, W.B. Saunders, 1987, with permission.)

39. Describe the four main elements of the HPA axis.

1. **Neural input into the hypothalamus:** The parvocellular CRH neurons are located primarily in the medial paraventricular neurons. They receive input from a variety of sources, including nociceptive pathways (e.g., pain, burn), limbic system (e.g., anxiety), and other hypothalamic nuclei (e.g., circadian rhythm, hunger, hypoglycemia), and via afferents from the nucleus of the tractus solitarius in the brain stem (hypotension, hypoxia).

2. **CRH** released into the portal circulation stimulates ACTH release.

3. **ACTH** released from the pituitary into the systemic circulation acutely stimulates cortisol synthesis and release. Long-term elevations in ACTH cause adrenal hypertrophy. Conversely, long-term suppression of ACTH (secondary adrenal insufficiency, corticosteroid therapy) leads to adrenal atrophy.

4. **Negative feedback:** Cortisol released from the adrenal gland exerts a variety of systemic effects. In addition, it limits its own release by inhibiting the ACTH sensitivity to CRH (at the pituitary), inhibiting CRH release (at the hypothalamus), and inhibiting input into the hypothalamus (e.g., via the limbic system).

40. Describe the circadian variation in cortisol.

In most humans with a diurnal lifestyle (awake during the day/asleep at night), cortisol peaks at or around 8 A.M. and is at its lowest at around midnight. The increase in cortisol early in the morning may be partly due to the overnight fast during sleeping. This pattern is shifted in humans with consistently nocturnal lifestyles (e.g., third-shift workers).

41. Can one classify the stimuli to the HPA axis?

The general term used to describe these stimuli is **stress.** Stress is difficult to define but can generally be divided into two categories: **neurogenic** (e.g., anxiety, pain, psychological disturbances) and **systemic** (hypotension, hypoglycemia, hypoxia). These categories are arbitrary, and it is often difficult to predict the magnitude of the ACTH response to specific stimuli.

42. Outline the general disorders of the HPA axis.

A. Adrenocortical insufficiency (not enough cortisol)
   1. Primary (loss of adrenal function; e.g., Addison's disease)
   2. Secondary (atrophy of adrenal gland as a result of long-term suppression of ACTH)

B. Cushing's syndrome (glucocorticoid excess)
   1. ACTH-dependent (ACTH induces hypertrophy of adrenal gland)
      a. Cushing's disease (pituitary source of ACTH usually from a microadenoma)
      b. Ectopic ACTH syndrome (nonpituitary source of ACTH; usually from a neoplasm)
   2. ACTH-independent
      a. Adrenal (autonomous secretion from adrenal adenoma or carcinoma)
      b. Iatrogenic/factitious (pharmacologic glucocorticoid therapy)

C. Adrenocortical enzyme deficiencies—congenital adrenal hyperplasia (CAH)
   1. 21-Hydroxylase (virilizing; salt wasting)
   2. 11β-Hydroxylase (hypertension)
   3. 3β-HSD (salt wasting)
   4. 17α-Hydroxylase (hypertension)

43. What are the most common symptoms of primary adrenal insufficiency?

Weakness	Weight loss
Fatigue	Hyperpigmentation
Anorexia	Hypotension

44. What is the cause of adrenal insufficiency?

Primary adrenal insufficiency is usually caused by an autoimmune destruction or by tuberculosis of the adrenal gland. **Secondary adrenal insufficiency** is usually caused by hypopituitarism. Abrupt withdrawal of long-term exogenous glucocorticoid therapy also leads to secondary adrenal insufficiency because of suppression of the HPA axis (negative feedback).

45. How is the diagnosis of adrenal insufficiency made?

If suspected, a rapid ACTH (cosyntropin) test is performed. If the patient has primary adrenal insufficiency, the cortisol response to exogenous ACTH is low. If the patient has **significant** secondary adrenal insufficiency, the cortisol response to exogenous ACTH is low because of adrenal atrophy owing to long-term loss of tropic action of ACTH. To differentiate between primary and secondary adrenal insufficiency, measurement of plasma ACTH is usually sufficient (ACTH elevated in primary; low or normal in secondary).

The fact that ACTH can be within the normal (reference) range in secondary adrenal insufficiency is an **extremely important** concept that has implications in other consequences of hypopituitarism (e.g., hypogonadotropic hypogonadism, secondary hypothyroidism). The best way to think about it is that if cortisol were low in a normal person, ACTH should be elevated. The fact that the ACTH **is not elevated** means that it is inappropriately low for the low cortisol and that there is something wrong with the hypothalamus, pituitary, or both.

46. What are the general symptoms of Cushing's syndrome (glucocorticoid excess)?

- Obesity (truncal distribution)
- Facial plethora (red cheeks) and moon face
- Hirsutism
- Hypertension (owing to mineralocorticoid action of cortisol)
- Myopathy (muscle weakness)
- Striae (purple stripes on the abdomen because of skin thinning and stretching and easy bruisability)
- Psychological symptoms (usually depression)

47. How does one screen patients to make the diagnosis of spontaneous Cushing's syndrome, and distinguish between ACTH-dependent and independent Cushing's?

One or more of the following is usually found in patients with any form of Cushing's syndrome:

- A 24-hour collection of urine for cortisol is elevated (index of adrenal secretion of cortisol).
- Bedtime salivary cortisol is elevated (due to loss of circadian rhythm; salivary cortisol reflects free [bioactive] plasma cortisol).
- A low dose of dexamethasone given at bedtime indicates that plasma cortisol not fully suppressed in Cushing's syndrome (test of negative feedback).

To distinguish ACTH-dependent from ACTH-independent Cushing's syndrome, the measurement of plasma ACTH by immunometric assay is *usually* sufficient. It is low in ACTH-independent Cushing's syndrome (because of cortisol feedback on a normal pituitary) and within or above the normal range in ACTH-dependent Cushing's syndrome. The logic here is similar to that for the normal ACTH in secondary adrenal insufficiency. Pituitary adenomas used to be normal corticotrophs and retain some responsiveness (albeit diminished) to glucocorticoid feedback. Therefore, although within the normal range, ACTH is inappropriately elevated for the increase in cortisol.

48. Is there a simple way to distinguish between Cushing's disease (pituitary) and ectopic ACTH?

Sometimes it is obvious (big pituitary tumor by magnetic resonance imaging or a lung tumor on radiograph). Occult (radiologically hidden) pituitary and ectopic ACTH-secreting tumors, however, are common. Biochemical testing (e.g., different doses of dexamethasone) is notoriously inaccurate. The only method with sufficient precision involves the measurement of ACTH in the venous outflow from the pituitary (i.e., in the petrosal sinuses) in response to stimulation with exogenous CRH.

49. What is the logic behind the dexamethasone suppression test?

This test was originally designed to diagnose Cushing's syndrome (hypercortisolism). The logic is that a corticotroph adenoma, although arising from a normal corticotroph cell and expressing the glucocorticoid receptor, has lost sensitivity to cortisol negative feedback. Therefore, low doses of dexamethasone (e.g., 1 mg at bedtime) suppress ACTH and cortisol release in normal subjects but do not suppress cortisol release in patients with any form of Cushing's syndrome. Some ACTH-secreting pituitary adenomas express sufficient glucocorticoid receptor function to exhibit suppression even with low doses of dexamethasone.

This test has also been modified to attempt to differentiate pituitary from ectopic ACTH-dependent Cushing's syndrome. A higher dose of dexamethasone (e.g., 8 mg at bedtime) is used. The logic is that ACTH-secreting pituitary adenomas (Cushing's disease), because they arose from normal corticotrophs and express some glucocorticoid receptor function, diminish ACTH secretion if enough dexamethasone is used. In contrast, ectopic tumors, which did not arise from pituitary corticotrophs, do not express glucocorticoid receptors linked to ACTH secretion. This method also lacks precision because not all pituitary corticotrophs suppress ACTH secretion with high-dose dexamethasone, and some ectopic tumors suppress ACTH secretion with dexamethasone. Therefore, although still widely used, the dexamethasone suppression test lacks sensitivity and specificity and is used with caution.

50. What is congenital adrenal hyperplasia?

Congenital adrenal hyperplasia is caused by a mutation (usually inherited) in a gene for a steroidogenic enzyme leading to a defect (usually partial) in a step of the steroidogenic pathway. In general, the fetal adrenal cannot synthesize adequate cortisol, and the loss of negative feedback inhibition leads to an increase in ACTH. This drives the adrenal to hypertrophy and increases the activity of the enzymes before the enzyme step that is blocked.

51. Describe the consequences of the most common enzyme deficiency, 21-hydroxylase deficiency.

Because 17-OH-progesterone cannot be converted to 11-deoxycortisol (cortisol pathway) *and* progesterone cannot be converted to 11-deoxycorticosterone (aldosterone pathway), both cortisol and aldosterone are deficient. The elevation of ACTH increases production of the precursors, which can be converted to androgens. The excess androgens cause virilization in girls and can lead to ambiguous genitalia in XX fetuses (not sure if phenotype is girl or boy). These children can be salt wasting because of a deficiency in mineralocorticoid production.

52. Why do some inherited enzyme deficiencies cause salt retention and hypertension?

The best example is 11β-hydroxylase deficiency. Because cortisol synthesis is impaired, ACTH is elevated, which drives steroidogenesis and increases production of the precursor to cortisol, 11-deoxycortisol, and the precursor to corticosterone, 11-deoxycorticosterone. Although a weaker mineralocorticoid than aldosterone, 11-deoxycorticosterone has sufficient mineralocorticoid when elevated to increase renal sodium reabsorption and cause hypertension.

53. List the major controllers of aldosterone secretion.

Stimulatory	***Inhibitory***
Ang II	Plasma sodium
ACTH (acutely)	ACTH (chronically)
Plasma potassium	Atrial natriuretic peptide

54. Describe the control of plasma Ang II concentration.

Renin release from the kidney is stimulated by a decrease in plasma sodium and a decrease in extracellular fluid volume, blood volume, and blood pressure. Renin catalyzes the cleavage of Ang II from the substrate angiotensinogen (see figure, top of next page). Angiotensin I is converted to Ang II by the angiotensin-converting enzyme (ACE). Ang II also directly inhibits renin secretion (negative feedback; not shown in figure).

55. How does aldosterone help to prevent increases in plasma potassium (hyperkalemia)?

An increase in plasma potassium directly stimulates aldosterone synthesis and secretion from the adrenal zona glomerulosa. An increase in aldosterone stimulates renal potassium excretion, thereby lowering plasma potassium.

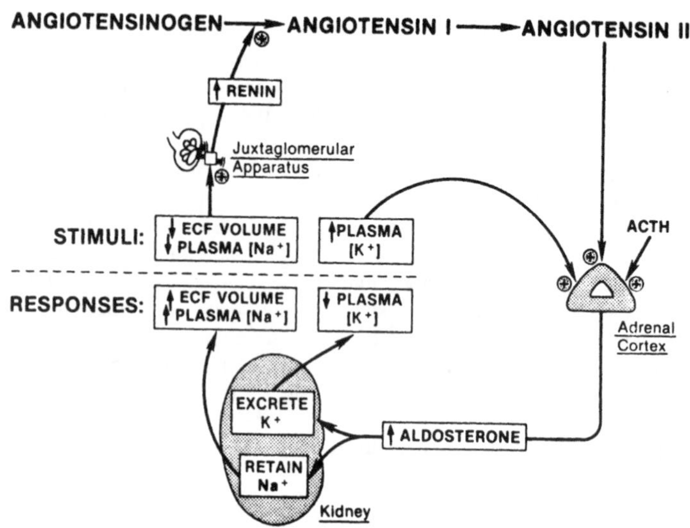

Highly simplified version of the renin-angiotensin-aldosterone system. + indicates that renin increases the conversion of angiotensinogen to angiotensin I and that plasma potassium and Ang II directly stimulate aldosterone release. ACTH is a potent acute stimulator of aldosterone release, but this effect wanes after several days. Notice that plasma potassium forms its own feedback loop independent of the renin-angiotensin system. Not shown is that the conversion of angiotensin I to Ang II is catalyzed by ACE. (From Hedge GA, Colby HD, Goodman RL: Clinical Endocrine Physiology. Philadelphia, W.B. Saunders, 1987, with permission.)

56. What are the other major renal effects of aldosterone?

Aldosterone is called a mineralocorticoid mainly because it increases reabsorption of sodium in the kidney. Therefore, when sodium intake is low, renin secretion is increased, which leads to an increase in plasma Ang II, which stimulates aldosterone secretion. Aldosterone increases sodium reabsorption to restore plasma sodium to normal.

57. List the major disorders of aldosterone production.

Hypoaldosteronism

- Primary (loss of zona glomerulosa function; e.g., Addison's disease)
- Secondary (hyporeninemic hypoaldosteronism; loss of renin secretion from the kidney)

Hyperaldosteronism

- Primary (hyporeninemic): usually caused by a solitary adrenal adenoma (Conn's syndrome) or nodular adrenal hyperplasia
- Secondary (hyperreninemic): usually caused by renal artery stenosis such that the perfusion pressure in the kidney is decreased and the intrarenal baroreceptor stimulates renin release

58. How does one make the biochemical diagnosis of primary hyperaldosteronism?

An increased ratio of plasma aldosterone to plasma renin activity, especially in the presence of hypokalemia (which usually decreases aldosterone secretion) with the appropriate clinical symptoms (e.g., hypertension), suggests an autonomous production of aldosterone.

ADRENAL MEDULLA

59. Why is the adrenal medulla analogous to a postganglionic sympathetic neuron?

The adrenal medulla is derived from neuroectoderm, is innervated by preganglionic sympathetic neurons, and synthesizes and releases catecholamines.

60. Describe the synthesis of adrenal catecholamines.

The relevant cells in the adrenal medulla are called chromaffin cells because they contain storage granules. These cells convert tyrosine to dihydroxyphenylalanine (DOPA) by the regulated enzyme tyrosine hydroxylase. DOPA is converted to dopamine. Dopamine is converted to norepinephrine by the enzyme dopamine-β-hydroxylase. Norepinephrine is converted to epinephrine by phenylethanolamine-*N*-methyltransferase (PNMT).

61. Which of these enzymatic steps are regulated?

The major regulated step is tyrosine hydroxylase, which is inhibited by the products of the pathway (end-product inhibition). Although somewhat controversial, it is also thought the PNMT activity in the adrenal medulla is increased by cortisol release from the adrenal cortex via a paracrine action within the adrenal gland.

62. What are the major effects of catecholamines, and what adrenergic receptor mediates these effects?

Responses of Target Tissues to Catecholamines

TARGET TISSUE	RECEPTOR TYPE	RESPONSE
Liver	β_2	Glycogenolysis, lipolysis, gluconeogenesis
Adipose tissue	β_2	Lipolysis
Skeletal muscle	β_2	Glycogenolysis
Pancreas	α_2	Decreased insulin secretion
	β_2	Increased insulin secretion
Cardiovascular system	β_1	Increased heart rate, increased contractility, increased conduction velocity
	α	Vasoconstriction
	β_2	Vasodilation in skeletal muscle arterioles, coronary arteries, and all veins
Bronchial muscle	β_2	Relaxation
Gastrointestinal tract	β_2	Decreased contractility
	α	Sphincter contraction
Urinary bladder	α	Sphincter contraction
	β_2	Detrusor relaxation
Uterus	α	Contraction
	β_2	Relaxation
Male sex organs	α	Ejaculation, detumescence
	β_2	Erection?
Eye	α_1	Radial muscle contraction
	β_2	Ciliary muscle relaxation
Central nervous system	α	Stimulation
Skin	α	Piloerection, sweat production
Renin secretion	β_1	Stimulation

Adapted from Hedges GA, Colby HD, Goodman RL: Clinical Endocrine Physiology. Philadelphia, W.B. Saunders, 1987.

63. What are the primary stimuli to catecholamine secretion?

- Hypoglycemia
- Trauma
- Hemorrhage
- Illness
- Hypoxia
- Cold exposure

64. Is there a disease of the adrenal medulla?

The best appreciated is pheochromocytoma, which is a catecholamine-secreting tumor. These tumors are usually located within the adrenal gland but can be extra-adrenal (along the sympathetic chain).

65. What are the most common symptoms of pheochromocytoma?

Hypertension
Headache
Excessive perspiration
Palpitations

Absence of all four of these symptoms virtually excludes pheochromocytoma.

THYROID PHYSIOLOGY

66. Describe the functional anatomy of the thyroid gland.

- **Follicles:** formed by cells that synthesize, store (extracellularly), and secrete thyroid hormone
- **Colloid:** central space in the follicle where thyroid hormone is stored as a component of thyroglobulin
- **Parafollicular (C) cells:** synthesize and secrete the hormone calcitonin

67. What are the main thyroid hormones?

- $\mathbf{T_4}$ (3,5,3′,5′-tetraiodo-L-thyronine) is the main secretory product of the thyroid gland.
- $\mathbf{T_3}$ (3,5,3′-triiodo-L-thyronine) can also be produced by the thyroid gland. Most T_3 is produced by monodeiodination of T_4 in peripheral tissue including target cells. Because T_3 is significantly more potent than T_4, T_4 can be considered a circulating prohormone.
- **Reverse** $\mathbf{T_3}$ (3,3′,5′-triiodothyronine) is found in the blood, although little if any is secreted by the thyroid. This hormone is essentially devoid of biologic activity and is produced primarily by peripheral monodeiodination of T_4.

68. What is the source of the iodine used by the thyroid gland to synthesize thyroid hormone?

Organic iodine or inorganic iodide (food supplement) in the diet is absorbed into the blood from the gastrointestinal tract. The follicular cell has an iodide (ionic form of iodine) pump, which traps iodine within the thyroid gland.

69. Describe the synthesis of thyroid hormone.

1. Trapping of iodide—iodide [I^-] pumped from the plasma to the intracellular compartment.
2. Oxidation and organification of iodide (on colloidal side of follicular cell). This is probably the conversion of I^- to I^0 and is catalyzed by the enzyme thyroperoxidase. I^0 is highly reactive and binds quickly to the ring of a tyrosyl residue of thyroglobulin (see later).
3. Exocytosis of thyroglobulin, which has been synthesized within the cell, into follicular lumen.
4. Iodination of tyrosine residues within thyroglobulin. This occurs within the **follicular lumen** and is therefore an extracellular reaction. If one carbon of the tyrosine ring is iodinated, this results in 3-monoiodotyrosine (MIT). If two carbons of the tyrosine ring are iodinated, this results in 3,5 diiodotyrosine (DIT).
5. Coupling of iodotyrosines (**on thyroglobulin molecule**) occurs when MIT and DIT come in contact while still part of the thyroglobulin molecule. If MIT and DIT are coupled, T_3 results. If DIT and DIT are coupled, T_4 results.
6. Endocytosis of thyroglobulin-containing thyroid hormone. If thyroid hormone is needed systemically, TSH from the pituitary is increased and stimulates recovery of thyroglobulin from its storage space in the colloid.

7. Proteolysis of thyroglobulin. The liberation of T_4 and T_3 from thyroglobulin occurs intracellularly.
8. Selective release of T_3 and T_4 from the intracellular to the plasma compartment.
9. Deiodination of MIT and DIT such that iodide and tyrosine can be recycled.

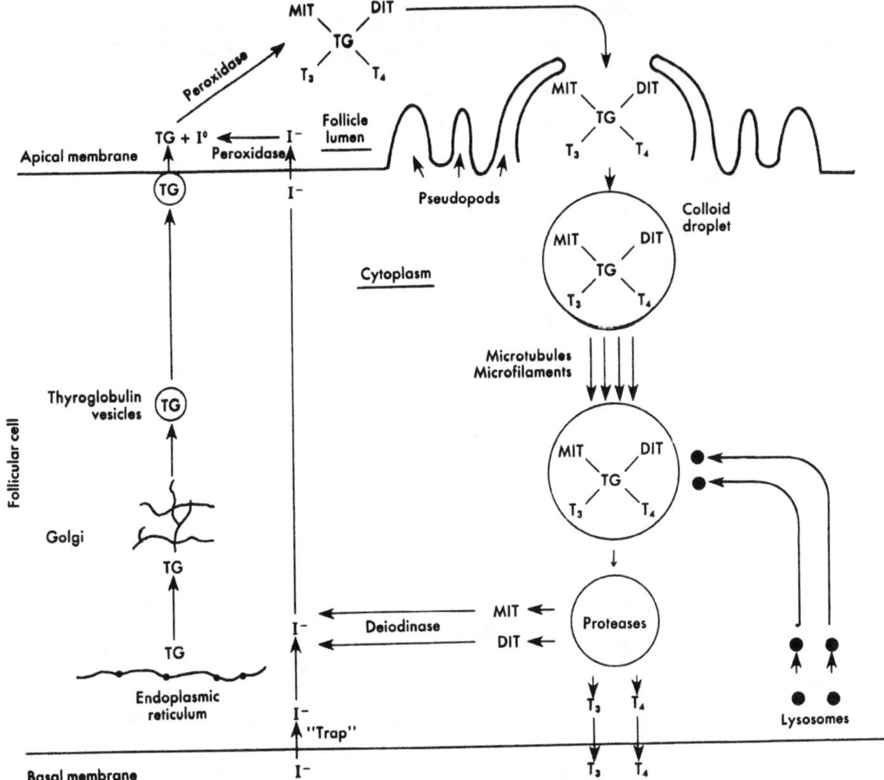

Thyroid hormone biosynthesis and secretion. Notice that iodination (iodide incorporation) of tyrosine and synthesis and storage of thyroid hormone as a component of thyroglobulin (TG) occur extracellularly (in the follicular lumen [colloid]). For detailed description of each step, see text. (From Genuth SM: The endocrine system. In Berne RM, Levy MN (eds): Physiology, 3rd ed. St. Louis, Mosby, 1993, with permission.)

70. Why do the thyroid hormones have such a long half-life?

The half-life of T_4 (6 days) and T_3 (1 day) is long primarily because thyroid hormones circulate bound to carrier proteins. T_4 circulates more than 99.9% bound to thyroid-binding globulin (TBG), transthyretin, and albumin. T_3 is slightly less tightly bound (99.7%) and apparently does not bind appreciably to transthyretin. Because little of the total circulating thyroid hormone is free, little is available for metabolism, hence the long half-life.

71. List the systemic effects of thyroid hormones.

- **Metabolism:** increase basal metabolic rate and oxygen consumption (and therefore increase minute ventilation, cardiac output, food intake, carbohydrate metabolism, and heat production)
- **Growth and maturation:** required for normal skeletal growth probably by allowing normal effects of IGF-1 on bone and normal GH secretion

- **Central nervous system:** necessary for perinatal maturation and normal reflexes
- **Autonomic nervous system:** increase sympathetic activity
- **Temperature regulation:** increase thermogenesis

72. How is the circulating thyroid hormone regulated?

The main feedback loop in this system is T_4-T_3 inhibition of TSH and TSH stimulation of T_4-T_3. Although probably not a major mechanism, T_3 and T_4 inhibit TRH secretion. TRH increases the set-point for T_4-T_3 negative feedback.

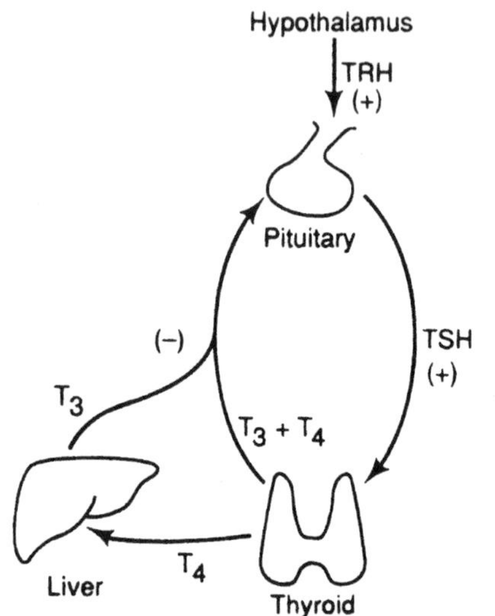

Regulation of the hypothalamic-pituitary axis. + indicates that TRH stimulates TSH and that TSH stimulates thyroid hormone release. T_4 is converted to the more potent T_3 in the liver and target tissue. − indicates that both T_3 and T_4 inhibit TSH release (negative feedback). (From Goodman HM: Basic Medical Endocrinology, 2nd ed. New York, Raven Press, 1994, with permission.)

73. Other than TSH, are there other factors that regulate thyroid function?

- **Thyroid-stimulating immunoglobulins (TSI):** These are antibodies produced under abnormal conditions (e.g., Graves' disease) that are directed against TSH receptors but result in activation by mechanisms similar to TSH.
- **Thyroid nerves:** These may modulate the sensitivity to TSH.
- **Iodine:** Although chronic iodine deficiency leads to a decrease in thyroid hormone and a TSH-mediated increase in thyroid size, an increase in iodine can also decrease thyroid hormone secretion by the paradoxical **Wolff-Chaikoff effect.** This is due to a decrease in the organification of iodide and may be protective against iodine-induced hyperactivity of the thyroid gland. Excess iodine may also decrease the secretion of thyroid hormone possibly by decreasing the sensitivity to TSH.

74. Outline the general disorders of thyroid gland function.

A. Hypothyroidism (too little thyroid hormone)
   1. Primary
      a. Hashimoto's thyroiditis (autoimmune)
      b. Iodine deficiency
   2. Secondary—Hypopituitarism

B. Hyperthyroidism (too much thyroid hormone secretion)
   1. Primary (thyrotoxicosis)
      a. Endogenous (Graves' disease—TSI)
      b. Iatrogenic (overuse of exogenous thyroxine)
   2. Secondary—TSH secreting tumors (very rare)

75. What is a goiter?

A goiter is an enlargement of the thyroid gland. It can be due to **hyperthyroidism** (e.g., TSI in Graves' disease) or **hypothyroidism** (e.g., iodine deficiency causing decreased T_4 production leading to elevated TSH, which induces thyroid hypertrophy).

76. What are the symptoms of hypothyroidism?

Reduced basal metabolic rate	Hoarse voice	Weight gain
Cold intolerance	Fatigue	Constipation
Cool, dry skin	Slow reflexes	Myxedema
Coarse hair	Muscle cramps	

77. Define myxedema.

An infiltration of the skin and subcutaneous tissue with mucopolysaccharides occurs leading to a puffy appearance, usually of the face, hands, and feet.

78. Is there a specific concern if hypothyroidism occurs in the neonate?

Yes, congenital hypothyroidism (cretinism) when untreated is characterized by dwarfism, mental retardation, and a puffy face with protruding tongue. The mental retardation can be prevented or minimized when thyroid hormone is administered in the neonatal period (and continued throughout life). Testing of all newborns for hypothyroidism (elevated TSH) is the standard of care.

79. If a patient is suspected of having hypothyroidism, is there a simple way to distinguish primary thyroid dysfunction from hypopituitarism?

Measurement of TSH using a third-generation supersensitive assay reliably distinguishes primary (elevated TSH) from secondary (normal or low) hypothyroidism.

80. Why can hypopituitarism lead to hypothyroidism if TSH is in the normal range?

As in secondary adrenal insufficiency, this is an **important** concept. If the hypothalamic-pituitary-thyrotroph function were normal, a low circulating T_4 should lead to an elevated TSH. If TSH is **not elevated,** the low thyroid hormone is due to hypothalamic-pituitary dysfunction.

81. How does one assess functional hypothyroidism if most of the circulating thyroid hormone is bound (not biologically active)?

Measure free T_4.

82. Is there a common condition that causes a discrepancy between free and total T_4?

The most common explanation is a change in circulating TBG concentration. For example, in **pregnancy** (or with **estrogen therapy**), TBG is elevated, which increases total T_4. Because the hypothalamic-pituitary system is normal in most pregnant women, once the new binding sites are saturated, free T_4 is properly regulated and maintained within the normal range.

83. List the symptoms of hyperthyroidism.

- Elevated basal metabolic rate
- Heat intolerance
- Warm skin
- Excessive perspiration
- Weight loss (despite an increase in the intake of food)
- Loss of muscle mass
- Hypertension
- Tachycardia (a sympathomimetic effect)
- Exophthalmos (protruding eyeballs; occurs in Graves' disease)

84. Is there a simple method to diagnose hyperthyroidism?

Because TSH-secreting tumors are exceedingly rare, suppressed TSH is used as a screening test. The current TSH assays available can distinguish normal from suppressed TSH, obviating the need for TRH testing.

85. What are the treatment options for patients with Graves' disease?

- Surgical removal of thyroid gland (thyroidectomy)
- Radioactive iodine administration (ablation)
- Interruption of thyroid hormone secretion with drugs (e.g., methimazole [Tapazole])

86. Summarize the thyroid findings in primary hyperthyroidism, primary hypothyroidism and pregnancy.

	NORMAL	HYPERTHYROID	HYPOTHYROID	PREGNANT
Total T_4	N	↑	↓	↑
TBG	N	N	N	↑
Free T_4	N	↑	↓	N
TSH	N	↓	↑	N

87. Discuss the thyroid findings in primary hyperthyroidism.

The main defect is excess secretion of T_4 and hence an increase in total and free T_4. TSH is suppressed in primary hyperthyroidism because of negative feedback inhibition by free T_4.

88. Discuss the thyroid findings in primary hypothyroidism.

The main defect is a failure to produce T_4 normally. Therefore, total and free T_4 are decreased. TSH is increased because of the loss of the negative feedback inhibition by free T_4.

89. Discuss the thyroid findings in pregnancy.

The increase in estrogen during pregnancy is probably due to an increase in TBG synthesis in the liver. (Oral contraceptives can cause a similar effect.) Total T_4 is increased because of an increase in the number of available binding sites on TBG. Assuming normal thyroid and pituitary function, free T_4 and TSH levels are regulated and maintained within the normal range. **Hyperthyroidism** may occur during pregnancy and postpartum, and it is extremely important that true endogenous hyperthyroidism be distinguished from a normal elevation of total T_4 during pregnancy because of an increase in TBG.

ENDOCRINE CONTROL OF GROWTH AND DEVELOPMENT

90. Summarize the hormonal regulation of growth.

Prenatal growth is not well understood. It is thought that insulin or insulin-like factors may be involved because women with increased blood glucose (diabetic hyperglycemia) tend to have larger infants (possibly as a result of fetal hyperinsulinemia). Clearly, other unknown factors influence fetal growth. Hormonal control of growth up to about 1 year of age is also not well understood.

Juvenile growth (from age 1 year to puberty) is thought to be influenced by the GH axis (and its intermediates), thyroid hormone, and insulin. Much of the effect of thyroid hormone appears to be due to its maintenance of normal GH secretion.

Puberty is a time of dramatic changes in growth and development. The increase in sex steroid production (androgens in males and estrogens in females) stimulates the pubertal growth spurt. The major mechanism appears to be sex steroid–induced growth hormone secretion, although many other factors are involved. Sex steroids also terminate the pubertal growth spurt by induction of fusion of the epiphyseal (growth) plates of long bones.

91. Itemize the hormones influencing normal growth.

- **GH** stimulates IGF-1, the major controller of somatic growth.
- **Thyroid hormone** is necessary for normal central nervous system development and for normal action of IGF-1; it stimulates GH secretion.
- **Gonadal steroids** stimulate and terminate pubertal growth spurt. They are necessary for normal GH secretion (particularly androgens).
- **Insulin** stimulates fetal and postnatal growth.
- **Cortisol** inhibits somatic growth by inhibiting GH release and decreasing effects of growth factors on growth plates of bone.

92. Does GH directly increase growth velocity in children?

The current theory is that most of the growth-promoting effects of GH are mediated by **IGF-1.** The synthesis and release of IGF-1 from the liver and its local production in GH-target tissues are stimulated by GH. IGF-1 was originally called sulfation factor because it increased incorporation of chondroitin sulfate into bone. It was then called somatomedin C because it mediates the effects of somatotropin (GH). Because somatomedin C was subsequently found to have sequence homology with insulin, the currently accepted name is IGF-1. IGF-1 circulates in the blood bound to insulin-like growth factor binding proteins (IGFBPs).

93. Describe the control of GH secretion.

Hypothalamic control of GH secretion involves stimulatory and inhibitory hypophysiotropic factors. Neurons in the hypothalamus synthesize GHRH, which stimulates GH release, and somatostatin, which inhibits GH. These neurons receive inputs from higher brain centers and stress pathways much like the HPA axis. An increase in GH secretion can be ascribed to an increase in GHRH release or a decrease in somatostatin release. GH then stimulates IGF-1 release, which can inhibit GH release directly at the pituitary, inhibit GHRH release, or stimulate somatostatin release, each of which is a negative feedback loop. It has been suggested that GH can also act as a negative feedback signal within the hypothalamus.

94. Describe the hypothalamic-pituitary-IGF-1 axis.

The figure at right demonstrates regulation of the hypothalamic-pituitary-IGF-1 axis. Notice that GHRH stimulates (+) whereas somatostatin inhibits (−) release of GH from the pituitary. Multiple feedback loops include inhibition of GHRH, stimulation of somatostatin, or glucose-induced inhibition of GH.

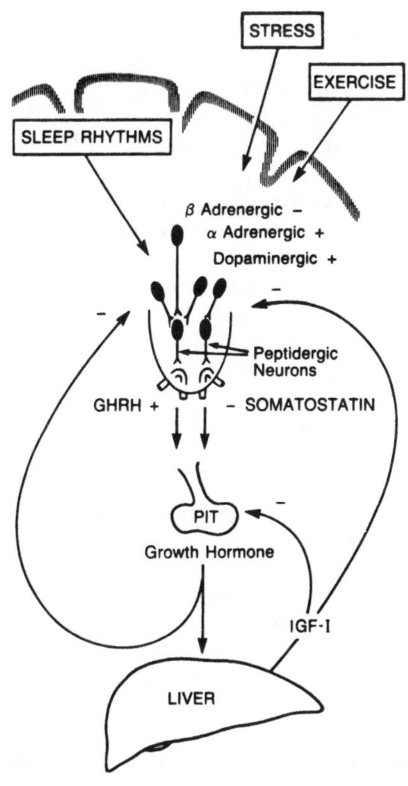

(Modified from Reichlin S: Neuroendocrinology. In Wilson JD, Foster DW, Kronenberg H, Larsen PR (eds): Williams Textbook of Endocrinology, 9th ed. Philadelphia, W.B. Saunders, 1998.)

95. List some potential negative feedback loops.

- GHRH stimulates GH, which inhibits GHRH, which decreases GH.
- GHRH stimulates GH, which stimulates IGF-1, which stimulates somatostatin, which inhibits GH release.
- Somatostatin decreases, which increases GH release, which increases IGF-1, which stimulates somatostatin release, which decreases GH release.

96. What central and systemic factors are involved in the control of GH release?

Stimulation of GH	*Inhibition of GH*
Decrease in plasma glucose (hypoglycemia)	Increase in plasma glucose (hyperglycemia)
Decrease in plasma free fatty acids	Increase in plasma free fatty acids
Increase in amino acids (e.g., arginine)	Cortisol (exogenous or endogenous)
Fasting	Pregnancy
Stage 4 (deep) sleep	
Exercise	

97. Place factors involved in the control of GH release into context.

GH has direct effects on intermediate metabolism. It is a counterregulatory hormone to insulin and stimulates glucose production. Therefore, it makes sense that plasma glucose would inhibit GH release because this forms yet another feedback loop: GH stimulates plasma glucose, which inhibits GH release, *or* a decrease in glucose stimulates GH, which increases plasma glucose.

- Because one of the main effects of GH (via IGF-1) is to increase linear growth, it makes sense that ingestion of the building blocks of protein (amino acids) stimulates GH release.
- Fasting and prolonged caloric deprivation require mobilization of endogenous fuel stores to mobilize glucose and fatty acids.
- GH secretion is stimulated during deep sleep. This is extremely important in children and may be one reason why sleep deprivation may lead to short stature.
- It is well known that endogenous Cushing's syndrome (hypercortisolism) and exogenous glucocorticoid therapy decrease growth velocity in children. Children receiving high doses of potent glucocorticoids (prednisone therapy) for rheumatoid arthritis or to prevent transplant rejection are often much shorter than predicted.

98. Classify the direct biologic actions of GH.

- In **adipose tissue:** GH decreases glucose uptake and increases lipolysis, leading to a decrease in adiposity.
- In **muscle:** GH decreases glucose uptake and increases amino acid uptake and protein synthesis, leading to an increase in lean body mass.
- In the **liver:** GH increases gluconeogenesis (glucose secretion) and increases IGF-1 release.

99. Summarize the direct biologic actions of GH.

Most of the **direct** actions of GH are on intermediate metabolism. GH results in hyperglycemia because of decrease in glucose uptake and increase in glucose production (counteracts effects of insulin). GH also stimulates increase in muscle mass. The net results of these two effects are a decrease in adiposity and increase in muscle mass. This explains the abuse of GH by bodybuilders and competitive athletes. GH may also directly increase epiphyseal growth, although most of this effect is mediated by local production of growth factors (such as IGF-1).

100. What are the direct effects of IGF-1?

IGF-1 stimulates an increase in organ size and function. For example, it ensures that as a child grows rapidly, the heart, lungs, kidneys, and other structures grow as well. IGF-1 also has dramatic effects on the chondrocytes in bone; it increases transcription, protein synthesis, chondroitin sulfate incorporation, and cell size and number, all of which lead to an increase in linear growth.

101. Briefly outline the pattern of linear growth from conception to adulthood.

A. Fetal growth
  1. Peaks at about 4–6 months' gestation
  2. Peaks at as high as 12 cm per month

B. Juvenile growth
  1. Declines from prenatal peak until about 2 years of age
  2. With adequate GH and thyroid hormone levels, continues at a fairly constant rate (about 4–8 cm/year) until the onset of puberty

C. Pubertal growth spurt
  1. Stimulated by increased gonadal steroids (which stimulate GH secretion)
  2. Usually starts at about 10 years of age in girls and 13 years of age in boys
  3. **Variable** between subjects even within the same family
  4. Usually peaks at about 12 years of age in girls and 14–15 years of age in boys
  5. Most females reach adult height by 15–16 years of age and most males by 17–18 years of age
  6. Termination of the pubertal growth spurt caused by gonadal steroid-induced fusion of the epiphyseal (growth) plates of the long bones

102. List the general disorders involving GH.

GH deficiency:
- Hypopituitarism, isolated GH deficiency—leads to short stature in children (dwarfism) and is treated with recombinant human GH injections
- Old age—controversial subject
- GH insensitivity—Laron dwarfism (high GH, low IGF-1)

GH excess—GH-secreting pituitary adenoma:
- Childhood—gigantism
- Postpubertal—acromegaly (acral enlargement, soft tissue overgrowth, insulin resistance leading to hyperglycemia and hyperinsulinemia)

103. Why does GH excess have two different names depending on the age of onset?

Although the cause is the same (almost always a GH-secreting pituitary adenoma), the physical appearance is quite different. GH excess before puberty leads to greatly increased growth velocity and a greatly increased final adult height (**gigantism**). If GH excess commences after pubertal fusion of the epiphyseal plates, linear growth is not restarted and final adult height does not change. **Acromegaly** (from the Greek *akron* ["extremity"] and *megas* ["large"]) is characterized by connective tissue proliferation.

104. List some of the features of acromegaly.

- Soft tissue swelling, particularly in hands and feet
- Skin thickening
- Increased sweating
- Bony changes (cortical thickening, osteophyte proliferation, mandible enlargement leading to a protrusion of the lower jaw [prognathism])
- Nerve entrapment (owing to bone and connective tissue overgrowth)
- Organomegaly (large liver and kidneys)
- Insulin resistance

105. How does one diagnose GH deficiency?

Because of the episodic nature of GH secretion, a single plasma measurement is not particularly helpful. Usually, some kind of stimulation test is performed, such as an arginine infusion or a GHRH infusion, or a sleep study to measure GH during stage 4 sleep.

106. How does one diagnose acromegaly?

Measurement of several elevated plasma IGF-1 levels is probably the most common current approach. Comparison of photographs from different ages is often helpful.

107. What is the treatment for acromegaly?

- Pituitary surgery to remove the GH-secreting tumor
- Treatment with somatostatin analogue
- Radiation therapy of the pituitary

ENDOCRINE PANCREAS

108. Describe the anatomy of the endocrine pancreas.

The pancreas is both an exocrine (secretes digestive enzymes into the gastrointestinal tract) and an endocrine organ. The endocrine component of the pancreas consists of several million clusters (islets) of cells called the **islets of Langerhans.**

109. What are the *major* hormones secreted by the islets and from what cell type?

- **Insulin** is secreted by B cells (also known as β cells)—approximately 75% of islet
- **Glucagon** is secreted by A cells (also known as α cells)
- **Somatostatin** is secreted by D cells (also known as δ cells)

110. What is the major secretory product of the islets of Langerhans, and how is it synthesized?

The protein insulin, the **storage hormone,** is synthesized as a prohormone called **proinsulin.** Posttranslational cleavage of proinsulin produces insulin and C-peptide (connecting). Although C-peptide has minimal, if any, biologic activity, its measurement is generally used as a marker for islet cell function because it is released with insulin.

111. List the major components of intermediate metabolism under endocrine control.

Glucose production	Glycogenolysis (breakdown of glycogen to glucose) Gluconeogenesis (synthesis of new glucose from precursors)
Glucose consumption	Glycolysis (burning of glucose for energy production)
Fat storage	Lipogenesis
Fat breakdown	Lipolysis
Ketone production	Ketogenesis (oxidation of fatty acids to ketone bodies)

112. Categorize the effects of insulin.

Generally, insulin promotes the storage (**anabolic effect**) of circulating sugar, amino acids, and fat *and* prevents the breakdown (**anticatabolic effect**) of these stores.

	ANABOLIC	ANTICATABOLIC
Effect on liver	Increases glycogen storage, synthesis of very low-density lipoproteins (VLDL), glycolysis	Inhibits glycogenolysis, ketogenesis, glucogenesis
Effect on muscle	Increases amino acid uptake and protein synthesis and increases glucose transport and glycogen synthesis	Inhibits glycogen phosphorylase
Effects on fat	Increases glucose uptake and triglyceride storage	Inhibits lipolysis

113. In question 112, why was hepatic glycolysis (glucose consumption) listed as anabolic?

The main effect of insulin within the hepatocyte is to increase glucose uptake and then to store it as efficiently as possible. Therefore, one of the goals of insulin is to maintain free intracellular glucose concentration within the hepatocyte as low as possible. If glucose cannot be stored quickly enough, the hepatocyte has no other option but to burn the glucose (glycolysis). Because this process is linked to glucose uptake, it is considered anabolic.

114. If one had to pick one primary effect of insulin, what would it be?

Insulin increases glucose uptake and leads to a decrease in blood glucose (plasma glucose).

115. How is the release of insulin controlled?

Factors that directly stimulate insulin release:

- Food metabolites (glucose, amino acids, fatty acids, ketones)
- Gastrointestinal hormones (increase sensitivity of B cell to glucose)
- Glucagon
- Acetylcholine

Factors that indirectly increase insulin release:

- Counterregulatory hormones (cortisol and GH induce peripheral resistance to insulin leading to increases in blood glucose [which stimulates insulin release])

Factors that inhibit insulin release:

- Somatostatin (paracrine effect, which may prevent insulin overshoot)
- Catecholamines (epinephrine and norepinephrine)

116. Describe the effects of glucagon.

Glucagon opposes (counterregulates) insulin and is therefore catabolic. The main role of glucagon is to prevent hypoglycemia by stimulating hepatic glycogenolysis and gluconeogenesis Glucagon also promotes the conversion of circulating free fatty acids to ketoacids.

117. Are the factors that regulate glucagon secretion basically the opposite of those that regulate insulin?

Yes, with notable exceptions. Glucose, ketones, and free fatty acids all inhibit glucagon release, as one would expect. Amino acids, however, actually stimulate glucagon release. A way to remember this is to consider a carnivore in the wild. The hyena can ingest up to 30% of its body weight when it eats, for example, a zebra. This represents a huge protein (and potassium) load. As the metabolites of protein digestion (amino acids) are absorbed (without concomitant glucose absorption), massive insulin release would lead to hypoglycemia and, possibly, loss of consciousness. Therefore, amino acid stimulation of glucagon makes sense to counteract the hypoglycemic effect of insulin when consuming a protein meal. Glucagon also increases amino acid uptake in the liver (for gluconeogenesis), so it makes sense that glucagon is stimulated by amino acids.

118. What is the derivation of the name *somatostatin* as it refers to an islet cell hormone?

The 14-amino-acid peptide somatostatin was first identified as a neurohormone in the hypothalamus that inhibits GH (somatotropin) release—hence the name somatostatin. The identical hormone was subsequently identified from the D cells of the islets of Langerhans and found to inhibit both insulin and glucagon release.

119. Describe the hormonal maintenance of blood glucose.

At one end of the spectrum is a state of total glucose consumption (**fed state**), and at the other end is a state of total glucose production (**fasted state**). Insulin and the counterregulatory hormones regulate the balance between glucose consumption and glucose production. In the fed state, insulin is stimulated and promotes glucose uptake in muscle and adipose tissue (storage). In the fasted state, insulin is low, allowing catabolism. Furthermore, the counterregulatory hormones (GH, cortisol, glucagon, and catecholamines) are elevated in the fasted state, which (1) decreases glucose uptake (decreases insulin sensitivity in muscle and fat) and (2) increases hepatic glucose production (gluconeogenesis).

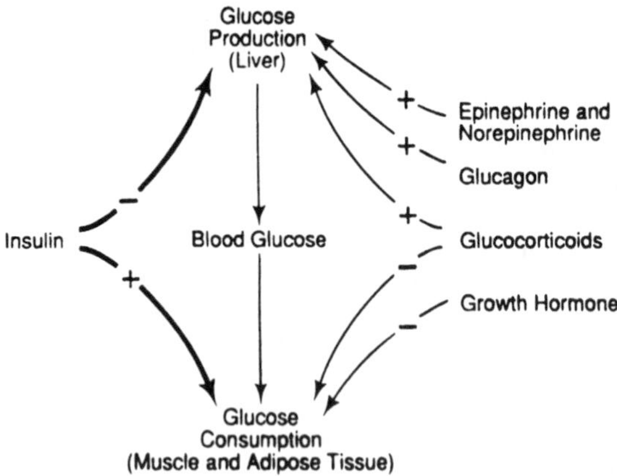

Integration of the regulatory (insulin) and couterregulatory hormones. In the fasted state (upward), insulin is low, which uninhibits glucose production; and the counterregulatory hormones are elevated, which stimulates glucose production (net increase in gluconeogenesis). In fed state (downward), insulin, the storage hormone, is increased, which inhibits glucose production while encouraging glucose intake (consumption). The counter-regulatory hormones are inhibited in the fed state, which unstimulates glucose production. (From Goodman HM: Basic Medical Endocrinology, 2nd ed. Philadelphia, Lippincott-Raven, 1994, with permission.)

120. What is the insulin-to-glucagon ratio?

In the normal individual, this reflects degree of fed versus fasted state. If the individual is in the fed state, the insulin-to-glucagon ratio is high, which induces anabolic enzymes and inhibits catabolic enzymes. If the individual is in the fasted state, the insulin-to-glucagon ratio is low, and catabolic enzyme activity predominates.

121. Describe the pattern of glucose, glucagon, and insulin during a typical day in a normal person.

A mixed meal (carbohydrate, protein, fat) increases glucose. Insulin increases in response, which stimulates glucose uptake and lowers blood glucose. After some meals, insulin levels actually decline while blood glucose is still elevated. This decrease in insulin may be due to paracrine actions of somatostatin within the islet cells and probably prevents too large a decrease in glucose after a meal (reactive hypoglycemia). That is, if insulin stayed high for too long, glucose would continue to decrease from its peak after a meal to below baseline. The attenuation of the insulin response after a meal allows plasma glucose to normalize gradually without going significantly below basal levels.

122. What is the flow of fuel during a prolonged fast, and what hormones are responsible?

In a prolonged fast, insulin is low, and the counterregulatory hormones are increased. Hepatic gluconeogenesis is the prime source of glucose (180 g/day), which is consumed by the central nervous system (which does not require insulin to maintain glucose uptake); blood cells; and, to some extent, muscle, heart, kidney, and other organs. The substrate for hepatic gluconeogenesis is supplied by cortisol-induced muscle catabolism, which can break down as much as 75 g of protein a day, thus supplying amino acids to the liver to be used in glucose synthesis. GH-induced and catecholamine-induced lipolysis supplies glycerol for hepatic gluconeogenesis and fatty acids. These fatty acids can be used by the heart, kidney, and muscle for fuel and are also converted to ketones in the liver.

123. What would be the consequence of either an inability to secrete insulin or an inability to respond properly to circulating insulin?

Diabetes mellitus (too much sweet urine):

- Type 1: the absence of insulin itself
- Type 2: a resistance to insulin action

Either form can result in a failure in glucose uptake leading to hyperglycemia and a glucose-induced (osmotic) diuresis.

124. Characterize the two forms of diabetes mellitus.

Type 1 diabetes mellitus (T1DM) has also been called juvenile-onset or insulin-dependent (IDDM) diabetes mellitus because its onset is usually (but not always) manifest before adulthood. It results from the autoimmune destruction of the B cells of the islets that normally produce insulin. (Other islet cell types can also be destroyed.) Without insulin, blood glucose is elevated, and, paradoxically, gluconeogenesis and fat breakdown continue. Therefore, although there is excess fuel (glucose, fatty acids, amino acids) available in the plasma compartment, the lack of an insulin signal prevents their uptake. This is why T1DM can be considered "tissue starvation in the face of plenty."

Type 2 diabetes mellitus (T2DM) has also been called adult-onset or non–insulin-dependent (NIDDM) diabetes mellitus because it usually occurs after puberty and is not due to a lack of insulin, at least early in the onset of the syndrome. NIDDM is currently thought to be an inadequate definition at best or a confusing one at worst because type 2 diabetes mellitus can be treated with pharmacologic doses of insulin under certain circumstances. Although the pathogenesis of T2DM is complicated, it generally can be considered a syndrome of severe insulin resistance. That is, the insulin-dependent glucose transporter has a decreased sensitivity to insulin, particularly in skeletal muscle and fat. Therefore, although the insulin signal is present, the response to it is inadequate, and glucose uptake is decreased.

125. Define diabetes mellitus.

Diabetes mellitus is generally defined as fasting hyperglycemia and an exaggerated plasma glucose response to oral glucose that is unexplained by other factors.

126. Discuss an example of diabetes mellitus as formally defined.

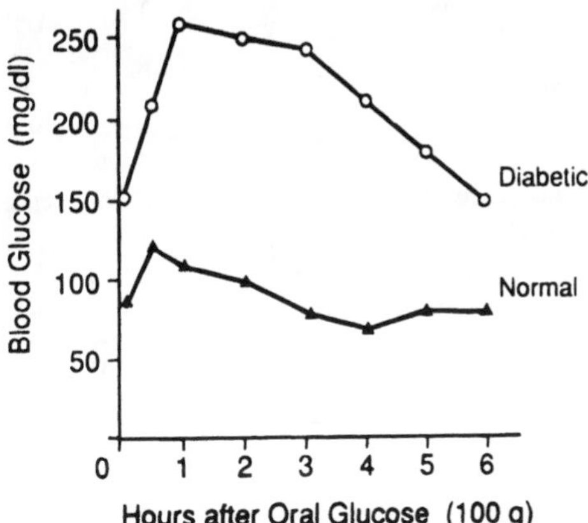

Typical oral glucose tolerance test in normal and diabetic subjects. The diabetic subject has fasting (0 hour) hyperglycemia. The normal subject responds to an oral glucose load by increasing insulin, which lowers blood glucose to (but usually not below) control. The diabetic subject's response to an oral glucose load is characterized by hyperglycemia because of a failure to release insulin (type 1 diabetes mellitus) or the failure to respond adequately to the insulin released (type 2 diabetes mellitus). (From Goodman HM: Basic Medical Endocrinology, 2nd ed. Philadelphia, Lippincott-Raven, 1994, with permission.)

127. How is T1DM treated?

Insulin therapy is the mainstay of treatment. Various preparations of insulin are available with different pharmacokinetics, such that the patient can fairly accurately duplicate a normal pattern of insulin action during the day. Nothing substitutes for a normal endocrine pancreas as of yet; so, eventually, most type 1 diabetics exhibit morbidity from the disease.

128. What happens if insulin therapy is not given to a patient with type 1 diabetes?

Carbohydrate. Glucose transport and glycogen synthesis are decreased, while glycogenolysis and gluconeogenesis are maintained. This leads to hyperglycemia, glucosuria, polyuria (osmotic diuresis), dehydration, and a failure of the circulatory system to maintain systemic perfusion.

Lipid. Lipogenesis is decreased, and lipolysis is increased. This leads to hyperlipemia. Insulin is not present to inhibit conversion of fatty acids to ketones, so ketonemia and ketonuria occur. This leads to severe metabolic acidosis.

Protein. A decrease in amino acid uptake and protein synthesis and an increase in protein degradation lead to increased amino acids in the blood and urine. This is manifest as a negative nitrogen balance.

The end result is the patient loses large quantities of calories, amino acids, water, and bicarbonate in the urine. This is manifest as extreme weight loss, weakness, hyperglycemic shock, coma, severe acidosis, and, if not treated, death.

129. What is the pathogenesis of type 2 diabetes mellitus?

The first defect is probably a decrease in the sensitivity to insulin (insulin resistance), which appears to be an inherited propensity. If this occurs without weight gain, the islet cell can usually compensate by increasing insulin secretion. If the patient gains weight and insulin resistance worsens, the islet cell response is inadequate, and hyperglycemia occurs. Eventually the insulin response to hyperglycemia wanes, and the symptoms worsen. There is usually adequate insulin secretion to prevent ketogenesis in the liver, although there is not sufficient insulin to shut off hepatic gluconeogenesis.

130. Compare and contrast type 1 and type 2 diabetes mellitus.

	TYPE 1 DIABETES MELLITUS	TYPE 2 DIABETES MELLITUS
Pathogenesis	Loss of islet cell function	Resistance to insulin
Age of onset	Usually < 30 years	Usually > 40 years
Ketoacidosis	Common	Uncommon
Body weight	Very thin	> 80% obese
Prevalence	0.5%	2–4% (may be higher)
Genetics	Approximately 50% concordance in twins	> 95% concordance in twins
Autoimmune	Yes	No
Treatment	Insulin	Diet, hypoglycemia agents, appetite suppression, weight loss, exercise, insulin (sometimes)
Symptomatic	Usually	Not usually (at least, at first)

131. List other conditions that can resemble diabetes mellitus.

Secondary diabetes

- Pancreatic disease
- Excess in the counterregulatory hormones such as GH (acromegaly), cortisol (Cushing's syndrome), catecholamines (pheochromocytoma)
- Drugs

Syndrome X (also known as syndrome of insulin resistance, subclinical diabetes, or the metabolic syndrome)

Gestational diabetes

- Glucose intolerance (hyperglycemia) usually only manifest during pregnancy. It is probably due to placental hormones (e.g., human chorionic somatomammotropin, placental steroids).

HORMONAL CONTROL OF CALCIUM HOMEOSTASIS

132. Why is calcium flux so tightly regulated?

Calcium is an extremely important cation in many intracellular and extracellular processes. **Extracellular** calcium is necessary for normal mineralization of bone, blood clotting, and plasma membrane function. **Intracellular** calcium is necessary for a large number of processes, including skeletal and cardiac muscle function; the secretion of hormones, neurotransmitters, and digestive enzymes; normal action potentials and retinal function; maintenance of transport of ions across membranes; regulation of enzyme function; and cell growth and division.

133. In what form does calcium circulate in the plasma?

- Bound to protein (primarily albumin)
- In the free ionized state

134. Describe daily calcium balance.

The extracellular fluid (including plasma) is the central compartment with which all other compartments exchange calcium. The other important compartments and their hormonal controllers are as follows:

Gastrointestinal tract. This is the primary site of calcium **absorption.** For example, out of 1000 mg of dietary calcium, about 400 mg (40%) is absorbed. The absorption of calcium in the gastrointestinal tract is stimulated by 1,25$(OH)_2$D, the biologically active component of the vitamin D pathway. Production of 1,25$(OH)_2$D is stimulated by PTH. About 300 mg (out of 1000 mg/day) of calcium is lost from the extracellular fluid compartment to the gastrointestinal tract via secretions. Therefore, the typical net calcium absorption per day is about 10% of the calcium intake, although this can be changed dramatically by vitamin D excess or deficiency.

Bone. Bone is the primary storage site for calcium (approximately 1 kg; ~99% of total body calcium). Calcium in bone is actively exchanged with the plasma compartment. Bone accretion (formation) is an ongoing process. Reclamation of calcium from bone is a process called **resorption** and is stimulated by PTH. In the long term (steady state), bone formation and resorption are generally in equilibrium. Any state in which calcium resorption is increased without an increase in formation or formation is decreased without a decrease in resorption ultimately results in loss of bone (e.g., osteoporosis).

Kidney. Calcium is filtered (about 10,000 mg/day) as part of the glomerular filtrate. The kidney has developed efficient mechanisms for reclaiming this filtered calcium from tubular fluid—**reabsorption**—which is stimulated by PTH.

Therefore, PTH increases extracellular calcium concentration directly by increasing calcium resorption from bone and increasing calcium reabsorption from renal tubular fluid and indirectly by increasing calcium absorption in the gastrointestinal tract via 1,25$(OH)_2$D.

135. How is the secretion of PTH controlled?

PTH, produced by the parathyroid glands, is one of the only hormones whose secretion is inhibited by an increase in extracellular calcium. In a simple feedback loop, a decrease in plasma calcium results in an increase in PTH, which increases bone resorption, calcium reabsorption, and calcium absorption (via 1,25$(OH)_2$D), all acting to restore plasma calcium. The converse is also true in that an increase in plasma calcium suppresses PTH release, which decreases the resorption, reabsorption, and absorption (via 1,25$(OH)_2$D) of calcium, allowing plasma calcium to decrease. PTH is the most important acute controller of plasma calcium.

136. How do the parathyroid cells detect small changes in extracellular (plasma) calcium?

These cells express a receptor with an extracellular calcium-sensing component and a 7-transmembrane spanning domain; the receptor is G-protein coupled. This receptor acts via phospholipase-C and also by inhibiting adenylate cyclase. Parathyroid hormone is one of the few whose secretion is **inhibited** by an increase in calcium.

137. Other than PTH and 1,25$(OH)_2$D, is there another hormonal controller of plasma calcium?

Calcitonin, produced by the parafollicular cells of the thyroid gland, inhibits bone resorption.

138. Describe the pathway that produces 1,25$(OH)_2$D.

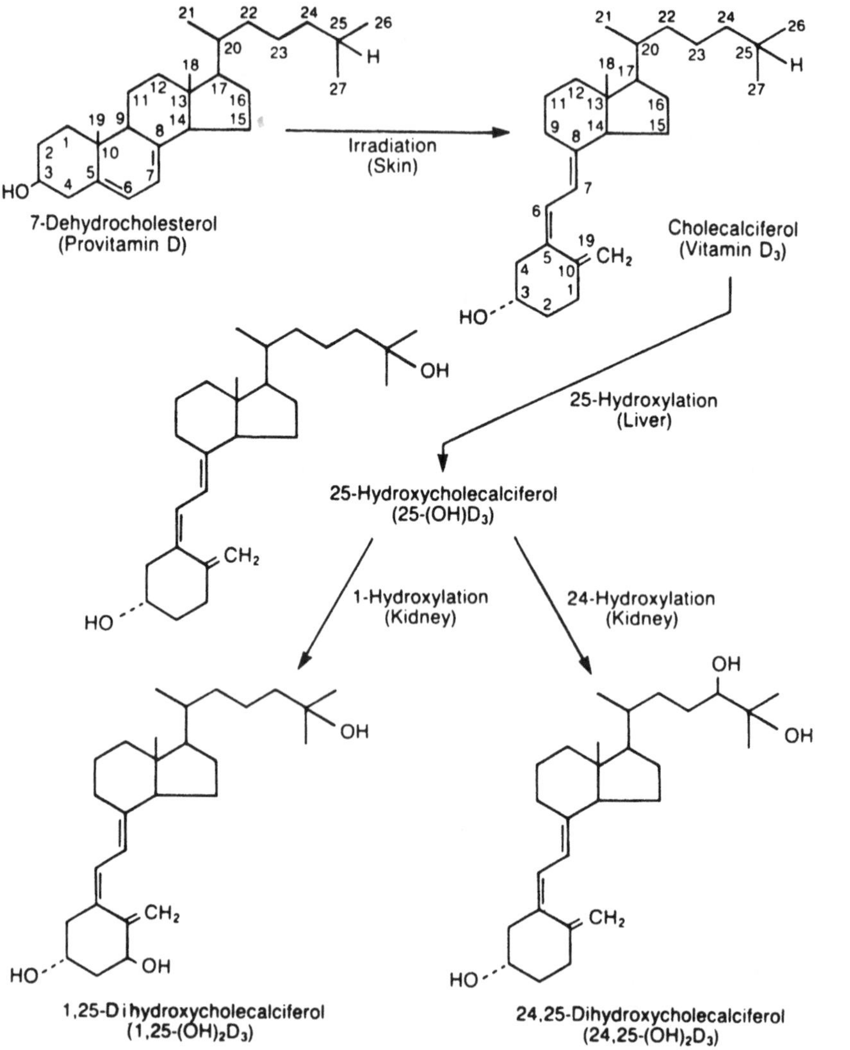

7-Dehydrocholesterol
(Provitamin D)

Irradiation
(Skin)

Cholecalciferol
(Vitamin D_3)

25-Hydroxylation
(Liver)

25-Hydroxycholecalciferol
(25-$(OH)D_3$)

1-Hydroxylation
(Kidney)

24-Hydroxylation
(Kidney)

1,25-Dihydroxycholecalciferol
(1,25-$(OH)_2D_3$)

24,25-Dihydroxycholecalciferol
(24,25-$(OH)_2D_3$)

The endogenous vitamin D steroidogenic pathway. Conversion of vitamin D to 25(OH)D in the liver is relatively unregulated while activation of 25(OH)D to 1,25$(OH)_2$D in the kidney is highly regulated (e.g., stimulated by PTH). Vitamin D can also be obtained in the diet as cholecalciferol (animal vitamin D_3) or ergocalciferol (plant vitamin D_2). (From Griffin JE, Ojeda SR (eds): Textbook of Endocrine Physiology, 3rd ed. New York, Oxford University Press, 1996, with permission.)

1. The vitamin D (calciferol) pathway is a steroidogenic pathway catalyzed by a series of cytochrome P-450 enzymes. There are two forms of vitamin D in the diet: animal vitamin D_3 (cholecalciferol) and plant vitamin D_2 (ergocalciferol). In addition, vitamin D_3 can be liberated from the skin from 7-dehydrocholesterol via the action of ultraviolet light.

2. Once vitamin D_2 or D_3 reaches the plasma compartment, it is converted to 25(OH)D by the action of 25-hydroxylase enzyme in the liver. This is a relatively unregulated step, although elevated 1,25$(OH)_2$D is thought to inhibit this step (end-product inhibition). In physiologic concentrations, 25(OH)D has little biologic activity, whereas it may have calciotropic effects when elevated.

3. 25(OH)D is activated to the active form, 1,25$(OH)_2$D, by 1-hydroxylase enzyme located in the kidney. The activity of 1-hydroxylase is increased by PTH and inhibited by plasma phosphate and 1,25$(OH)_2$D (end-product inhibition). 25(OH)D can also be inactivated to 24,25$(OH)_2$D by 24-hydroxylase in the kidney.

139. What is the best method to assess the activity of the vitamin D pathway?

Measurement of serum 1,25$(OH)_2$D, the active component of the pathway.

140. What is the best method to assess vitamin D intake and stores?

Measurement of serum 25(OH)D because it reflects the summation of vitamin D from dietary and skin sources available for activation to 1,25$(OH)_2$D.

141. Summarize the actions of the major calcium-regulating hormones.

HORMONE	SITE	ACTION
Parathyroid hormone	Bone	↑ Calcium and phosphate resorption
	Kidney	↑ Calcium reabsorption
		↓ Phosphate reabsorption
		↑ Conversion of 25(OH)D to 1,25$(OH)_2$D
Calcitonin	Bone	↓ Calcium and phosphate resorption
	Kidney	↓ Calcium and phosphate reabsorption
Vitamin D [1,25$(OH)_2$D]	Bone	Maintains calcium transport system
	Gastrointestinal tract	↑ Calcium and phosphate absorption

142. Discuss other hormones that affect bone and calcium metabolism.

Gonadal steroids. Androgens and estrogens are necessary for the pubertal growth spurt and closure of the epiphyseal (growth) plates in bone and, therefore, before adulthood, favor bone formation. In the adult, estrogen decreases bone resorption (probably PTH-mediated) and therefore protects bone density. Loss of estrogen at menopause (or loss of testosterone in men because of hypogonadism) is characterized by a loss of bone mineral density (osteoporosis).

Glucocorticoids. Although cortisol is necessary for normal skeletal growth, cortisol in excess produces severe osteoporosis. There are several mechanisms for glucocorticoid-induced osteoporosis, including hypercalciuria and an inhibition of 1,25$(OH)_2$D-mediated calcium absorption in the gastrointestinal tract. The resultant secondary hyperparathyroidism accelerates bone resorption. Furthermore, cortisol in excess appears to inhibit osteoblastic bone formation directly. Finally, excess glucocorticoid may induce secondary hypogonadism.

Thyroid hormone. Lack of adequate thyroid hormone delays ossification of bone growth centers and can retard bone development in children. Excess thyroid hormone may cause increased bone resorption.

GH. GH stimulates IGF-1, which increases bone formation.

143. Describe the overall regulation of calcium balance.

In the steady state, calcium intake should roughly equal calcium loss via the gastrointestinal tract and the urine. Calcium absorption is increased by 1,25$(OH)_2$D, whose production is increased by PTH. PTH also increases calcium resorption from bone and calcium reabsorption from the urine. If plasma calcium is high, calcitonin may decrease bone resorption.

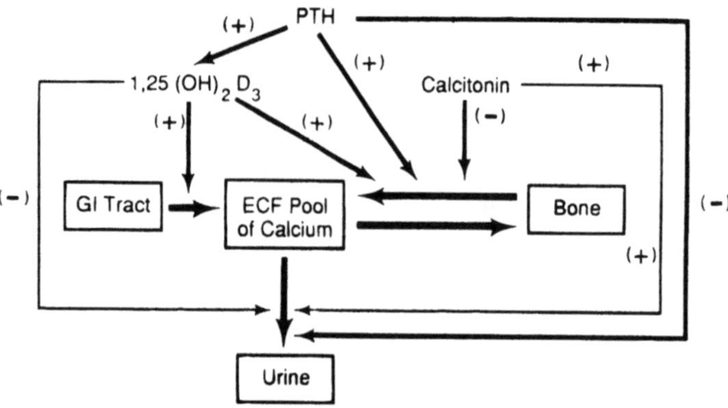

Integration of the hormonal regulation of calcium balance. PTH increases plasma (ECF) calcium by increasing bone resorption, increasing reabsorption of calcium in the kidney, and by increasing renal production of $1,25(OH)_2D$, which stimulates gastrointestinal absorption of calcium. Although calcitonin does decrease bone resorption at pathophysiologic concentrations and with pharmacologic doses, its physiologic role is minor. (From Goodman HM: Basic Medical Endocrinology, 2nd ed. Philadelphia, Lippincott-Raven, 1994, with permission.)

144. Briefly explain phosphate balance.

Phosphate resorption in the gastrointestinal tract accompanies calcium and is increased by $1,25(OH)_2D$. Phosphate resorption also accompanies calcium and is increased by PTH. The main difference between calcium and phosphate balance occurs in the kidney, where PTH **increases** phosphate excretion. This is why patients with elevated PTH have hypercalcemia and hypophosphatemia—they reclaim calcium from the urine while allowing phosphate to be excreted.

145. Discuss the pathogenesis of PTH-dependent hypercalcemia.

PTH-dependent hypercalcemia is defined as **primary hyperparathyroidism** and is usually due to a parathyroid adenoma. These tumors produce intact PTH in excess and are not suppressed by small increases in plasma calcium (as opposed to normal PTH-producing cells). Therefore, plasma calcium increases but fails to shut off PTH adequately. This increases calcium (and phosphate) resorption from bone, increases calcium reabsorption and decreases phosphate reabsorption in the kidney, and increases $1,25(OH)_2D$ production from the kidney to increase calcium absorption in the gastrointestinal tract. The result is hypercalcemia without a suppression of PTH or with frankly elevated PTH, hypophosphatemia (owing to the phosphaturic effects of PTH), and hypercalciuria.

146. Explain why a patient with elevated PTH has hypercalciuria if PTH increases renal calcium reabsorption.

When plasma calcium is elevated, the filtered load of calcium in the kidney increases. Although PTH does increase tubular calcium reabsorption of calcium, the filtered load of calcium may exceed the renal reabsorptive capacity, and calcium spills into the urine.

147. What are PTH-independent causes of hypercalcemia?

- Vitamin D intoxication
- PTH-related peptide (PTHrP) secretion from a malignancy

148. Discuss the pathogenesis of vitamin D intoxication.

Hypercalcemia is not necessarily due to an elevation in $1,25(OH)_2D$ but may be due to small but significant biologic activity of 25(OH)D, and that elevated 25(OH)D (index of increased vitamin D stores) may displace $1,25(OH)_2D$ from its plasma carrier protein, increasing its free, biologic activity. The increase in gastrointestinal absorption of calcium increases plasma calcium and suppresses PTH. This allows increased calcium excretion and results in marked hypercalciuria.

149. Discuss the endocrine causes of hypocalcemia.

A loss of parathyroid gland function leads to **primary hypoparathyroidism.** Lack of PTH results in a failure to increase $1,25(OH)_2D$ and a decrease in gastrointestinal absorption of calcium. In addition, the lack of PTH activity in the kidney prevents the renal response to hypocalcemia to increase calcium reabsorption. Also, without PTH to inhibit phosphate reabsorption, hyperphosphatemia may ensue.

Hypocalcemia may also result from a failure to take in adequate vitamin D (**rickets** in children; **osteomalacia** in adults).

Gastrointestinal malabsorption of calcium and vitamin D may also lead to hypocalcemia. This is called **secondary hyperparathyroidism** because PTH is elevated in response to hypocalcemia. This increases calcium resorption from bone and calcium reabsorption in the kidney in an attempt to restore plasma calcium. Secondary hyperparathyroidism is also often a consequence of renal failure because of the inability to generate $1,25(OH)_2D$ and, perhaps, a loss of renal calcium reabsorptive capacity.

150. List the symptoms of hypocalcemia.

- Neurologic: peripheral (tetany) and central (seizures) nerve
- Cardiovascular: abnormal electrocardiogram (prolonged Q-T interval)

151. How can one distinguish between hypercalcemia caused by a PTH-secreting adenoma and hypercalcemia caused by PTHrP?

The best way is to measure intact PTH. Although PTH and PTHrP have sequence homology, most currently used assays for intact PTH do not measure PTHrP. PTH does not have to be above the reference range to suggest primary hyperparathyroidism. PTHrP-induced hypercalcemia should suppress intact (normal) PTH.

152. How can one distinguish between vitamin D intoxication and hypercalcemia of malignancy caused by PTHrP since they both have suppressed intact PTH?

Assays for PTHrP provide accurate results. Furthermore, patients with vitamin D intoxication usually have elevated 25(OH)D levels (an index of vitamin D stores). Measurement of nephrogenous (urinary) cAMP has been done in the past because this is an index of PTH **activity** and is increased by both intact PTH and PTHrP.

FEMALE REPRODUCTION (EXCEPT FOR PREGNANCY AND LACTATION)

153. Discuss the factors controlling fetal sexual differentiation.

Under most circumstances, genotype (genetic sex) and phenotype (sexual characteristics) are the same. That is, an XX conceptus develops into a female baby and an XY conceptus develops into a male baby. The presence of a Y-chromosome (H-Y antigen) induces development of testes, whereas the absence of a Y-chromosome (no H-Y antigen) allows the development of ovaries. The testes secrete testosterone, which induces development of the male reproductive tract from the wolffian ducts. Testosterone is also converted to dihydrotestosterone (DHT) by 5α-reductase in target tissue, which induces development of male genitalia. In addition, the testes secrete müllerian-inhibiting factor (MIF), which causes regression of the müllerian ducts. The absence of testes, and hence the absence of testosterone, DHT, and MIF, allows wolffian ducts to regress, the development of female genitalia, and the formation of the female reproductive tract from the müllerian ducts.

154. Can the histology of the ovary give insight into its function?

Yes.

Oogonia. The number of germ cells (potential oocytes) peaks at approximately 6 million at about 6 months of gestational age and decreases thereafter via a process called **atresia.** By menopause (approximately 50 years of age), almost no viable germ cells remain.

Primary follicles. These have the potential to start maturation.

Maturing follicles. These begin to develop intrafollicular fluid and proliferating steroidogenic cells (theca and granulosa cells).

Graafian follicle. The dominant follicle is filled with fluid and contains a mature oocyte ready for ovulation. It produces large amounts of estrogen and is primed to produce large amounts of progesterone after ovulation.

Corpus luteum. This develops from the ruptured follicle after ovulation. It is full of steroidogenic cells, which produce large amounts of progesterone (and estrogen, to a lesser extent).

Atretic follicle. This is a follicle whose oocyte was not ovulated but regressed during maturation (nondominant follicle).

Retrogressive corpus luteum. If conception does not occur, the corpus luteum "dies."

155. List the general female endocrine changes throughout life.

- HCG (from trophoblast and placenta) and fetal FSH and LH stimulate development of ovarian germ cells.
- LH and FSH burst approximately 4 months postpartum (sexual differentiation of the brain?).
- Adrenarche—increase in adrenal androgens at about 8 years of age.
- At onset of puberty (8–10 years old), GnRH pulses from hypothalamus increase, which stimulates LH and FSH and increases ovarian function.
- Increase in ovarian steroids induces development of secondary sex characteristics.
- Menstrual cycles (menarche) start at approximately 12 years of age.
- In addition to development of secondary sex characteristics, pubertal estrogens stimulate growth spurt (assuming presence of adequate GH).
- Estrogens also stop growth spurt by causing fusion of epiphyseal plates in bone.
- At menopause (at approximately 50 years of age), ovaries stop producing steroids. This leads to the absence of menses as well as other physiologic (hot flashes) and psychological changes. Lack of steroid negative feedback leads to an increase in FSH and LH.

156. How are ovarian steroids synthesized?

The pathway is essentially the same as that outlined in the adrenal cortex section, particularly with respect to progesterone production. After 17-hydroxylation and androgen production, androstenedione is converted to estrone, and testosterone is converted to estradiol by the enzyme aromatase. It is generally believed that this process requires the two follicular cell types—theca and granulosa cells—to work in what has been called the "two-cell hypothesis of ovarian steroidogenesis" (see figure, next page).

The **theca cell** expresses primarily LH receptors. LH stimulates steroidogenesis and large amounts of androgen production. The theca cell is relatively devoid of aromatase activity.

Androgens diffuse through the basal lamina into the **granulosa cell.** The granulosa cell expresses primarily FSH receptors, although it can express LH receptors just before ovulation. Androgens from the theca cell are aromatized to estrogens primarily in the granulosa cell.

157. Since the gonadal hormones are steroids, do they circulate bound to carrier proteins similar to cortisol?

Estradiol and estrone, because they have undergone the 17,20 lyase reaction, do not resemble cortisol very much and therefore do not bind to CBG. There is another carrier protein called sex hormone–binding globulin (SHBG) that carries estradiol (approximately 38%). Progesterone does circulate bound to CBG (approximately 18%).

158. If progesterone only binds about 18% to CBG and estradiol only binds about 38% to SHBG, do these gonadal steroids circulate mostly in the free form?

No, because they are bound significantly by plasma albumin, with estradiol having about 60% binding with albumin, and progesterone about 80% binding with albumin. Therefore, estra-

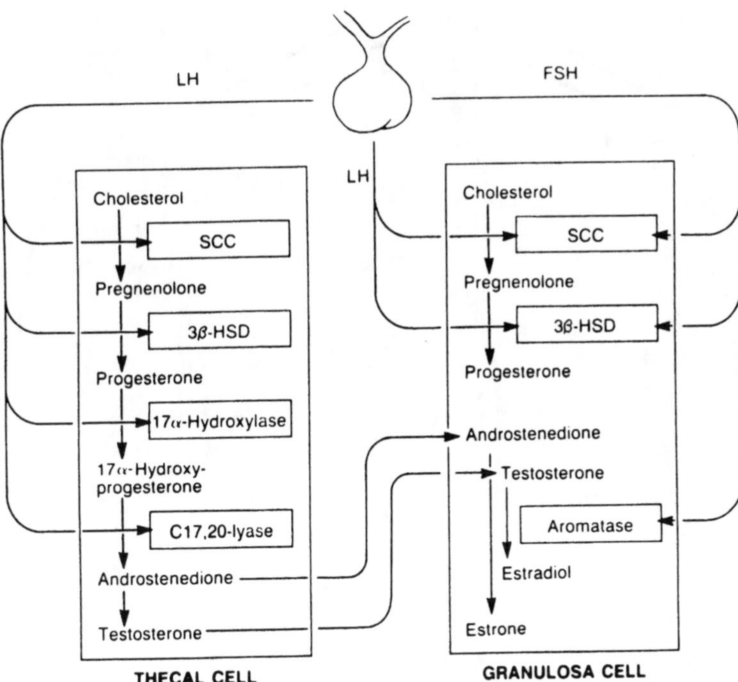

The two-cell hypothesis of ovarian steroidogenesis. LH primarily stimulates theca cell production of androgens, which diffuse into the granulosa cell where they are converted to estrogens by FSH-stimulated aromatase activity. Granulosa cells also produce progesterone but do not have adequate enzymatic machinery to convert progesterone to androgens. (From Griffin JE, Ojeda SR (eds): Textbook of Endocrine Physiology, 3rd ed. New York, Oxford University Press, 1996, with permission.)

diol and progesterone circulate approximately 2% free, with about 98% percent bound to carrier proteins or albumin.

159. Do the ovaries produce peptide hormones?

Relaxin: relaxes pelvic ligaments
Inhibin: selective inhibition of FSH
Activins: selective stimulation of FSH

160. How is the hypothalamic-pituitary-ovarian control system similar to and different from the HPA axis?

In the prepubertal and postmenopausal state, they are similar. Increases in GnRH pulses from the hypothalamus stimulate the secretion of the pituitary gonadotropins LH and FSH. These two hormones stimulate ovarian steroidogenesis, which, via negative feedback, decreases the secretion of GnRH and LH and FSH. Therefore, if ovarian steroids are deficient, LH and FSH are increased (hypergonadotropic hypogonadism analogous to primary adrenal insufficiency); and if hypopituitarism exists, LH and FSH are inappropriately low (analogous to secondary adrenal insufficiency).

Between menarche and menopause, there are quite a few differences. The ovaries produce a second hormone, called inhibin, which inhibits the release of FSH. Therefore, there are parallel negative feedback pathways: gonadal steroids inhibiting LH and inhibin inhibiting FSH. Another major difference is the existence of **positive feedback.** During a specific time (midcycle) in the menstrual cycle, estrogen actually stimulates LH and FSH release. This results in a surge in gonadotropins, which stimulates ovulation. (See figure, next page.)

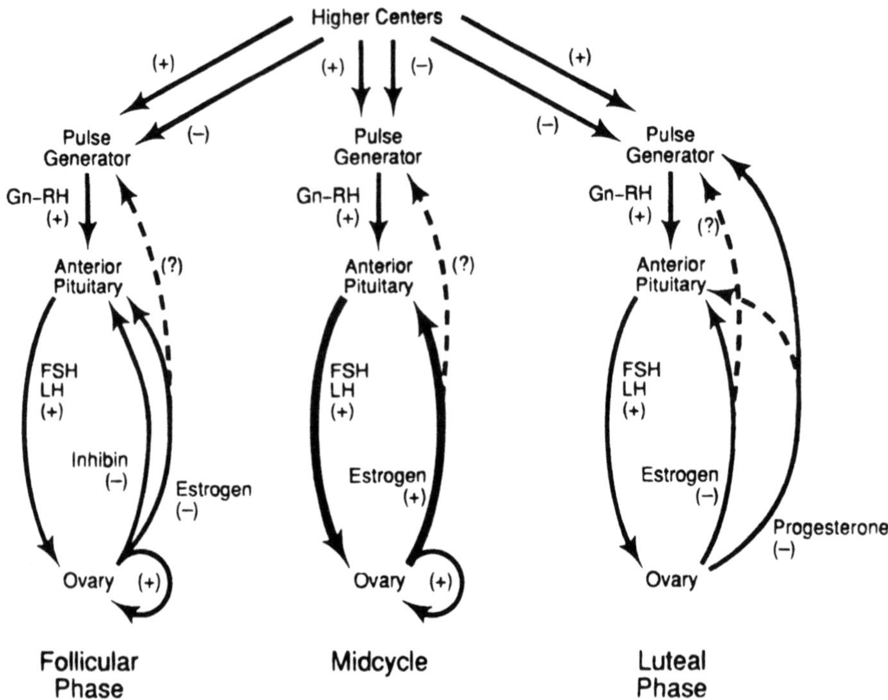

The hypothalamic-pituitary-ovarian system at different phases of the menstrual cycle. +, stimulation; −, inhibition. Dashed lines indicate hypothetical relationships. Line thickness indicates the intensity of stimulation. (From Goodman HM: Basic Medical Endocrinology, 2nd ed. Philadelphia, Lippincott-Raven, 1994, with permission.)

161. Outline a typical menstrual cycle.

Because this is truly a cycle, **day 1** is somewhat arbitrary. Because the major physical sign is the onset of menses, however, this is considered day 1.

Follicular phase: The emergence of the dominant follicle.

1. Menses are induced by decreases in estrogen and progesterone.
2. Increase in FSH on day 28 is induced by loss of steroid negative feedback. Increase in FSH on day 28 promotes the maturation of 6–12 primary follicles.
3. Increase in FSH on day 28 followed by LH on days 2–5 increases estrogen production.
4. One (usually) follicle becomes dominant and increases estrogen production. This estrogen inhibits FSH secretion by negative feedback. Estrogen concentration may correlate with the size of the dominant follicle.
5. The nondominant follicles cannot survive the decrease in FSH and undergo atresia. The dominant follicle survives this decrease in FSH because it has increased expression of LH and FSH receptors.
6. The system shifts from negative to positive feedback so that the large increase in estrogen from the dominant follicle induces the LH surge. ↑ estrogen causes ↑ LH causes ↑ estrogen causes ↑ LH.
7. Preovulatory increase in progesterone potentiates estrogen positive feedback on LH.
8. LH surge (and FSH surge) occurs, with the ratio of LH to FSH increasing dramatically. This induces resumption of meiosis in the oocyte of the dominant follicle.
9. FSH surge induces LH receptors on granulosa cells to prepare the follicle for transformation into the corpus luteum.

10. Estrogen starts to decrease as LH reaches its peak. This is hypothesized to be due to down-regulation of the LH receptor on the theca/granulosa cells.

11. The loss of estrogen positive feedback stimulation of LH terminates the LH surge. The increasing ratio of progesterone to estrogen may be a negative feedback signal.

Ovulation: The expulsion of the ovum from the dominant follicle.

12. Ovulation occurs owing to prior LH surge.

Luteal phase: Progesterone (and estrogen) secretion from the corpus luteum.

13. Corpus luteum is formed primarily by granulosa cells primed by LH and FSH surge.

14. Corpus luteum secretion of progesterone and estrogen increases; the process is dependent on low (but adequate) LH levels.

15. Progesterone and estrogen decrease owing to finite life of corpus luteum in the absence of significant gonadotropin levels. (If fertilization occurs, HCG from the trophoblast rescues the corpus luteum and prevents menstruation.) The corpus luteum dies unless fertilization occurs and HCG production from the trophoblast rescues the corpus luteum.

16. **Go to** step 1.

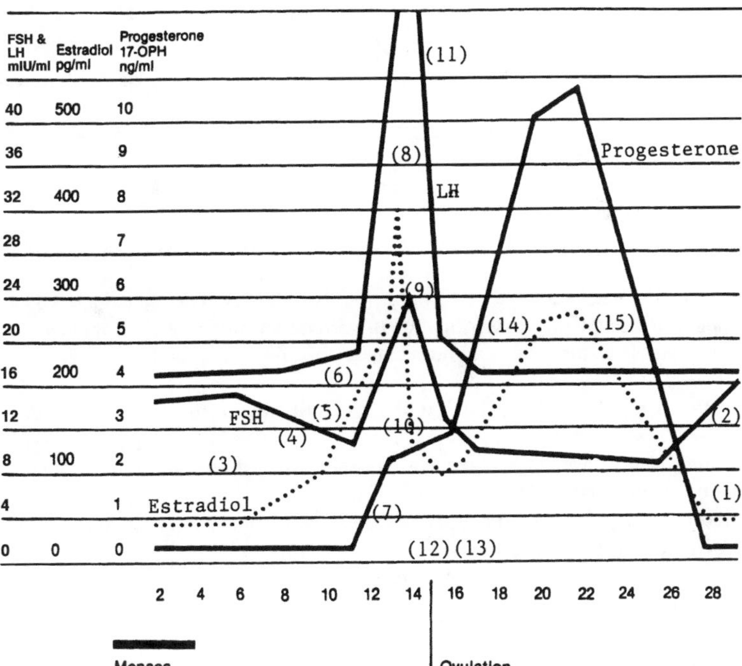

Idealized human menstrual cycle. Days of the cycle are shown across the bottom. Menses start at day 1; ovulation usually occurs around day 15. Each step is identified numerically in the text. (Adapted from Speroff L, Glass RH, Kase NG: Clinical Gynecologic Endocrinology and Infertility. Baltimore, Williams & Wilkins, 1983.)

162. Describe the proliferation of granulosa cells during follicular development.

As the dominant follicle grows, it secretes more and more estrogen despite decreases in FSH in the early follicular phase. Local estradiol production within the dominant follicle increases the expression of FSH receptors. Positive feedback of estrogen from the dominant follicle stimulates FSH release, which induces LH receptor expression on granulosa cells. By the later follicular phase (just before ovulation), the granulosa cells of the dominant follicle have increased greatly in number and express FSH and LH receptors in great number.

163. How do changes in the endometrium of the uterus correlate with the phases of the menstrual cycle?

The **endometrial cycle** is in synchrony with the menstrual cycle and is a hallmark of the extraovarian actions of gonadal steroids.

- **Proliferative phase** occurs during the follicular phase of the menstrual cycle. Estrogen stimulates the growth of the epithelial and stromal layers. The thickness of the endometrium increases, and the uterine glands increase in size. The spiral arteries, which are the primary blood supply for the endometrium, elongate.
- **Secretory phase** occurs during the luteal phase of the menstrual cycle and prepares the endometrium for implantation of the conceptus. Progesterone stimulates secretory activity of the uterine glands, and glycogen production increases. The stroma becomes edematous, and the spiral arteries coil.
- **Menstrual phase** correlates with the end of the luteal phase of the menstrual cycle. The loss of gonadal steroid secretion from the corpus luteum induces vasoconstriction (spasm?) of the spiral arteries and necrosis of the endometrium. The endometrial lining is sloughed off in the form of menstrual bleeding.

164. Are there other extraovarian actions of estrogen and progesterone?

Oviducts—Estrogen increases cilia formation and contractility, and progesterone increases secretory activity and decreases contractility.

Myometrium—Estrogen increases growth and contractility, and progesterone decreases contractility.

Cervix—Estrogen induces a watery secretion, and progesterone stimulates the production of dense, viscous secretions.

Vagina—Estrogen induces epithelial proliferation, and progesterone induces epithelial differentiation.

Breasts—Estrogen stimulates development of the duct system and adipose tissue (e.g., at puberty), and progesterone induces formation of secretory alveoli (e.g., during pregnancy).

Bone—Estrogen stimulates *and* terminates pubertal growth spurt. Estrogen inhibits bone resorption.

Other—Estrogen increases SHBG, CBG, and TBG. Estrogen alters lipid profile.

165. List and briefly describe fertilization of the ovum and implantation of the conceptus.

- **Ovum transport:** Ovulated oocyte collected by fibrial end of fallopian tube
- **Sperm transport and capacitation:** Contact with female tract activates sperm function
- **Fertilization:** Usually occurs in fallopian tube
- **Implantation and placentation:** Blastocyst usually implants on endometrial lining approximately 7 days after ovulation

166. What is menopause?

Menopause is the age-related cessation of regular menses during the female climacteric when reproductive cyclicity gradually disappears. Usually, menstrual cycles become irregular before they completely stop. Menopause is characterized by a loss of ovarian function probably as a result of exhaustion of available follicles lost because of atresia. Because of the decrease in estrogen production from the ovary, LH and FSH increase owing to loss of negative feedback. In that sense, menopause can be defined as **hypergonadotropic hypogonadism.**

167. What is amenorrhea?

- **Primary amenorrhea:** the failure to have menarche (the onset of menstrual cycles at puberty). It is currently believed that the failure to have normal menstrual cycles by the age of 16 should be evaluated.
- **Secondary amenorrhea:** the premature cessation of normal menstrual cycles. Causes include pregnancy, hyperprolactinemia, premature menopause, excessive exercise, and weight loss.
- **Oligomenorrhea:** irregular menstrual cycles.

MALE REPRODUCTION

168. In the male (XY genotype), is there a relationship between gonadal function and physiologic changes throughout life?

As opposed to the female, the development of a male phenotype requires a signal from the developing gonads. The secretion of müllerian inhibitory factor (MIF) induces regression of the müllerian ducts and allows the wolffian ducts to develop into the internal male genitalia. The secretion of testosterone from the fetal testes induces somatic sex differentiation and the male phenotype. If testosterone is absent or if there is resistance to the action of testosterone (testicular feminization), a female (external) phenotype develops.

After parturition, LH and FSH increase at about 6 months of age (analogous to a similar event in females). The subsequent increase in testicular steroidogenesis and androgen secretion may result in the sexual differentiation of the brain.

Adequate testosterone secretion is necessary before puberty to maintain normal growth. Adrenarche (increase in adrenal androgens), which usually occurs at approximately 8 years of age, is a harbinger of the onset of puberty.

At 10–14 years of age, LH and FSH increase, leading to a marked increase in testicular steroidogenesis and spermatogenesis. The increase in testosterone leads to the outward signs of male puberty (deepening of the voice, axillary and pubic hair, increased sweat glands).

The existence of a male climacteric in the elderly is a controversial topic. Although testosterone secretion decreases as men age into their forties to sixties, this may not represent clinical hypogonadism, and spermatogenesis can be maintained.

169. Summarize testicular steroidogenesis.

This is essentially the same as adrenal androgen production, in which pregnenolone and progesterone are converted to DHEA and androstenedione by P450c17. DHEA and androstenedione can be converted to testosterone. Although testosterone is the primary androgen produced by the testes, it is not the most potent. Dihydrotestosterone (DHT) is produced from testosterone by 5α-reductase primarily in target tissue (peripheral activation). In addition, testicular androgens can be converted to estrogens in males primarily by peripheral conversion by aromatase.

170. Review the circulating gonadal steroids in the male and state their sources.

- > 95% of circulating **testosterone** is from the testes.
- > 80% of the circulating **DHT** is from peripheral conversion of testosterone.
- > 80–90% of circulating **estrogen** is from peripheral conversion of precursors.
- > 90% of circulating **DHEA** (sulfate) is from the adrenal cortex.

171. List the hormonal and somatic changes during male puberty.

1. GnRH pulses from the hypothalamus increase FSH and LH secretion.
2. LH stimulates testosterone production, which induces development of secondary sex characteristics.
3. FSH stimulates spermatogenesis.
4. ACTH (or some other pituitary factor) increases adrenal androgen production (adrenarche).
5. GH maintains linear growth.
6. Testosterone enhances the secretion of GH and initiates the pubertal growth spurt. Testosterone then causes epiphyseal fusion (termination of the pubertal growth spurt).

172. What is the significance of the pulsatility of GnRH release from the hypothalamus?

One of the hallmarks of the gonadotropin control system in males and females is pulsatility. LH in males is usually released in pulses with about a 90-minute frequency, although this is variable between and within subjects and by time of day (and even seasons of the year). GnRH pulses are necessary to maintain LH pulses. Constantly high levels of GnRH, although stimulating LH at first, lead to down-regulation of pituitary gonadotrophs and a decrease in LH. This is the basis for using GnRH analogs to induce hypogonadotropic hypogonadism in men with testosterone-sensitive prostate cancer.

173. Describe the overall regulation of testicular function.

The hypothalamic-pituitary-testicular (HPT) axis is, for the most part, similar to the HPA axis.

1. Neural input into the brain regulates the release of pulses of GnRH from the hypothalamus into the long portal veins, which drain into the anterior pituitary. GnRH pulses stimulate LH and FSH release.

2. LH stimulates steroidogenesis (testosterone production) from the Leydig (interstitial) cells in the testes.

3. FSH stimulates Sertoli cells (in concert with local testosterone) to increase spermatogenesis, androgen binding protein (a local factor), and inhibin production.

4. **Negative feedback:** Testosterone inhibits GnRH and LH release. Inhibin decreases FSH release.

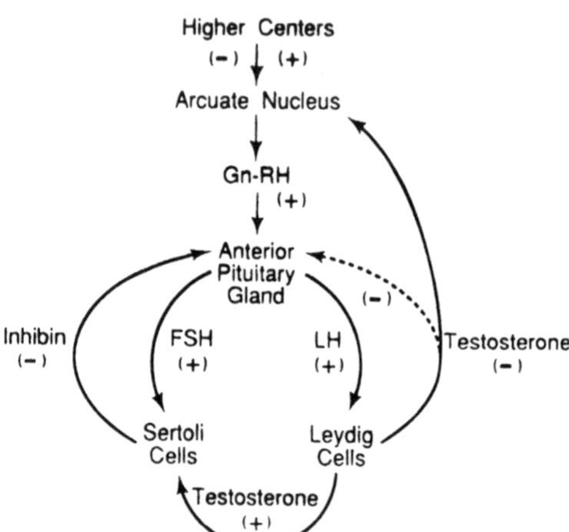

HPT axis. + indicates that GnRH stimulates FSH and LH, that FSH stimulates Sertoli cells while LH stimulates Leydig cells, and that Leydig cells stimulate Sertoli cells (paracrine). − indicates that inhibin produced from Sertoli cells inhibits FSH release while testosterone inhibits GnRH release (negative feedback). Direct inhibition of LH by testosterone has not been firmly established (dotted line). (From Goodman HM: Basic Medical Endocrinology, 2nd ed. Philadelphia, Lippincott-Raven, 1994, with permission.)

174. What is the main difference between the HPT and HPA axes?

The testes produce two negative feedback signals: Testosterone inhibits LH (and FSH); inhibin inhibits FSH release.

175. Categorize the actions of FSH and LH on the testes.

LH stimulates steroidogenesis (testosterone synthesis and release) from the Leydig (interstitial) cells. Although LH was named for its luteinizing action in the female, its effect in males (increase in androgen) is analogous. In fact, in the past, LH has been called interstitial cell-stimulating hormone.

FSH stimulates androgen binding protein from Sertoli cells into the lumen of the seminiferous tubule. Androgen binding protein acts as a local testosterone sink, which dramatically increases the local concentration of testosterone that is necessary for sperm maturation. FSH also stimulates spermatogenesis. (See figure, next page.)

176. Why are LH and FSH necessary?

LH is necessary to stimulate testosterone, which has systemic effects and local effects. FSH stimulates spermatogenesis and increases local testosterone concentration by increasing androgen binding protein release from Sertoli cells into tubular lumens.

177. What are the major actions of androgens?

Fetal development: Testosterone stimulates internal genitalia and testosterone metabolite (DHT) stimulates external genitalia.

Puberty: Testosterone and DHT increase secondary sex characteristics (musculature, lar-

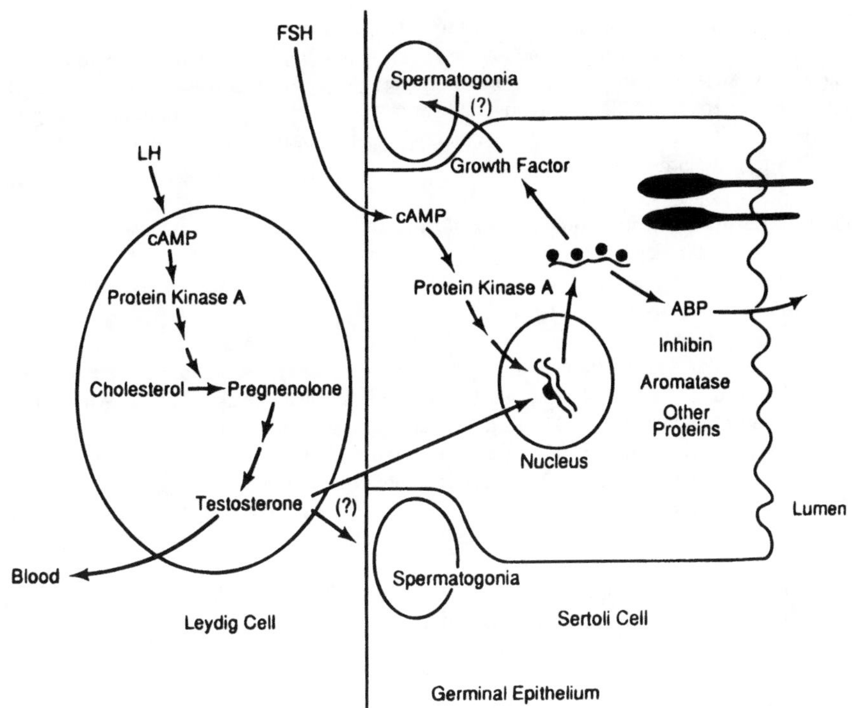

Control of testicular steroidogenesis and spermatogenesis. LH stimulates testosterone production, which exerts actions on target organs via the blood and exerts actions on the Sertoli cell via diffusion (paracrine effect). FSH stimulates Sertoli cells directly to increase androgen binding protein (ABP) production which acts as a testosterone "sink," increasing the testosterone concentration in the fluid bathing the developing sperm. (From Goodman HM: Basic Medical Endocrinology, 2nd ed. Philadelphia, Lippincott-Raven, 1994, with permission.)

ynx, sexual hair, sebaceous glands), spermatogenesis, and prostatic secretion. Androgens also stimulate the pubertal growth spurt (with adequate GH) and terminate the pubertal growth spurt by inducing closure of epiphyseal plates.

Adulthood: Actions include maintenance of normal skeleton, libido, spermatogenesis, and the other secondary sex characteristics.

178. Outline the profile of male puberty.

AGE (YEARS)	PHYSIOLOGIC CHANGES
About 8	Adrenal androgens (DHEA and androstenedione) induce subtle increases in secondary sex characteristics (e.g., light mustache).
About 9–10	GnRH pulses increase, which stimulates LH and FSH release. This stimulates testicular growth and increases in testosterone.
About 12	The pubertal increase in pubic and axillary hair starts followed by an increase in penile growth.
13	The pubertal growth spurt has usually started with a peak growth velocity at about age 14–15 years.
About 16	The growth spurt starts to wane.
18	Final adult height is usually achieved (although growth until age 20 is not uncommon).

179. Is there an event in males analogous to menopause in females?

Total testosterone levels do tend to decrease as men age but usually remain within the normal range. More importantly, free (bioactive) testosterone may decrease due to changes in SHBG binding characteristics. Although hypogonadism in aging men is not a ubiquitous finding (like menopause), it is amenable to testosterone therapy. Spermatogenesis has been reported to be adequate for fertility in men in their eighties.

180. What is the most common disorder of the HPT axis?

Hypogonadism (a decrease in testicular function).

181. Discuss the causes of male hypogonadism.

Hypogonadism in males can be generally classified as two types:

1. **Testicular dysfunction** is due to a decrease in testosterone production from the testes. LH and FSH increase because of a loss of negative feedback. Therefore, this is called **hypergonadotropic hypogonadism** and is analogous to primary adrenal insufficiency.

2. **Hypopituitarism** is called **hypogonadotropic hypogonadism** and can be due to an idiopathic decrease in LH and FSH or due to panhypopituitarism. "Hypogonadotropic" may be misleading because LH concentrations are often in the normal range in patients with hypogonadotropic hypogonadism. The LH levels are **inappropriately** low for the low testosterone.

Another cause of hypogonadotropic hypogonadism is **hyperprolactinemia,** which is usually due to a prolactin-secreting pituitary adenoma. Elevated prolactin levels inhibit gonadotropin secretion and induce hypogonadism in males (and amenorrhea in females).

182. What are the symptoms of hypogonadism in males?

Symptoms depend on the age of onset.

- Androgen deficiency or insensitivity to androgens in **early fetal development** leads to varying degrees of ambiguity of the genitalia and male pseudohermaphroditism.
- **Prepubertal** androgen deficiency leads to limited secondary sex characteristics and eunuchoid skeletal proportions because, even though there is no androgen-mediated pubertal growth spurt, there is also failure to close the epiphyseal plates and the long bones continue to grow. Therefore, the arm span of these individuals is longer than a typical man.
- Androgen deficiency **after puberty** usually results in decreased libido, impotence, and low energy levels. If androgen deficiency continues for longer periods of time, there can be a decrease in facial or body hair.

183. What is the most common cause of male hypogonadism?

Klinefelter syndrome, which occurs in about 0.2% of male births.

184. Describe the genotype and phenotype of Klinefelter syndrome.

The most common genotype is XXY (an extra X chromosome). An XXY genotype usually results from meiotic nondisjunction during gametogenesis. The phenotype usually appears at puberty and includes increased lower-to-upper body segment ratio, gynecomastia, small penis, and sparse upper body hair. The testes do not develop normally and are usually small and fibrotic. The decreased testosterone production usually leads to elevated LH and FSH concentrations.

BIBLIOGRAPHY

1. Ganong WF: Review of Medical Physiology, 20th ed. New York, McGraw-Hill, 2001.
2. Genuth SM: The endocrine system. In Berne RM, Levy MN (eds): Physiology, 4th ed. St. Louis, Mosby, 1998.

3. Goodman HM: Basic Medical Endocrinology, 2nd ed. Philadelphia, Lippincott-Raven, 1994.
4. Greenspan FS, Gardner DG (eds): Basic and Clinical Endocrinology, 6th ed. New York, McGraw-Hill, 2001.
5. Griffin JE, Ojeda SR (eds): Textbook of Endocrine Physiology, 4th ed. New York, Oxford University Press, 2000.
6. McDermott MT (ed): Endocrine Secrets, 3rd ed. Philadelphia, Hanley & Belfus, 2001.
7. Porterfield SP: Endocrine Physiology, 2nd ed. St. Louis, Mosby, 2001.
8. Reichlin S: Neuroendocrinology. In Wilson JD, Foster DW, Kronenberg H, Larsen PR (eds): Williams Textbook of Endocrinology, 9th ed. Philadelphia, W.B. Saunders, 1998.

9. BONE PHYSIOLOGY

Hershel Raff, Ph.D., and Joseph L. Shaker, M.D.

1. Describe the general composition of bone.

Bone is composed of an organic matrix (primarily type 1 collagen fibers) into which calcium and phosphate are deposited and precipitate to form the salt hydroxyapatite crystals. Other ions are also present within the bone, and the organic matrix is also composed of proteoglycans and glycoproteins. The process of deposition of calcium and phosphate in bone is called **mineralization.** Collagen is the primary source of tensile strength, whereas the deposited minerals are the primary source of the ability to withstand compression. Bone is the main storage site for calcium and phosphate in the body. These minerals are in a constant state of flux with the plasma compartment.

2. What are the general types of bone?

Cortical bone (~ 80% of bone mass)—e.g., long bones
Trabecular bone (~ 20% of bone mass)—e.g., skull, ribs, vertebrae, pelvis

3. Compare and contrast cortical and trabecular bone.

Cortical bone provides the external surface of bones and is dense. Trabecular bone is composed of a network of thin calcified trabeculae. In cortical bone, about 80–90% of the volume of bone is calcified; in trabecular bone, 15–25% of the bone is calcified. The remainder of trabecular bone is marrow, blood vessels, and connective tissue. Cortical bone serves a mechanical and protective function. Trabecular bone is more metabolically active than cortical bone.

4. Is bone mass constant?

No. Bone minerals are constantly being renewed by the coupling of bone formation and bone resorption. This coupling is tightly regulated and occurs in basic multicellular units (BMUs). Bone mass increases in childhood and teenage years and probably reaches a peak in the third decade of life. As described in Chapter 8, bone growth occurs at the growth (epiphyseal) plates.

5. What cell types are involved in bone remodeling.

- **Osteoblasts** are responsible for bone formation (arise from stromal mesenchymal cells).
- **Osteoclasts** are responsible for bone resorption (arise from hematopoietic stem cells).
- **Osteocytes** are mature osteoblasts that have been trapped in mineralized bone. They may serve a mechanosensory function.

6. Describe the process of bone remodeling.

Bone remodeling helps repair fatigue damage and occurs at the level of the BMU. Approximately 20% of the trabecular surface is undergoing remodeling at any given time. The process is as follows (see figure, next page):

- Local and circulating hormones, cytokines, and growth factors influence the origination of BMUs.
- Activation is followed by osteoclastic bone resorption. The osteoclasts tunnel into bone by release of enzymes (e.g., collagenase) and hydrogen ions (acid).
- After resorption has occurred, there is a reversal phase followed by bone matrix formation. Osteoblasts synthesize osteoid (unmineralized bone matrix).
- Mineralization, the process of deposition of calcium phosphate into unmineralized matrix, occurs next. Mineralization is completed with the deposition of hydroxide and bicarbonate to form hydroxyapatite crystals.
- The osteoblasts surrounded by mineralized bone transform into osteocytes.

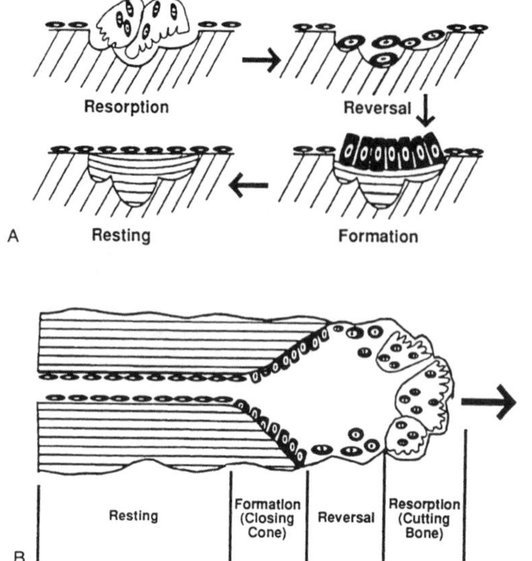

Principal phases of the adult bone remodeling cycle in trabecular (cancellous) bone (*A*) and cortical bone (*B*). Large multinucleated cells are osteoclasts; small, mononucleated cells are osteoblasts. (From Dempster DW: Bone remodeling. In Coe FL, Favus MJ (eds): Disorders of Bone and Mineral Metabolism. New York, Raven Press, 1992, with permission.)

7. List the steps in the development and growth of long bone.

1. Initial (fetal) step is cartilage deposition after which the shaft of the bone is ossified (endochondral bone formation).
2. Epiphyses (end of long bones) are separated from the shaft by epiphyseal (growth) plates.
3. Bone length increases as the epiphyseal plate lays down new bone at the end of the shaft of the bone. Bone growth is accelerated by a variety of endocrine and local growth factors stimulated by growth hormone (including insulin-like growth factor 1 [IGF-1], as described in Chapter 8, Endocrine Physiology).
4. Long bones stop growing when the epiphyses are closed, usually after puberty. The closure of the growth plates is mediated by gonadal steroids (see Chapter 8).

8. How are calcium and phosphates readily exchanged between the interior bone and extracellular fluid?

Fluid-filled channels called **canaliculi** provide a large surface area and path for exchange of ions.

9. Describe the coupling of bone formation and resorption in more detail.

- Bone resorption and formation are normally coupled in the remodeling process.
- The factors that are responsible for this coupling are not completely understood.
- If resorption exceeds formation, bone mass will decrease.

10. What are lamellae and haversian canals?

Orientation of collagen fibrils in bone alternates from layer to layer, resulting in a lamellar structure. Lamellae may be parallel to each other on a flat surface (trabecular and periosteum) or concentric if around a channel for blood vessels (haversian canal).

11. When does bone mineral mass usually reach its peak?

After puberty and the closure of epiphyseal plates, bone width increases by addition to the surfaces of cortical bone (periosteum). Bone mass continues to increase and usually reaches its peak toward the end of the third decade of life.

12. What controls the attainment of peak bone mass?

Many factors are involved in the achievement of peak bone mass. One important factor is **genetics.** Genes are important in determining the maximal predicted peak bone mass, although the specific genes involved are not yet understood. Another major factor is **weight-bearing,** which increases bone mass. This is one reason why weight-bearing exercise is often recommended to prevent bone loss. Many **humoral factors** are also involved. Gonadal steroids (estrogen and testosterone) inhibit bone resorption and encourage an increase in bone mass. This is why hypogonadism in men and women can lead to loss of bone mass.

13. Does bone mass decline with aging?

Yes. After the peak in bone mass, resorption exceeds accretion, and bone mass decreases. This process accelerates with menopause in women because of the decline in estrogen (an antiresorptive hormone). Osteoporosis also occurs in men but is less common and occurs on average at an older age. A moderate decrease in bone mass is called **osteopenia,** or low bone mass. A more severe decrease in bone mass is called **osteoporosis.**

14. Other than osteoporosis, name one other metabolic bone disease.

Osteomalacia is a softening of bone due to failure to mineralize osteoid adequately. It may be due to vitamin D deficiency caused by inadequate intake or malabsorption. Conditions that result in phosphate wasting in the kidney or inability to properly metabolize vitamin D also may cause osteomalacia. When it occurs in children, osteomalacia is called **rickets.**

15. How is bone mineral mass assessed clinically?

The most common method of assessment of bone mineral density (BMD) is by **dual energy x-ray absorptiometry (DEXA).** It is a simple painless technique that exposes the patient to very low levels of radiation.

16. How can osteoporosis be prevented?

An important factor is to attain maximal genetically determined peak bone mass. In general, adequate calcium and vitamin D intake and weight-bearing exercise are useful. Avoidance of tobacco and excess alcohol is also recommended. Antiresorptive drugs (see question 17) also may be used to prevent bone loss after menopause. Eating disorders (e.g., anorexia or bulimia) may prevent attainment of optimal peak bone mass.

17. How can osteoporosis be treated?

As in prevention, adequate calcium and vitamin D are important. Avoidance of tobacco and excess alcohol is advisable. Currently, several drugs that decrease bone resorption are used, including estrogen, selective estrogen receptor modulators (SERMs), bisphosphonates, and calcitonin. In the future, drugs that directly stimulate bone formation may be used (e.g., intermittent exposure to parathyroid hormone).

BIBLIOGRAPHY

1. Bilezikian JP, Raisz LG, Rodan GA (eds): Principles of Bone Biology, 2nd ed. San Diego, Academic Press, 2002.
2. Favus MJ (ed): Primer on the Metabolic Bone Diseases and Disorders of Mineral Metabolism, 4th ed. Philadelphia, Lippincott Williams & Williams, 1999.
3. Ganong WF: Review of Medical Physiology, 20th ed. New York, McGraw-Hill, 2001.
4. Genuth SM: Endocrine regulation of calcium and phosphate metabolism. In Berne RM, Levy MN (eds): Physiology, 4th ed. St. Louis, Mosby, 1998, pp 848–871.
5. Guyton AC, Hall JE (eds): Textbook of Medical Physiology, 10th ed. Philadelphia, W.B. Saunders, 2000.

III. Integrative Physiology

10. ENDOCRINE-METABOLIC INTEGRATION

Lauren Jacobson, Ph.D.

1. What are the two main determinants of body weight?

Body weight, or energy stored in the body, is the difference between **energy intake** and **energy expenditure.**

2. What determines energy intake?

Energy intake depends largely on food consumption. The **calorie** content of food is determined by its **macronutrient** composition (carbohydrate, protein, or fat). Complete oxidation of each type of macronutrient yields the following number of calories:

Carbohydrate	4 kcal/g
Protein	4 kcal/g
Fat	9 kcal/g

The standardized adult Western diet is 2000 kcal/day, of which 15–20% is recommended to come from protein, and no more than 30% is recommended to come from fat. However, calorie and nutrition requirements to maintain metabolic balance will depend on the size, activity, and health of an individual.

3. What other physiologic processes influence energy intake? Give examples.

Energy intake also depends on normal **digestion, absorption,** and cellular **uptake** of nutrients. For example, lactase deficiency (lactose intolerance) prevents breakdown of lactose into its component sugars, glucose and galactose, for absorption by the small intestine. Instead, lactose calories are lost through the stool. Loss of intestinal surface area from surgery or disease (such as opportunistic infections in AIDS) or excessively rapid transit of digestive products through the intestine (as in severe diarrhea) will decrease intestinal nutrient absorption even when digestion is normal. Once nutrients enter the bloodstream, they also must be capable of being transported into cells. Untreated type 1 diabetes mellitus causes severe wasting because muscle and fat lack insulin-mediated glucose uptake.

4. Besides appropriate calorie levels, what else must the diet provide to maintain metabolic balance?

The diet must contain sufficient amounts of substrate and energy to replace molecules that are damaged or destroyed as part of normal cellular functions. **Essential amino acids** and **essential fatty acids** cannot be synthesized from other molecules and must be supplied by the diet. If intake of these nutrients is inadequate, body stores will be broken down to obtain the needed molecules.

Dietary **vitamins** and **minerals** are not a significant source of calories, but are required for activity of enzymes and other proteins involved in normal macronutrient metabolism. These dietary components are called **micronutrients** because daily requirements are in the milligram range. Some minerals (Ca^{2+}, PO_4^{3-}, Mg^{2+}) are required in larger than milligram quantities per day and are known as macrominerals. Vitamin and mineral deficiencies can be caused by inadequate intake, absorption, or retention.

5. How does the body store energy?

Fat is the largest energy store, representing approximately 75% of total calorie reserves in the body. Its high caloric density, combined with its low water content, make fat a lightweight, efficient form of energy storage. Adult fat stores usually contain up to 2 months' worth of calories. **Glycogen** (carbohydrate) stores are an important energy source during short periods of fasting (meal-to-meal and overnight) but represent only about 1%, or less than 24 hours' worth, of calories. Glycogen is not an efficient form for long-term energy storage, because it is heavier (highly hydrated) and less calorically dense than fat. Protein is not a significant source of energy except in extreme starvation or disease, when glycogen and fat stores are gone.

6. What are the three main determinants of energy expenditure (metabolic rate)?

1. **Resting energy expenditure** (REE), also known as **basal metabolic rate** (BMR) is the fewest number of calories necessary to maintain all life processes when the body is at rest. REE is determined by lean (fat-free) body mass and body surface area, and accounts for **60–70% of total energy expenditure.** BMR is lower in women than men, and lower in older than in younger individuals.

2. **Thermogenesis** includes **diet-induced thermogenesis** (thermic effect of food), representing the calories used to digest, absorb, and store nutrients, and **nonshivering thermogenesis,** representing the calories used to produce heat or prevent heat loss, without physical activity. This accounts for **10–20% of total energy expenditure.**

3. **Physical activity** is highly variable, accounting for **20–30% of total energy expenditure**. This may include aimless activity (**fidgeting**) as well as **deliberate** activity.

7. Can total energy expenditure change?

Yes, although physical activity is the component most susceptible to voluntary control. Resting energy expenditure can be increased by hormones (thyroid hormone, progesterone), infection, and increases in the proportion of muscle to fat mass (secondary to physical activity). Nonshivering thermogenesis can be increased (although not always efficiently) by chronic increases in calorie intake, by leptin, and by drugs that activate β-adrenergic receptors on adipocytes (discussed below).

8. What is malnutrition?

Malnutrition occurs when ingestion, absorption or retention of macro- and micronutrients is insufficient to meet the body's needs. Malnutrition usually occurs when protein intake is inadequate, either because the diet contains enough calories but not enough protein (**protein malnutrition,** or **kwashiorkor**) or because total food consumption is too low to provide sufficient protein or calorie intake (**protein-calorie malnutrition,** or **marasmus**). In the latter case, ingested proteins are metabolized for energy rather than used for new protein synthesis.

9. Does malnutrition occur outside of developing nations?

Yes. Protein malnutrition can occur in individuals undertaking vegetarian diets. **Anorexia nervosa** is a psychiatric disease of self-imposed starvation and distorted body image, in which patients, typically young women, lose dangerous amounts of weight because they believe themselves to be too fat. **Infection, injury,** and **chronic disease** can cause *symptoms* of malnutrition (discussed in Chapter 11, Endocrine-Immune Interactions).

10. What are the endocrine effects of chronic malnutrition?

STIMULATION OF ENERGY-MOBILIZING HORMONES	INHIBITION OF ENERGY-STORING AND ENERGY-REQUIRING HORMONES
Glucocorticoids (cortisol)	Insulin
Glucagon	IGF-1
Growth hormone (lipolysis favored over growth because IGF-1 is decreased)	Thyroid axis Reproductive axis Sympathoadrenomedullary system

IGF-1 = insulin-like growth factor 1.

11. How do the endocrine effects of chronic malnutrition differ from those of short-term fasting?

During fasts of less than 3 days, **sympathetic nervous system** and **adrenomedullary activity** increases, leading to increased release of epinephrine (from the adrenal medulla) and norepinephrine (from postganglionic nerve terminals). However, during prolonged starvation or malnutrition, **sympathoadrenomedullary activity decreases to conserve energy**. This decrease is mediated by falling leptin levels (see questions 18–20).

12. What common clinical symptoms are associated with malnutrition?

Growth failure in children (failure to thrive) indicates a serious underlying problem with nutrition, metabolism, or disease and results from inhibition of both growth hormone (GH)–induced insulin-like growth factor 1 (IGF-1) secretion and IGF-1–induced protein synthesis. Malnutrition or overexercise can cause **amenorrhea** (cessation of menstruation) in adult women of reproductive age. Amenorrhea occurs in highly trained athletes and dancers and is the *primary* complaint bringing women with anorexia nervosa to a physician.

13. Describe the effects of malnutrition on the thyroid axis.

Peripheral deiodination of tetraiodothyronine (T_4) to triiodothyronine (T_3) is inhibited, leading to a **decrease in circulating T_3.** Thyroid-stimulating hormone (TSH) does not increase despite loss of feedback inhibition by T_3. These changes are thought to reflect inhibition of thyrotropin-releasing hormone (TRH) at the hypothalamic level.

14. How does malnutrition inhibit the reproductive axis?

The reproductive axis is inhibited by malnutrition at the level of the hypothalamus. This effect was deduced by the finding that administration of gonadotropin-releasing hormone (GnRH) would reinstate gonadal steroid and pituitary gonadotropin secretion in undernourished individuals.

15. What are the main determinants of total food intake?

Total food intake is the product of **meal size** and **meal number.** Meal size and meal number can vary widely depending on food availability, food palatability, activity schedules, and associated cues but typically change inversely to one another to maintain a constant body weight. Meal size is reduced by **gastric distention** and by the release of **intestinal satiety peptides.** However, these short-term signals do *not* affect meal number or total food intake.

16. Which intestinal peptides act as satiety factors?

Cholecystokinin (CCK) is the best characterized of the satiety peptides. CCK is secreted by I cells in the **duodenum** in response to protein and fat digestion products entering the small intestine. CCK has a number of roles in digestion, including the stimulation of gall bladder contraction and stimulation of pancreatic enzyme secretion, in addition to its function as a satiety factor. Administration of CCK decreases the size of a meal, whereas CCK antagonists increase meal size. CCK synergizes with the effects of gastric distention in inhibiting **short-term food intake,** but has little effect on subsequent meal number or total food intake. Other possible intestinal satiety factors include bombesin-related peptides and glucagon-like peptide 1 (GLP-1).

17. Is anything that decreases food intake a satiety factor?

No. Nausea, drowsiness, and fear can inhibit food intake but are not what normally control satiety and meal termination. Drugs that impair motor control can interfere with the ability to approach, manipulate, chew, and swallow food. CCK has been shown to increase satiety and decrease meal size in humans without any of these adverse effects.

18. What is leptin and why is it a good index of long-term metabolic balance?

Leptin is a peptide hormone secreted by adipocytes. Leptin is secreted in proportion to fat mass. Because fat can be stored only when energy intake exceeds short-term needs, leptin levels are an indicator of the body's energy reserves.

19. What are the physiologic effects of leptin?

Leptin **inhibits food intake** and **increases energy expenditure.** Leptin is derived from a Greek wording meaning "thin" because its actions produce weight loss. Leptin-induced weight loss differs from that produced by food restriction in that metabolic rate does not fall and leptin selectively stimulates **fat mobilization** (rather than water or protein loss).

20. What is the physiologic role of leptin in body weight regulation?

Leptin is more important for indicating when the body is "fat enough" than for protecting against obesity. This theory derives from studies in *ob/ob* mice, which are genetically deficient in leptin. These mice show endocrine and metabolic effects of starvation, even though they are actually hyperphagic (overeating) and obese. *Ob/ob* mice are growth-stunted, infertile, underactive, and unable to increase metabolic rate normally. These functions can be restored by leptin treatment while the mice are still relatively obese. These observations have been interpreted as showing that lack of leptin, rather than excessive body mass, interferes with normal physiology. Leptin also normalizes the hormonal changes and decreases in metabolism caused by starvation in normal, lean animals. Thus, leptin signals when the body can afford to devote energy to relatively expensive processes not strictly needed for individual survival.

21. Does leptin deficiency account for most human obesity?

No. Most overweight individuals have high plasma leptin levels proportional to their greater total fat mass, indicating that their leptin production is normal. Only a handful of obese individuals worldwide have been found to have mutations in the leptin gene.

22. Can leptin treatment help overweight individuals lose weight?

Yes, but no more effectively than other weight loss drugs or regimens. Virtually all cases of excess weight are thought to be due to **leptin resistance.**

23. Is leptin resistance in human obesity due to leptin receptor mutations?

Rarely. Only one case of obesity has been linked to a mutation in the long (biologically active) form of the leptin receptor. Leptin resistance, like insulin resistance, is a **polygenic** syndrome (caused by many genes) that is influenced by **environmental factors.**

24. Where does leptin act?

The **brain** is a major target of leptin action. The **hypothalamus** expresses the highest levels of the signaling form of the leptin receptor. Several shorter isoforms of leptin receptor lacking the intracellular signaling domain have been found; these are thought to function in leptin transport.

Leptin receptors are present in neurons in both the **medial hypothalamus,** a **satiety area** where lesions cause animals to overeat and gain weight, and the **lateral hypothalamus,** a **feeding area** where lesions inhibit food intake. Although these regional distinctions are only rough generalizations, they remain useful for characterizing the overall influence of hypothalamic areas controlling body weight.

25. What is the relationship between satiety factors and leptin in the control of food intake?

Inhibitory effects of short-term satiety factors on meal size are mediated by structures in the **brainstem** such as the **nucleus of the tractus solitarius** (NTS), which receives **vagal afferents** signaling gastric filling and contains neurons responsive to CCK. **Leptin enhances satiety factor effects on meal size.** However, **regulation of total food intake** in response to metabolic status signaled by leptin **requires connections with the forebrain** (presumably the hypothalamus). These anatomic distinctions were demonstrated in rats whose connections between the forebrain and the brainstem were severed at the level of the inferior colliculus. Such animals show normal regulation of meal size when fed passively but do not initiate meals or exhibit compensatory increases in passive intake if they have been previously food-deprived. These deficits are not attributable to the severity of their brain lesion, because they are still capable of voluntary activities such as grooming and climbing.

26. What is neuropeptide Y?

Neuropeptide Y (NPY), so named because of its high number of tyrosine (Y) residues, is a potent **orexigen** (stimulator of food intake) when administered into the brain, even in sated animals. NPY is concentrated in the **arcuate hypothalamus** but is also present at lower levels in the caudal medulla.

27. What is the role of NPY in leptin action?

NPY is required for the increases in food intake when leptin levels are low. NPY expression is increased by food deprivation (which decreases plasma leptin), and in models of leptin deficiency, such as the *ob/ob* mouse. Mice deficient in both NPY and leptin, produced by breeding *ob/ob* and NPY knockout mice, eat and weigh less than mice lacking only leptin.

28. NPY stimulates feeding but is expressed in the medial (arcuate) hypothalamus. Doesn't this contradict the role of the medial hypothalamus in mediating satiety?

No. Satiety and feeding areas of the hypothalamus are functional generalizations, meaning that the effects of factors promoting satiety predominate over those of orexigenic (appetite-stimulating) factors in the medial hypothalamus. The opposite situation occurs in the lateral hypothalamus.

29. What is the role of pro-opiomelanocortin in leptin action?

Pro-opiomelanocortin (POMC) is expressed by **arcuate hypothalamus** neurons. POMC neurons process the POMC precursor peptide more completely than do the adrenocorticotropic hormone (ACTH)–secreting corticotrophs of the anterior pituitary, liberating the first 11 amino acids of the ACTH molecule as α-melanocyte–stimulating hormone (**α-MSH**). α-MSH inhibits food intake, and leptin stimulates POMC expression and POMC neuron activity. POMC neurons do *not* express NPY.

30. What are melanocortin receptors?

Melanocortin (MC) receptors bind POMC-derived peptides and related molecules. The melanocortin-1 (MC-1) receptor mediates pigmentation effects in skin, the melanocortin-2 receptor is the adrenocortical receptor for ACTH, and the melanocortin –3 and –4 receptors are expressed almost exclusively in the brain and have been implicated in body weight homeostasis. In particular, **MC-4 receptor** knockout mice have been found to have increased food intake, increased body weight, and decreased sensitivity to leptin.

31. Do melanocortin receptors bind anything besides POMC-derived peptides?

Yes. At least one other neuropeptide, **agouti-related peptide** (AgRP), competes for α-MSH binding to the MC-4 receptor. This competition blocks the anorectic effect of α-MSH. AgRP is so named because it is related to agouti, a pigment protein in mice. Brain overexpression of agouti in a natural mouse mutant, transgenic overexpression of AgRP in a normal mouse, or AgRP injection into the brain induces hyperphagia and obesity by antagonizing α-MSH action. AgRP is expressed by NPY neurons in the arcuate hypothalamus; thus, activation of these neurons produces a "2-for-1" stimulus to food intake by engaging both NPY and melanocortin receptor systems.

32. What is the *clinical* evidence that melanocortins are important for regulating body weight?

Two obese humans have been identified with POMC gene truncations that prevent α-MSH synthesis. One human patient has been found with a mutation in the MC-4 receptor. This individual is also obese and constantly hungry.

33. How does leptin regulate energy expenditure?

Leptin increases thermogenesis by **increasing sympathetic nervous system activity.** Norepinephrine released by sympathetic nerves binds β-adrenergic receptors on adipocytes. White and brown adipose tissues express a fat-specific β receptor, the **β_3 adrenergic receptor,** although β_1 and β_2 receptors are also present. β-Adrenergic receptor activation in white as well as brown adipocytes contributes to whole-body thermogenesis and energy expenditure. Compounds that selectively stimulate the fat-specific β_3 receptor are currently a focus of drug development.

34. What are uncoupling proteins?

Uncoupling proteins (UCP) are a family of proteins structurally related to uncoupling protein 1 (UCP-1), an inner mitochondrial membrane protein found exclusively in brown fat. Brown fat gets its characteristic dark appearance from high numbers of mitochondria. UCP-1 in brown fat mitochondria acts as a proton transporter, allowing the energy gradient built up by the electron transport chain to dissipate as heat (**thermogenesis**) without being stored through adenosine triphosphate (ATP) synthesis. UCP-1 is stimulated by leptin and by β-adrenergic receptor activation.

35. How do uncoupling proteins contribute to body weight homeostasis?

Uncoupling electron transport prevents energy from being stored as fat. Sustained increases in calorie intake induce increases in thermogenesis. The extent to which increased thermogenesis compensates for increased intake contributes to an individual's susceptibility to weight gain. Conversely, when intake is reduced, the body conserves energy by reducing thermogenesis. Such reductions in energy expenditure account for slower rates of weight loss after the first 1–2 weeks of dieting.

36. Do thinner individuals have higher levels of UCP-1?

Probably not. UCP-1 is expressed only in brown fat, and humans do not have significant amounts of brown fat after infancy. Other related proteins, some of which (e.g., UCP-2, UCP-3) have been found in white fat and skeletal muscle, are more likely to account for thermogenesis in humans.

37. What are the risks of being overweight?

Overweight and obese individuals have a higher risk of several chronic diseases, including hypertension, cardiac failure, stroke, and type 2 diabetes mellitus. These diseases shorten life span. The inference that excess body fat, by increasing these diseases, also increases mortality has been supported by epidemiologic studies correlating increased longevity with lower weight gain during aging. Other disorders associated with being overweight include arthritis, gallstones, sleep apnea, and an increased risk of colon cancer.

38. How is obesity defined?

Obesity is defined as a **body mass index** (BMI, expressed as body weight in kilograms divided by the square of height in meters) above 30 kg/m^2. A person is **overweight** if his or her BMI is 25.0–29.9 kg/m^2.

39. What are the risks of *negative* metabolic balance?

When energy expenditure exceeds energy intake, body energy stores are mobilized in the following order: glycogen, fat, and finally protein. Such conditions can occur in starvation, or in severe disease states (AIDS, cancer, sepsis, major trauma) in which decreased food intake may be combined with increased metabolic demand. When fat stores drop below a given set point, endocrine abnormalities result, including infertility in adults and reduced growth in children. When fat stores are exhausted and protein breakdown decreases lean body mass below 60%, death occurs, usually due to infections that overwhelm the body's weakened defenses.

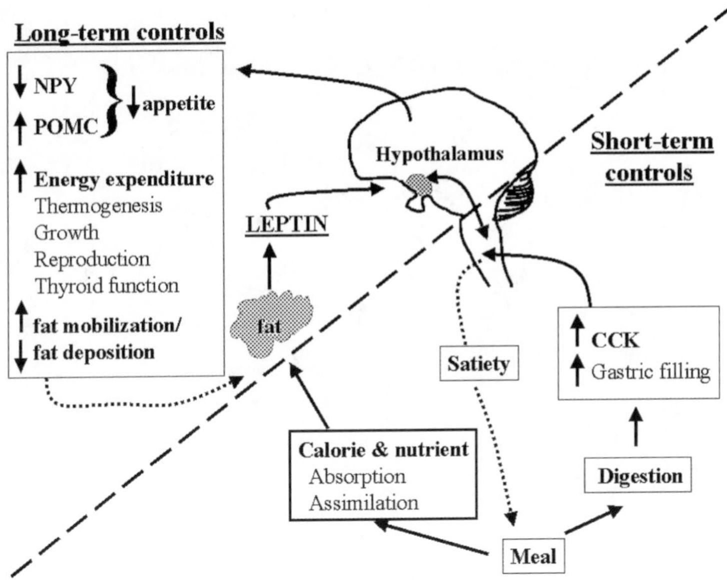

Relationship between short-term satiety controls and long-term, leptin-related controls on food intake and metabolism. The dashed diagonal line delineates short-term (*right*) from long-term factors (*left*) and the general brain regions (brainstem vs. forebrain) subserving their effects. The double-headed arrow spanning this line represents connections between the forebrain and brainstem that are also required for leptin action. Solid lines are used to indicate stimulatory influences, while dotted lines represent inhibition.

BIBLIOGRAPHY

1. Dananberg J, Caro JF: Obesity. In DeGroot LJ, Jameson JL (eds): Endocrinology, 4th ed. Philadelphia, W.B. Saunders, 2001, pp 615–630.
2. Harper ME, Himms-Hagen J: Mitochondrial efficiency: Lessons learned from transgenic mice. Biochim Biophys Acta 1504:159–172, 2001.
3. Heber D: Starvation and nutritional therapy. In DeGroot LJ, Jameson JL (eds): Endocrinology, 4th ed. Philadelphia, W.B. Saunders, 2001, pp 642–653.
4. Woods SC, Seeley RJ, Porte D Jr, Schwartz MW: Signals that regulate food intake and energy homeostasis. Science 280:1378–1383, 1998.

11. ENDOCRINE-IMMUNE INTERACTIONS

Lauren Jacobson, Ph.D.

1. What are cytokines?

Cytokines are soluble molecules released by cells of the immune system. Cytokines act as growth, activation, and chemotactic factors for other immune cells and are an essential part of normal immune function. Cytokines include **interleukins, tumor necrosis factor** (TNF), **interferons, hematopoietic growth and colony-stimulating factors,** and **chemokines.**

2. How are cytokines like hormones?

Cytokines can enter the bloodstream and affect cells and tissues distant from their source of production. Cytokines are also produced by some endocrine tissues. Cytokines produced by immune cells during injury, infection, or inflammation have direct effects on many endocrine tissues (see figure).

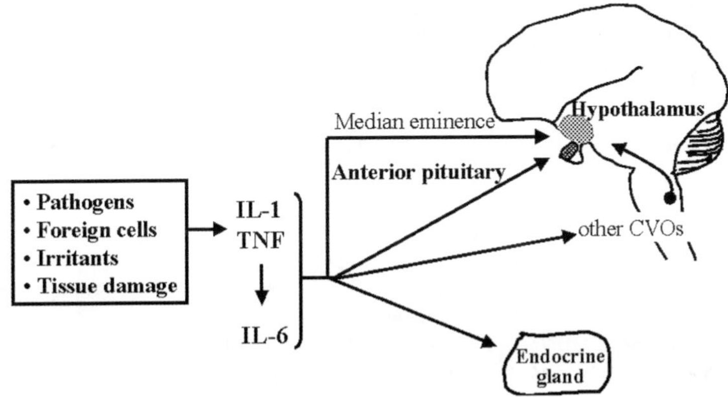

Schematic of endocrine-immune interactions after systemic infection, inflammation, or injury. The cytokines typically produced in response to these stimuli can act at the brain to regulate neuroendocrine releasing factors in the hypothalamus (gray-shaded area), probably via the median eminence or afferent connections from other circumventricular organs (CVOs). Cytokines can also act directly at both the anterior pituitary and the endocrine gland itself to influence hormone secretion.

3. What is the acute-phase response?

The acute phase response is a characteristic sequence of **immune, endocrine,** and **metabolic** responses to tissue injury or immune challenge:

1. Exposure to foreign substances, organisms, cells, or products of tissue injury first stimulates production of the cytokines **interleukin 1** (IL-1) and **TNF.**
2. IL-1 and TNF have 3 main actions:
   a. Fever induction (by increasing hypothalamic **prostaglandins**)
   b. Appetite inhibition
   c. Stimulation of a third cytokine, **interleukin-6** (IL-6)
3. IL-1, TNF, and IL-6 stimulate glucocorticoid secretion by activating the **hypothalamic-pituitary-adrenocortical axis.**
4. Glucocorticoids and IL-6 act together on the liver to induce synthesis of acute phase proteins (complement-related proteins, globulins, and fibrinogen) involved in tissue repair and antimicrobial defenses.

4. In addition to acute-phase protein induction, what other important effects do glucocorticoids have on the response to injury or infection?

Glucocorticoids also have potent **immunosuppressive** and **anti-inflammatory** actions that function as negative feedback controls restraining the immune response. Glucocorticoid-deficient humans and animals are much more susceptible to shock induced by immune or inflammatory stimuli.

Synthetic glucocorticoids (such as prednisone) are widely used to treat a variety of inflammatory diseases, such as asthma and arthritis, and to suppress tissue rejection in transplant patients. Anti-inflammatory and immunosuppressive therapies are the most common clinical uses of glucocorticoids. These therapeutic benefits are not without risk, because immune suppression also renders individuals treated with high levels of glucocorticoids highly susceptible to opportunistic infection.

5. Which three main aspects of the inflammatory response are inhibited by glucocorticoids?

1. Glucocorticoids **inhibit production of cytokines** (including IL-1, TNF, and IL-6) and **other inflammatory mediators** (prostaglandins, histamine).
2. Glucocorticoids **reduce immune cell response** to inflammatory mediators. The most dramatic example of this effect is glucocorticoid-induced apoptosis (programmed cell death) in lymphocytes.
3. Glucocorticoids **reduce vasodilation** in response to inflammatory mediators, thereby reducing accumulation of immune cells and fluid (edema) at the site of injury or infection.

6. How do cytokines stimulate the hypothalamic-pituitary-adrenocortical axis?

IL-1, TNF, and IL-6 can act directly at all three levels of the hypothalamic-pituitary-adrenocortical axis to increase glucocorticoid secretion:

1. At the **brain,** they stimulate secretion of corticotropin-releasing hormone, the main adrenocorticotropic hormone (ACTH)–releasing factor.
2. At the **pituitary corticotroph,** they stimulate secretion of ACTH.
3. At the **adrenocortical zona fasciculata,** they increase glucocorticoid (cortisol) secretion.

7. How do cytokines act on the brain?

Cytokine proteins are too large to cross the blood-brain barrier. However, cytokines can act at **circumventricular organs** such as the median eminence, where the blood-brain barrier is incomplete. Cytokine production by cerebrovascular endothelium, choroid plexus, and glial cells may represent another mechanism by which cytokine signals are transmitted across the blood-brain barrier.

8. How are the general metabolic and endocrine effects of cytokines *similar* to those of starvation?

Many cytokines cause **anorexia** (appetite inhibition), so food intake is decreased. Cytokines also reprioritize energy expenditure, promoting **energy mobilization** for tissue defenses and suppressing processes not required for immediate survival. Therefore, hormones important for energy mobilization (glucocorticoids, catecholamines, glucagon) are stimulated, whereas energy-requiring endocrine systems are inhibited (thyroid, growth, and reproductive axes).

9. How do cytokines affect the secretion and action of glucagon and insulin?

Cytokines promote **glucagon secretion,** resulting in **increased hepatic glucose output.** Cytokine effects on insulin and glucose tolerance vary depending on the stage and severity of the acute phase response. Typically, cytokines, particularly TNF, induce **insulin resistance.** This effect is both a direct effect of cytokines on muscle and fat and an indirect effect of cytokine-induced elevations in glucocorticoids and glucagon. In the early stages of sepsis or exposure to high levels of cytokines, hypoglycemia may occur if metabolic demand outstrips hepatic glucose output.

10. How do cytokines affect the growth hormone (GH) axis?

As with fasting or hypoglycemia, the metabolic stimulus of cytokine exposure is associated with increased growth hormone levels. However, as in prolonged starvation, there is **little anabolic effect** of elevated GH because growth-promoting responses to GH are inhibited. Cytokines inhibit the response of insulin-like growth factor 1 (IGF-1; somatomedin C) to GH and reduce tissue protein synthesis in response to IGF-1.

11. What effects do cytokines have on the thyroid and reproductive axes?

Both the thyroid and the reproductive axes are suppressed by cytokines. Teleologically, such effects can be viewed as shunting energy toward immune defenses and avoiding the additional metabolic demands imposed by elevated thyroid hormone levels or by having to bear and care for offspring. Cytokines act at the brain to **suppress thyrotropin-releasing hormone (TRH) and gonadotropin-releasing hormone (GnRH)** and at the **thyroid and gonads** to **inhibit thyroid hormone and sex steroid secretion**, respectively. The respective pituitary trophic hormones, thyroid-stimulating hormone (TSH), and the gonadotropins, luteinizing hormone (LH) and follicle-stimulating hormone (FSH), are generally unchanged or slightly reduced. The failure of these hormones to increase, despite loss of feedback inhibition by their target gland hormones, reflects inhibition of their respective hypothalamic releasing factors.

12. What is euthyroid sick syndrome (nonthyroidal illness)?

This condition is the most common thyroid problem found in hospitalized patients and refers to the association of "inappropriately normal" levels of TSH with reduced levels of thyroid hormones. Chronic malnutrition and disease, including wasting states associated with elevated cytokines, inhibit production of thyroid hormones, which are secreted primarily as tetraiodothyronine (T_4). Peripheral deiodination of T_4 to triiodothyronine (T_3) is also inhibited, causing reduced levels of T_3. The degree to which T_4 levels are normal or reduced depends on the extent to which decreased peripheral conversion of T_4 offsets decreases in T_4 secretion. However, because T_3 is more potent than T_4, TSH would be expected to increase with reductions in T_3 feedback inhibition. As discussed above, the lack of an increase in TSH indicates aberrant inhibition of the thyroid axis at the level of the brain.

13. How do the metabolic and endocrine effects of cytokines *differ* from those of starvation?

Unlike prolonged starvation, in which metabolic rate and sympathetic activity decrease in order to conserve energy, cytokines **increase metabolic rate** and catecholamine levels. Sepsis and severe injury are referred to as "hypermetabolic states" because the calorie expenditure required for fighting infection and tissue repair is disproportionately high relative to food intake and activity level. Much of the increase in metabolic rate is due to fever.

14. What is the net metabolic impact of cytokine effects on endocrine activity?

INCREASE IN	MEDIATED BY
Hepatic glycogenolysis	Increased glucagon, catecholamines
Gluconeogenesis	Increases in glucagon, glucocorticoids, and GH
Circulating glucose	Increases in glucagon, glucocorticoids, catecholamines, and GH
	Decreases in insulin sensitivity
Protein breakdown (catabolism)	Increases in glucocorticoids
	Decreases in responsiveness to insulin, GH, and IGF-1
Lipolysis	Increases in glucocorticoids, catecholamines, and GH

15. Why is the metabolic state associated with elevated cytokines, injury, or infection called cachexia?

As can be seen from the table of metabolic effects above, these conditions favor depletion of all energy stores in the body. Particularly, once body protein is lost, physical **wasting** (cachexia) is readily apparent. One of the first cytokines to be identified was isolated on the basis of its ability to cause wasting in experimental animals and was originally called *cachectin* (now known as TNF).

16. How can a vicious cycle develop between malnutrition and infection or injury?

If nutrient intake is inadequate to support normal protein synthesis, cytokine production, along with the immune and repair processes it supports, will be impaired. Poor tissue healing and lower immune defenses increase susceptibility to infection. Infection, by simultaneously increasing metabolic demands and decreasing food intake, can take a further toll on body protein stores, particularly because recovery will be slower when immune function is compromised. Almost 50% of all hospitalized patients show signs of malnutrition. Loss of more than 30% of body protein is inevitably fatal.

BIBLIOGRAPHY

1. Heber D: Starvation and nutritional therapy. In DeGroot LJ, Jameson JL (eds): Endocrinology, 4th ed. Philadelphia, W. B. Saunders, 2001, pp 642–653.
2. Reichlin S: Endocrine-immune interactions. In DeGroot LJ (ed): Endocrinology, 3rd ed. Philadelphia, W. B. Saunders, 1995, pp 2964–2989.

12. MATERNAL–FETAL PHYSIOLOGY

Maureen Keller-Wood, Ph.D., and Charles E. Wood, Ph.D.

PLACENTAL PHYSIOLOGY

1. How is the placenta formed in humans?

The placenta is formed by tissues derived from the embryo. The trophectoderm of the blastocyst forms the placenta by invading the endometrial layer of the uterus. This process, called **implantation,** causes modification and restructuring of the endometrium and its vasculature. This allows the chorion of the trophoblast to form villi, which project into pools of maternal blood in the intervillous spaces. Within the center of each villus are fetal arterioles, which perfuse a capillary network within the villus (see figure). The fetal blood vessels are surrounded by fetal connective tissue and macrophages; the surface of the villus is comprised of fetal trophoblast cells. The outer cell layer of the villus is composed of syncytiotrophoblast cells, which are multinucleate cells formed from fusion of the underlying layer of cells, the cytotrophoblasts. Together the tissues of the fetal villi and the maternal blood form the functional placenta.

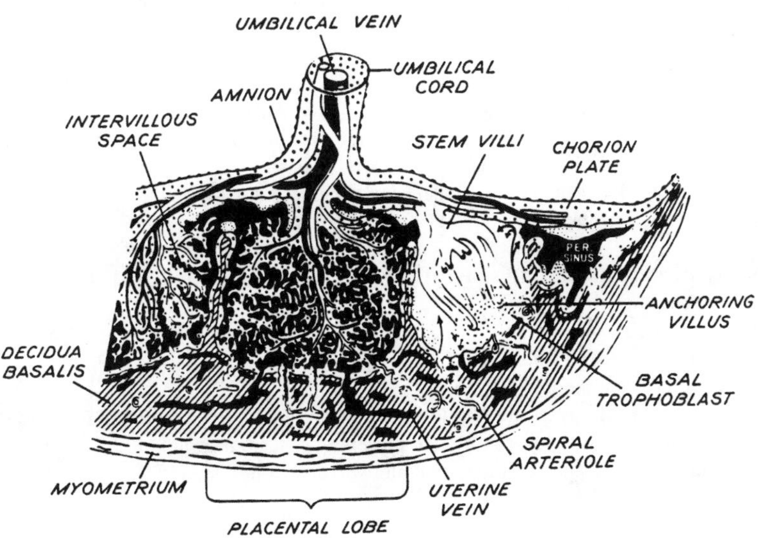

Structure of villus (dark areas show intervillous space filled with maternal blood). Fetal tissues are depicted as stippled areas. Maternal tissues (decidua) are depicted as hatched areas. (From Dawes GS: Foetal and Neonatal Physiology. Chicago, Year Book Medical Publishers, 1968, with permission.)

2. What form of placenta is found in humans?

Human placenta has several designations:

- **Chorioallantoic placenta.** The chorionic membrane is formed by the trophoblast and consists of a membrane around the embryo and the yolk sac cavity (see figure). The allantoic sac is formed as an outgrowth of the fetal gut caudal to the yolk sac. The allantoic membranes contact the chorionic membrane; in humans, the lumen of the allantois itself is small.
- **Discoid placenta.** Placenta has a disk-like shape.

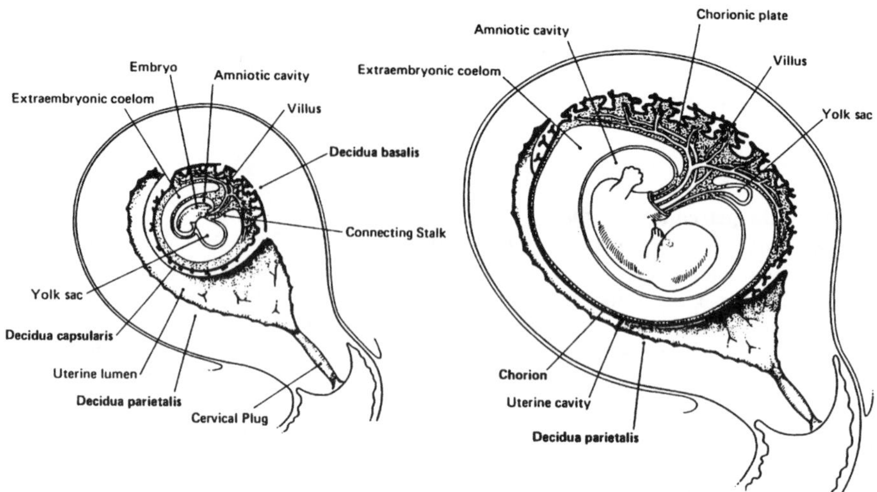

Anatomic relationships between fetus, chorion, amnion, and decidual layers in the human. (From Faber JJ, Thorburn KL (eds): Placental Physiology. New York, Raven Press, 1983, with permission.)

- **Deciduate placenta.** This designation refers to the invasion of the maternal endometrium by the trophoblast so that a portion of the endometrium, the decidua, is shed, along with the placental tissues, with delivery of the fetus.
- **Hemochorial placenta.** The maternal blood (hemo-) directly bathes the outermost trophoblastic (chorial) layer.

3. What layers make up the diffusion barrier between maternal and fetal blood in the primate and human placenta?

- Trophoblast cells
- Fetal connective tissue cells
- Fetal capillary endothelium

All three of these cell layers are within the villus and are derived from the fetus. Maternal capillary endothelium is not a layer in human placenta because maternal arterial blood empties directly into the intervillous pools of maternal blood that surround the villi.

4. List the functions of the placenta.

1. Acts as an exchanger of solutes, solvents, and heat between the mother and fetus
2. Maintains a barrier to most large protein molecules and immunoglobulins between mother and fetus
3. Secretes hormones
4. Is active in metabolizing many substances

5. List the substances exchanged across the placenta.

Essential for fetal growth and development:

Water
Ions
Glucose
Lipids
Amino acids
Calcium
Phosphorus
Oxygen

Fetal waste products:

Carbon dioxide
Creatinine
Bilirubin
Urea

Some of these substances, including water, most ions, glucose, and amino acids, pass through channels or use specific carrier molecules within the placenta. The placenta is a barrier to most large proteins, including most pituitary hormones and hormones such as insulin and glucagon, circulating binding proteins, and immunoglobulins. However, IgG appears to be passed from mother to fetus before birth. The placenta is also active in the metabolism of many hormones, including ACTH, insulin, thyroid hormones, and cortisol.

6. What determines the exchange of substances across the placenta?

- The arrangement of fetal and maternal blood vessels
- The blood flows in the maternal and fetal vessels
- The total membrane surface available for exchange
- The concentration, osmotic, and electrochemical gradients for the substance across the placenta
- The permeability of the substance (or diffusing capacity)
- The presence of carriers or pores (or both) for passage of the substance

7. What hormones are produced within and secreted by the placenta?

The placenta secretes **estrogens** and **progesterone.** In the case of the human placenta, progesterone is produced within the placenta, whereas estrogens are aromatized from androgens produced in other sites. The placenta also produces and secretes a number of hormones with similarities to pituitary and hypothalamic hormones, including human chorionic gonadotropin (hCG), human placental lactogen (hPL), corticotropin-releasing hormone (CRH), and proopiomelanocortin (POMC).

8. Are placental hormones secreted by the fetus or the mother?

The fetus.

9. What cell type(s) in the placenta secrete hormones?

The hormones are secreted by the fetal **cytotrophoblast,** which predominates in the first trimester, and the **syncytiotrophoblast,** which predominates thereafter. The secretion of hCG is thought to be primarily from cytotrophoblasts, whereas the secretion of hPL, placental corticotropin-releasing hormone (CRH), and the steroid hormones is thought to occur from syncytiotrophoblasts.

10. Discuss the role of hCG.

hCG is a glycoprotein hormone secreted by the trophoblastic cells of the human placenta. It is structurally similar to the glycoprotein hormones of the anterior pituitary. It has an α subunit identical to luteinizing hormone (LH), follicle-stimulating hormone (FSH), and thyroid-stimulating hormone (TSH) and a β subunit with about 80% homology with human LH. hCG acts on the LH receptors in the ovary to stimulate progesterone and estrogen secretion and prevents luteolysis. The production of progesterone and estrogen by the corpus luteum maintains the uterine endometrium and prevents menses. The secretion of hCG is essential for the maintenance of pregnancy for the first trimester in humans. The concentration of hCG in maternal blood peaks at approximately 10 weeks of gestation and then declines. Placental secretion of progesterone begins in the 6th week and is normally adequate by 10–12 weeks to prevent uterine involution. The secretion of hCG into fetal blood is also thought to stimulate the production of testosterone by the fetal testes.

11. Discuss the role of hPL.

hPL is the major protein hormone secreted by the human placenta. The majority of the hPL produced is secreted into the maternal circulation. hPL has sometimes also been called human chorionic somatomammotropin (hCS) because this hormone is structurally similar to the pituitary growth hormone (GH). Two structural variants of the protein are found in human placenta; these have approximately 85% sequence homology with GH protein but only 27% homology with prolactin. The mRNA for hPL are similar to that of GH, and the genes for hPL also appear to be related to GH and are found on the same chromosome as the gene for GH. As primate GH also acts on prolactin receptors, hPL can exert some prolactin-like actions; in fact, the hPL molecule appears to have a greater action at prolactin receptors than GH receptors. Despite this, hPL actually is thought to have little lactogenic action because it does not stimulate milk production during pregnancy. hPL, however, is thought to have mammotrophic actions on the mammary glands to cause ductal development.

hPL is also thought to have GH-like action on maternal metabolism. hPL has relatively little growth-promoting action but appears to act like GH to stimulate lipolysis, reduce insulin sensitivity, and increase glucose resistance. These metabolic effects of hPL are thought to increase maternal blood glucose levels and therefore increase supply of glucose to the fetus. hPL may have anabolic actions in the fetus. There is evidence that it acts at fetal fibroblasts, muscle, and liver. In fetal liver, it may stimulate insulin-like growth factor (IGF) release, increase fetal glycogen deposition by increasing the effects of insulin, and inhibit glycogenolytic actions of glucagon. In fetal muscle, it may increase amino acid uptake, which is not dependent on pituitary GH in the fetus.

The production of hPL is proportional to fetal growth and fetal weight. Therefore, its increased production as the fetus grows may allow for increased supply of glucose to the fetus. hPL is also increased with maternal hypoglycemia or fasting when it may also help to maintain fuel supply to the fetus.

In primates there is also production of a substance similar in structure to hPL by the decidua of the uterus. This prolactin-like hormone is stimulated by relaxin and progesterone and may be important for maintaining the decidua; in rats, terminating prolactin expression in decidua causes regression and degeneration of the decidua.

12. Discuss the role of placental CRH.

The role of placental CRH is unknown. CRH secretion from the human placenta appears to increase as pregnancy progresses and appears to increase more precipitously in pregnancies complicated by pregnancy-induced hypertension or preterm labor. By late gestation, circulating plasma CRH levels are high. The majority of CRH produced by the placenta is bound to a circulating binding protein, which is also produced by the human placenta. Most of this CRH is therefore rendered biologically inactive in terms of stimulation of ACTH release from the pituitary. Both ACTH and cortisol, however, are increased during pregnancy. This increase occurs by the second trimester and also occurs in species with no placental secretion of CRH, suggesting that placental CRH is not the primary factor causing an increase in maternal or fetal adrenocortical activity. The higher levels of CRH in maternal plasma during preterm and term labor have suggested that CRH may play a role in initiation of labor. CRH has effects on prostaglandin production in the placenta, and therefore on myometrial contractility, but also may vasodilate the uterine vasculature. Cortisol, prostaglandins, and oxytocin all stimulate placental CRH secretion; this suggests that placental CRH may play an autoregulatory role in modulating tone of myometrial and vascular smooth muscle.

13. Define relaxin and discuss its role.

Relaxin is a protein hormone made by the corpus luteum. It is highest in the first trimester but detectable for all of human pregnancy. Relaxin release from the corpus luteum may be stimulated by hCG. Relaxin has been shown to inhibit uterine contractions and to cause relaxation of the pubic symphysis.

14. What is the principal estrogen secreted by the human placenta?

Estriol. The ratio of estriol to estradiol in the urine of pregnant women is about 10:1. Estriol accounts for about 30% of the unconjugated estrogens in plasma and about 90% of the conjugated estrogens in urine.

15. What is the major progestational agent of human pregnancy?

Progesterone.

16. How is progesterone produced?

Progesterone is produced from cholesterol in the human placenta. The primary source of this cholesterol appears to be low-density lipoproteins (LDL), rather than de novo synthesis from acetate.

CHANGES IN MATERNAL PHYSIOLOGY DURING PREGNANCY

17. What changes in maternal physiology occur during pregnancy?

- Growth, development, and differentiation of estrogen-dependent and progesterone-dependent tissues
- Changes in the maternal cardiovascular system, respiratory function, renal function, and metabolism
- Increased levels of estrogens, progesterone, and placentally derived hormones
- Increased levels of hormones of the renin-angiotensin system, the thyroid, the adrenal, and the pancreas

18. What changes occur in the maternal cardiovascular system during pregnancy?

During pregnancy maternal blood volume is increased by approximately 40%. The increase in maternal plasma volume is not matched by an equivalent increase in red cell mass; therefore, maternal hematocrit usually decreases, resulting in the "anemia of pregnancy." Maternal cardiac output also dramatically increases, with a large increase in stroke volume and a small increase in heart rate. Despite the increase in maternal blood volume and cardiac output, maternal blood pressure falls by about 5–10 mmHg. This suggests that maternal vascular resistance is decreased and maternal vascular compliance is increased. Maternal baroreflex responses are also blunted during pregnancy so that heart rate, hormone, and renal responses to reduced pressures are also blunted. These changes occur relatively early in pregnancy, by the end of the first trimester. As pregnancy progresses, maternal venous return can be compromised by compression of the inferior vena cava, particularly if the woman lies on her back.

19. Describe the factors that might contribute to the pronounced changes in maternal volume and blood pressure in pregnancy.

The exact mechanisms for the change in maternal cardiovascular function is not known. However, several factors appear to contribute. Estrogens are known to increase the production of angiotensinogen in the liver during pregnancy. Progesterone and estrogen increase the release of renin from the kidney. These effects together increase the plasma concentrations of angiotensin II. Aldosterone concentrations are therefore increased in pregnancy and would increase plasma volume. Plasma ACTH and cortisol secretion also increase in pregnancy and may contribute to increased vascular volume; in addition, progesterone itself may increase volume.

Pregnancy appears to reduce the baroreflex response to changes in arterial pressure, which appears to allow the regulation of blood pressure at a new (lower) level. This effect may be mediated by a central action of progesterone.

Pregnancy also reduces the increase in vascular resistance and blood pressure in response to angiotensin II. The refractoriness of vascular beds, including the uterine bed, to angiotensin may be mediated by nitric oxide or by prostaglandins. Both of these appear to be stimulated by estrogens.

20. Discuss the changes in respiratory function that occur during pregnancy.

Tidal volume is increased, and there is a slight increase in respiratory rate. The increases in tidal volume and respiratory rate are thought to be stimulated by progesterone, which appears to increase sensitivity of the respiratory center to the partial pressure of carbon dioxide in arterial blood ($PaCO_2$). Maternal respiratory function is also altered by the growth of the fetus; functional reserve capacity is decreased in late gestation. The increased ventilation in pregnancy tends to cause a decreased arterial $PaCO_2$. Thus, pregnant women frequently have a respiratory alkalosis and a compensatory metabolic acidosis.

21. Discuss the changes in renal function that occur during pregnancy.

Renal blood flow and glomerular filtration rate are increased. Glucosuria can occur in pregnant women; more glucose is filtered as a result of increased glomerular filtration rate, and if the tubular maximal threshold is relatively low, this results in glucose in the urine. Plasma sodium levels are generally decreased in pregnant women, despite the increase in plasma aldosterone. Plasma vasopressin levels are elevated relative to the plasma sodium levels, suggesting that the relative hemodilution and sodium dilution are maintained by retention of water in excess of sodium. There is also evidence that progesterone may promote sodium excretion by opposing effects of aldosterone. When pregnant women are placed in the supine position, there is a decrease in sodium excretion, which follows from the decreased glomerular filtration rate, decreased renal blood flow, and decreased cardiac output caused by decreased venous return.

22. What changes in glucose metabolism occur in the mother during pregnancy?

Increased insulin secretion in response to glucose. This change may be related to increased plasma cortisol, since cortisol can stimulate pancreatic secretion of insulin; however, it may also be related to plasma estrogens and/or progesterone, since estrogen and progesterone receptors are also present in the pancreas. Despite the increase in insulin secretion, the pregnant woman has relative insulin resistance, causing increased plasma glucose concentrations. The relative insulin insensitivity is thought to be caused by human placental lactogen, hPL, and by the increase in cortisol secretion by the maternal adrenal.

23. What changes in calcium metabolism occur during pregnancy?

Maternal plasma calcium concentrations generally fall, as plasma albumin levels drop. Ionized calcium concentrations remain constant. The decidua and placenta appear to produce the active vitamin D metabolite, 1,25$(OH)_2$ vitamin D_3, which increases calcium and phosphorus absorption in the small intestine. The increase in calcium intake is offset by calcium influx into the fetus. Parathyroid hormone concentrations may also increase in pregnancy, although this increase is not always demonstrable.

24. Are there changes in maternal thyroid function during pregnancy?

- Basal metabolic rate increases in pregnant women, in part owing to increased metabolism by the placenta and increased maternal cardiac output.
- Total triiodothyronine (T_3) and thyroxine (T_4) levels increase in pregnancy; this may be in response to increases in hepatic production of the binding protein, thyroxine-binding globulin, which is stimulated by estrogen.
- Hypothyroid women may require more thyroid hormone during pregnancy, and the thyroid may increase in size during pregnancy.
- The placenta expresses a monodeiodinase enzyme that degrades T_4 to reverse triiodothyronine (rT_3) and deiodinates T_3 to inactive diiodothyronine, inactivating most of the maternal thyroid hormone before it can pass to the fetus.
- Some T_4 in maternal blood crosses the placenta to the fetus, where it is metabolized by the fetal brain to T_3. This occurs before the time of fetal thyroid production of T_3 and T_4, and thus may be important for early fetal neural development before the time of fetal thyroid hormone secretion.

25. How do changes in maternal metabolism affect fuel supply to the fetus?

The supply of nutrients across the placenta is increased by the changes in maternal metabolism of substrates in both the fed and fasted states. After a meal or oral glucose intake, the relative insulin insensitivity of maternal tissues results in a greater increase in plasma glucose relative to the nonpregnant or postpartum state. Glucose transfer across the placenta is concentration dependent; therefore, the increased plasma glucose concentration increases transfer of glucose to the fetus and provides glucose as a fuel source for placental metabolism. Plasma triglyceride concentrations also are greater in pregnant women and may provide an alternative fuel source for maternal tissues. With fasting, maternal plasma glucose levels are reduced. Normally, about 30% of maternal glucose production is used by the fetus and placenta; about 30% of that is used by the fetus itself; however, the fractional utilization of glucose by the placenta is kept constant even with maternal food deprivation. As fasting progresses, maternal lipolysis is stimulated, and free fatty acid concentrations and ketoacids are greatly elevated to supply fuel to both the mother and the fetus. This is referred to as the accelerated starvation response of pregnancy.

26. What hormones are important for uterine growth in pregnancy?

Estrogens:

- Stimulate proliferation of decidual layer of uterus
- Increase uterine blood flow

Progesterone:

- Causes endometrial glands to secrete nutrients to supply blastocyst before implantation
- Maintains decidua after implantation
- Inhibits production of prostaglandin
- Inhibits oxytocin receptor expression
- May inhibit local host-graft rejection of the embryo through its effects as an immune suppressant

27. What changes in the breast occur during pregnancy?

Breast Changes during Pregnancy

TRIMESTER	CHANGES
First	Within First month, ducts of the breast begin to branch Later, alveoli begin to form
Second	Arborization and proliferation of glandular structures in the developing lobules continues Later, secretory activity occurs within the alveoli
Third	Alveolar spaces and ducts begin to fill with colostrum Mammary blood flow increases Myoepithelial cells (cells that cause ejection of milk) hypertrophy

28. What hormones stimulate mammary development in pregnancy?

The proliferation of ducts and the development of the lobulo-alveolar structure in the breast is stimulated by **progesterone** and **estrogens.** These steroids are initially derived from the corpus luteum but later are secreted by the placenta.

Prolactin is also important for the proliferation of the stem cells that will become the myoepithelial cells and the secretory alveolar cells. Although prolactin also stimulates synthesis of milk fats and proteins in late gestation, milk production is limited until after delivery. Therefore, the mammotropic actions of prolactin on the breast predominate over lactotropic actions during pregnancy. There is evidence that the mammotropic actions of prolactin require the presence of cortisol, insulin, and growth hormone. However, in women hypophysectomy during pregnancy does not prevent mammary development. This suggests that the action of prolactin may also be produced in pregnant women by hPL working in concert with the placental steroids.

29. What is the origin of amniotic fluid?

Amniotic fluid results from the balance between fetal lung liquid production, fetal swallowing, fetal urination, and intramembranous flow of water from amniotic fluid to fetal blood and transmembranous flow of water from amniotic fluid to maternal blood.

30. Name two clinical conditions related to the amniotic fluid.

1. **Oligohydramnios:** condition of having too little amniotic fluid
2. **Polyhydramnios:** condition of having too much amniotic fluid

PHYSIOLOGIC CHANGES AT PARTURITION AND POSTPARTUM

31. What mechanisms allow the uterus to be quiescent until the end of pregnancy?

Uterine quiescence is thought to be achieved by action of progesterone on the myometrium to suppress prostaglandin synthesis and inhibit oxytocin receptor expression. Progesterone appears to reduce excitability of smooth muscle cells, perhaps as a result of hyperpolarization, and to prevent gap junction formation, resulting in reduced communication between smooth muscle cells.

32. Discuss mechanisms that stimulate an increase in uterine excitability.

Uterine excitability is thought to increase because of the increase in estrogen-to-progesterone ratio. In many species, this occurs because placental production of progesterone is decreased in late gestation. In women, however, there is no measurable decrease in progesterone levels in plasma until after delivery of the placenta. In women, there is an increase in estrogen production throughout pregnancy; however, the estrogen-to-progesterone ratio increases markedly during late gestation. In addition, there is evidence for a local increase in estrogen-to-progesterone ratio at the time of labor in women. The local production of progesterone within the chorion and decidua is decreased, and the conversion of sulfated estrogens to active free estrogens is increased after labor is initiated.

Estrogens increase the production of prostaglandin $F_{2\alpha}$. Estrogens also increase the synthesis of connexon, the protein that comprises gap junctions in the myometrium. Estrogen therefore increases the ability of the myometrium to act as a syncytium and produce waves of contraction, which spread from the fundus downward over the body of the uterus.

33. What mechanisms initiate the uterine contractions during labor and delivery?

It is still not completely understood what process initiates labor in humans. There are no pronounced changes in maternal plasma oxytocin concentrations before the start of labor. Studies in other primate species suggest that there may be increases in nocturnal secretion of oxytocin well in advance of the onset of perceived labor contractions. The nocturnal increases in oxytocin may increase the number and frequency of nonlabor contractures (Braxton-Hicks contractions). In advance of a measurable increase in maternal plasma oxytocin concentrations, an increase in the number of myometrial oxytocin receptors appears to occur. This may increase uterine sensitivity to oxytocin before a consistent increase in oxytocin levels is observed. As labor progresses, cervical stretch simulates oxytocin release. This occurs by a neuroendocrine reflex arc through spinothalamic tracts and the medial forebrain bundle to the hypothalamus. Oxytocin release is also stimulated during delivery by afferents from the vagina. Thus, myometrial contractions during the expulsive phase of delivery are thought to be stimulated by these increases in oxytocin.

34. What effects does oxytocin have on the myometrium?

Oxytocin stimulates contraction of the uterine smooth muscle directly. Oxytocin may also stimulate the smooth muscle indirectly by stimulating production of prostaglandin $F_{2\alpha}$ in decidual cells.

35. What hormones stimulate maternal milk production after delivery?

Milk production in the postpartum period is stimulated by prolactin, acting in concert with insulin and cortisol. Prolactin induces the differentiation of presecretory cells into active secretory cells and increases the synthesis of the fatty acids, phospholipids, and the milk proteins casein, lactalbumin and β-lactoglobulin. The enzymes necessary for production of lactose are also induced by prolactin. Prolactin synthesis is stimulated by estrogen and is therefore increased dramatically during pregnancy. Circulating concentrations of prolactin in the mother increase progressively during pregnancy.

36. How is milk production limited or prevented during pregnancy?

The lactogenic effects of prolactin are inhibited during pregnancy by estrogen and progesterone.

37. How is milk production stimulated in lactating women?

- Suckling increases prolactin release as a neurogenic reflex.
- Impulses from afferent nerves from the nipple travel through the spinothalamic tract to the midbrain; from there the impulses are carried through the medial forebrain bundle to the hypothalamus.
- Stimulation of the nipple causes release of prolactin either by inhibiting the release of dopamine, which acts as a prolactin-inhibiting factor, or by stimulating the release of a prolactin-releasing factor.

38. How is milk production maintained in lactation?

Milk production is maintained by the prolactin released in response to suckling. As the frequency of suckling decreases, however, the prolactin response to suckling also decreases. Milk production is thereafter maintained by the increased sensitivity to prolactin.

39. How is milk ejected from the breast?

The myoepithelial cells of the breast surround the alveoli. Contraction of smooth muscle component in the myoepithelial cells compresses the alveoli and expels milk under pressure into the lactiferous sinuses or out of the nipple. The contraction of the myoepithelial cells is caused by the hormone oxytocin. Oxytocin is, in turn, stimulated by suckling through a neuroendocrine reflex arc similar to that used to stimulate prolactin but terminating in the oxytocin-producing magnocellular neurons of the paraventricular nucleus of the hypothalamus.

40. List stimulants of oxytocin release in lactating women.

- Suckling
- Cues associated with nursing or presence of an infant
    - Auditory
    - Olfactory
    - Visual
- Vaginal stimulation

FETAL ENDOCRINOLOGY

41. What is the fetoplacental unit?

The term **fetoplacental unit** refers to the biosynthetic scheme for synthesis of estrogens during pregnancy in humans. The major steroidogenic tissues involved in the biosynthesis of estrogens include the placenta and the fetal adrenal cortex.

The **placenta** is incapable of making estrogens from cholesterol because it lacks the enzyme cytochrome P-450_{c17}, which has the activity of 17α-hydroxylase. This enzyme, which is normally present in adult adrenal cortex and adult gonad, converts progesterone to 17α-progesterone and pregnenolone to 17α-pregnenolone and is a requisite step in the synthesis of estrogen from cholesterol.

The **fetal adrenal gland** is divided into two general zones. The majority of the tissue in the fetal adrenal cortex is contained in the fetal zone, and the remainder is contained in the definitive zone or adult zone. Both zones are responsive to fetal pituitary ACTH, but the fetal zone lacks the enzyme 3β-hydroxysteroid dehydrogenase (3βHSD). This enzyme is required for conversion of progesterone to pregnenolone and is therefore also required for biosynthesis of glucocorticoids and mineralocorticoids. The fetal zone therefore secretes dehydroepiandrosterone (DHEA) and dehydroepiandrosterone sulfate (DHEAS).

42. Explain the process of biosynthesis of estrogens by the fetoplacental unit.

Together the fetal zone of the fetal adrenal and the placenta contain all of the enzymes needed to synthesize estrogens. Fetal ACTH stimulates the secretion of DHEA and DHEAS from the fetal zone of the fetal adrenal. These weak androgens circulate in fetal blood and can be taken up by the placenta, where they are converted into estrone or estradiol (after conversion to testosterone) (see figure, left). Some of the DHEA and DHEAS secreted by the fetal adrenal are taken up by the fetal liver, converted to 16-hydroxy-DHEA or 16-hydroxy-DHEAS, and released into the fetal blood. These steroids can also be taken up by the placenta and converted to estriol (see figure, right). Because the fetoplacental unit requires a functioning fetal pituitary, fetal adrenal, and placenta, the circulating concentrations of estriol in the plasma of the pregnant woman have been used to demonstrate viability of the fetus.

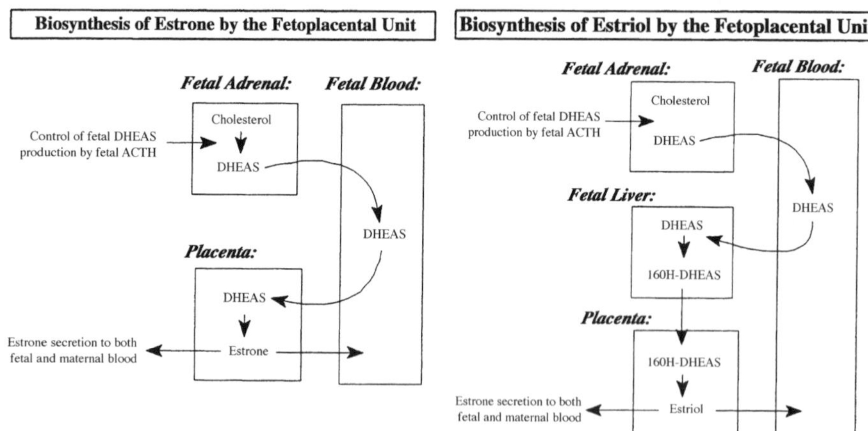

Left, Biosynthesis of estrone by the human feto-placental unit. *Right,* Biosynthesis of estriol by the human fetoplacental unit.

43. Do all species have functioning fetoplacental units?

It appears that all primate species have functioning fetoplacental units similar to that in the human being. Interestingly, some species appear to have variations in this biosynthetic scheme. For example, the horse has a fetoplacental unit that involves the fetal gonad and the placenta. Sheep and other ruminants do not have fetoplacental units. In these species, the fetal adrenal does not have a fetal zone, and the placenta contains cytochrome P-450_{c17} at the end of gestation.

44. Who determines when the fetus is born: the mother or the fetus?

Experiments have demonstrated that the signal initiating the process of parturition originates in the fetus. In human fetuses, natural conditions ("accidents of nature" such as anencephaly) that disrupt the function of the fetal hypothalamus-pituitary-adrenal axis also disturb the normal timing of parturition.

45. What is the mechanism of parturition in sheep?

In this species, which does not have a functioning fetoplacental unit, parturition is clearly initiated by an increase in the secretion of ACTH from the fetal pituitary. This peptide hormone stimulates the secretion of cortisol from the fetal adrenal cortex. The exponential increase in fetal plasma cortisol concentrations acts, in part, on the placental tissue, which is perfused by fetal blood. The placental steroidogenic tissue, before this preparturient increase in fetal plasma cortisol, lacks cytochrome P-450$_{c17}$, the enzyme that contains 17α-hydroxylase activity. The placenta therefore synthesizes mainly progesterone, a hormone that maintains uterine quiescence via an action on the myometrium. Cortisol in the fetal circulation induces the activity of cytochrome P-450$_{c17}$, therefore allowing the placenta to synthesize relatively large amounts of estrogen, which counteracts the effect of progesterone on uterine quiescence. Recent evidence suggests that the induction of cytochrome P-450$_{c17}$ might be dependent on the local generation of prostaglandins in the placenta. The resultant increase in the estrogen-to-progesterone ratio in the myometrium enhances the excitability of the cell membrane and initiates myometrial contractions. The initiation of myometrial activity increases intrauterine pressure and stretches the cervix. The cervix contains mechanoreceptors that, when stretched, send afferent signals to the hypothalamus and stimulate the secretion of oxytocin from the maternal posterior pituitary. The oxytocin, reaching the myometrium from the maternal blood, augments the contractile activity of the uterus. The mechanoreceptors and stimulated oxytocin secretion form a positive feedback loop by which uterine contractions are amplified. The process continues until the fetus is born, allowing intrauterine pressure to be reduced.

46. How does the process of parturition in the human differ from that in the sheep?

Many investigators believe that the critical step in the human being is, as in sheep, an increase in the estrogen-to-progesterone ratio in the myometrium. However, the biosynthesis of estrogen is more complex in the human being than in the sheep because of the fetoplacental unit. At present, there are much data supporting the hypothesis that at the end of human gestation, the fetus secretes ACTH from the pituitary and DHEA and DHEAS from the fetal zone of the fetal adrenal and that these steroidogenic intermediates act as precursors for estrogen biosynthesis by the placenta. Ultimately, the fetal neuroendocrine events that initiate parturition might be the same in both human beings and sheep.

47. What role is played by prostaglandins in parturition?

Prostaglandin $F_{2\alpha}$ is produced as an autacoid that stimulates or augments the contraction of the myometrial cells. During parturition in the sheep, for example, this prostaglandin is secreted in large amounts into the uterine vein. The action of prostaglandin $F_{2\alpha}$ is critical to the normal uterine contraction. Prostaglandin E_2 (PGE_2) is synthesized in the fetal brain and fetal pituitary and is a potent stimulator of the fetal hypothalamus-pituitary-adrenal axis. Increased activity of the fetal hypothalamus-pituitary-adrenal axis is an integral event in the initiation of parturition.

48. What are the ontogenetic changes in fetal plasma cortisol?

- Fetal plasma cortisol is relatively low throughout much of the latter half of gestation.
- Before term (the timing differs among various species), cortisol increases as a result of a spontaneous increase in fetal hypothalamic-pituitary-adrenal axis activity.

49. What is the significance of the ontogenetic increase in fetal plasma cortisol?

In the sheep, this increase in fetal plasma cortisol initiates parturition by inducing the synthesis of cytochrome P-450$_{c17}$ in the placenta. In all mammalian species, it is thought that cortisol accelerates the terminal maturation of the lungs and visceral organs, thought to be an important step in the process of readying the fetus for birth. Premature infants, born before the normal ontogenetic increase in fetal plasma cortisol, are more susceptible to respiratory distress syndrome (or hyaline membrane disease) and sometimes require ventilatory support for survival. This action of cortisol on the fetal lung is explored in more detail in the following section on fetal cardiopulmonary physiology.

50. What influence does the maternal adrenal have on the fetus?

The placenta is a relative diffusion barrier, which slows the passage of steroids between the maternal and fetal circulations. An important amount of cortisol gains access to the fetal blood from the maternal adrenal. In fetal sheep, approximately 1% of the maternal adrenal secretion passes from the mother to the fetal blood. This is a sufficient amount to alter fetal neuroendocrine function and, perhaps, alter other aspects of fetal physiology (such as fetal fluid balance). Increases in maternal plasma cortisol concentration, equal to those produced after maternal stress, effectively inhibit fetal ACTH responses to subsequent stresses.

In women, the passage of cortisol from mother to fetus is thought to be reduced by the presence of **11β-hydroxysteroid dehydrogenase** (11β-HSD) in the placenta. This enzyme catalyzes the conversion of cortisol to cortisone (which does not effectively bind glucocorticoid receptors and is therefore not biologically active).

FETAL CARDIOPULMONARY PHYSIOLOGY

51. Describe the anatomy of the fetal circulation.

The fetal circulation contains several shunts that allow blood to bypass the pulmonary circulation and allow perfusion of the umbilical-placental circulation (see figure).

Ductus arteriosus—connects the pulmonary artery to the descending aorta. This shunt allows the majority of the blood passing through the pulmonic valve to bypass the lungs and enter the descending aorta.

Foramen ovale—between the two atria. This shunt is actually much like a flap-valve that allows blood to pass from the right atrium to the left atrium (in the fetus, the hydrostatic pressure of the blood in the right atrium exceeds that in the left atrium).

Ductus venosus—from the portal vein to the inferior vena cava. This shunt allows highly oxygenated blood, ultimately from the umbilical vein, to bypass the liver and enter the inferior vena cava (see figure, below).

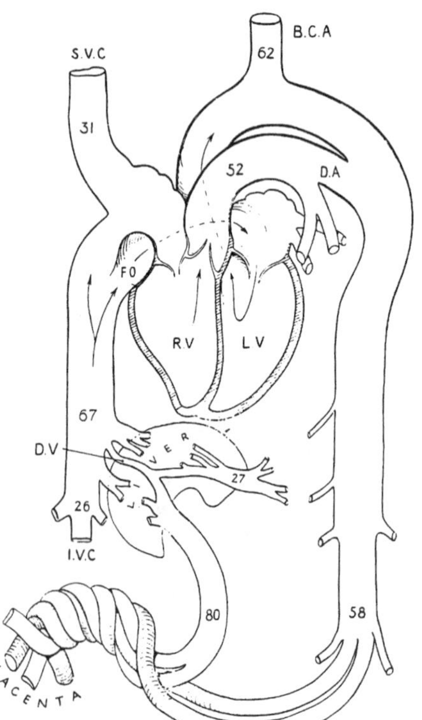

The fetal circulation. I.V.C., inferior vena cava; S.V.C., superior vena cava; D.V., ductus venosus; F.O., foramen ovale; D.A., ductus arteriosus; B.C.A., brachiocephalic artery. Numbers represent the percentage oxygen saturation of blood at those sites. (From Born, et al: Changes in the heart and lungs at birth. In Cold Spring Harbor Symposia on Quantitative Biology, vol XIX, The Mammalian Fetus: Physiological Aspects of Development. New York, Cold Spring Harbor, 1954, with permission.)

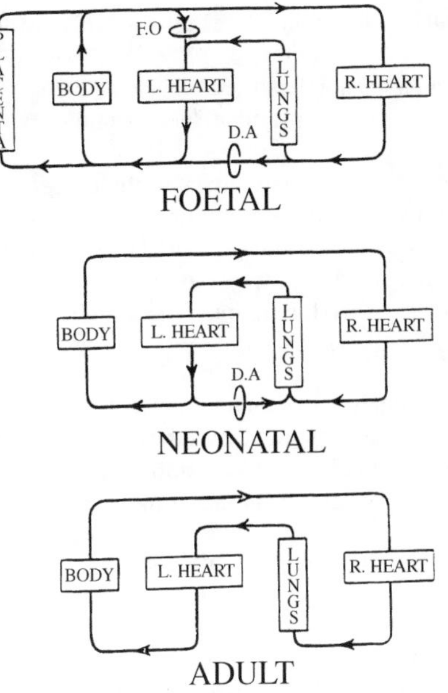

Blood flow within the fetal circulation. F.O., foramen ovale; D.A., ductus arteriosus. (From Born, et al: Changes in the heart and lungs at birth. In Cold Spring Harbor Symposia on Quantitative Biology, vol XIX, The Mammalian Fetus: Physiological Aspects of Development. New York, Cold Spring Harbor, 1954, with permission.)

52. What is combined ventricular output?

In the late-gestation fetus, the right ventricle pumps approximately twice the volume (approximately 130 mL/kg/minute) compared with the left ventricle (approximately 60 mL/kg/minute). **Combined ventricular output** describes the presence of the shunts within the fetal circulation, the inequality of the volume pumped by the right and left ventricles, and the admixture of blood exiting the heart through the aorta and pulmonary arteries.

53. How much blood flows through the umbilical-placental circulation?

Approximately 40% of the combined ventricular output. This is rather large compared with the 8% of combined ventricular output that perfuses the fetal lungs (which do not serve a gas exchange function in the fetus).

54. What controls umbilical-placental flow?

The rate of umbilical-placental blood flow is largely a function of fetal arterial blood pressure. There is little autoregulation of blood flow within this vascular bed, and there is no innervation of the resistance vessels by sympathetic nervous system efferent fibers. Nevertheless, vasoconstrictors do reduce the blood flow through the placenta (as studied in the fetal sheep). Reduction in umbilical-placental blood flow caused by α-adrenergic agonist drugs is mainly due to constriction of the main umbilical artery and not to the constriction of potential resistance vessels in the microvasculature.

55. How does the fetal circulation rearrange itself to become the newborn circulation?

At birth, the fetus becomes a neonate and starts to breathe:

- The increase in pulmonary volume and the increase in microvascular oxygen tension decrease pulmonary vascular resistance.
- This decrease in resistance allows relatively greater flow through the pulmonary circulation and decreases flow through the ductus arteriosus.
- The increased flow through the lungs also increases left atrial pressure relative to the right atrial pressure.

- The reverse in pressure gradient across the interatrial septum closes the flap-valve of the foramen ovale.
- At the same time, the increase in arterial oxygen tension from fetal levels of around 25 mmHg to neonatal levels of around 100 mmHg induces molecular changes in the ductus arteriosus that cause it to constrict.
- This constriction greatly reduces the flow from the pulmonary artery to the descending aorta and forces a greater proportion of the right ventricular output through the lungs.

In normal infants, complete closure of the ductus arteriosus can take several days. The umbilical cord, containing the umbilical arteries and vein, constricts when exposed to atmospheric oxygen tensions. This stops flow through the placenta and therefore through the umbilical vein. The reduced flow through the ductus venosus eventually allows it to close.

56. What molecular changes within the ductus arteriosus are involved in closure?

The ductus arteriosus remains open in the fetus because of continued synthesis of PGE_2. On exposure to elevated oxygen tensions, the biosynthesis of PGE_2 is reduced, allowing the ductus to close. The influence of PGE_2 on ductus tone appears to be greatest in full-term fetuses.

57. Name the condition in which the ductus arteriosus remains open after birth.

Patent ductus arteriosus.

58. Is there a treatment for patent ductus arteriosus?

Some infants, especially closest to full term, can be successfully treated with inhibitors of cyclooxygenase, such as indomethacin.

59. How do fetal blood pressure and heart rate in the fetus differ from that in the newborn and the adult animal?

Fetal blood pressure is lower and heart rate is higher than in the newborn or adult animal. The best available data were generated in studies on chronically catheterized fetal sheep. Throughout the latter half of gestation, fetal blood pressure slowly increases, from approximately 35 to approximately 50 mmHg. Fetal heart rate slowly decreases from approximately 190 to approximately 170 beats per minute. At birth, the rearrangement of the fetal circulation (see question 55) is associated with a rapid increase in fetal arterial blood pressure, to approximately 65 mmHg, and further decrease in fetal heart rate, to approximately 100 beats per minute. As the lamb matures, the arterial blood pressure slowly increases, and the heart rate slowly decreases throughout the life of the animal. These changes measured in sheep mirror the changes in blood pressure and heart rate in humans.

60. Why does the pulmonary circulation dilate at birth?

An important adaptation to neonatal life is the decrease in pulmonary vascular resistance at birth. Without this decrease in resistance to blood flow, the lungs would impede blood flow and tend to reduce the likelihood of closure of the ductus arteriosus. Persistent increases in pulmonary vascular resistance after birth produce a condition that is called **persistent pulmonary hypertension of the newborn.**

61. Discuss the molecular and physiologic determinants of pulmonary vascular tone.

In the normal lung, the physical stretching of the vasculature on lung inflation increases vascular dimensions and reduces resistance to blood flow. Several endocrine or paracrine events are also critical for reduction of vascular resistance. The increased oxygen tension in the pulmonary vasculature stimulates the release of dilator substances (and perhaps reduces the release of constrictor substances) within the vasculature. There is evidence for the release of nitric oxide from the vascular endothelium, providing the impetus for dilation during the first breath of life. There is also evidence that prostanoids (e.g., PGI_2 and leukotrienes) and peptides (e.g., endothelin) are involved in the process. This process is likely multifactorial and involves the coordination of various locally produced mediators of tone. The high vascular tone which defines persistent pulmonary hypertension of the newborn can be overridden by inhaled nitric oxide, demonstrating the potential importance of the vascular endothelium in the generation of tone within this vascular bed in the perinatal period.

62. What function does the lung have in the fetus?

The placenta, not the lung, is the organ of gas exchange in the fetus. The lungs are the source of **lung liquid,** an exudate of plasma that contains electrolytes but few proteins. Lung liquid exits the lungs continuously during fetal life. Some of the lung liquid exits the mouth and nares of the fetus and therefore contributes to the volume and electrolyte content of amniotic fluid. Some of the lung liquid (as much as half, as estimated in some experiments on fetal sheep) is swallowed by the fetus and is reabsorbed in the fetal gastrointestinal tract. The lung might also serve an endocrine function because the lung contains hormone-containing cells (the so-called **pulmonary neuroendocrine cells**) within the bronchial epithelium and within the parenchyma of the lung.

63. What is the significance of bradycardia in the fetus?

Rapid decelerations of fetal heart rate are sometimes observed during the process of birth. Fetal hypoxia (reduced arterial oxygen tension) and hypotension (reduced fetal arterial blood pressure) stimulate decreases in fetal heart rate that are rapid and easily recognized during fetal monitoring. Reductions in fetal heart rate, indicating what physicians term **fetal stress,** are caused by stimulation of the fetal peripheral chemoreceptors. Arterial chemoreceptors, located in glomus tissue in the carotid sinuses and aortic arch, increase afferent neural traffic to the nucleus of the tractus solitarius of the medulla when the arterial oxygen tension is reduced. Reductions in fetal arterial blood pressure also cause these chemoreceptors to fire, most likely because the reduction in blood pressure reduces the blood flow through the chemoreceptors. The reduced flow through the glomus tissue does not provide sufficient oxygen delivery to this tissue, which has a high metabolic rate. Consequently the intracellular oxygen tension is reduced and the chemoreceptors fire.

64. What is pulmonary compliance and what controls it?

Pulmonary compliance is defined by the following equation:

$$c = \Delta V/\Delta P$$

where C is compliance, ΔV represents a change in volume, and ΔP represents a change in pressure. The surface tension of the pulmonary alveoli would be relatively high if the alveolar surface were simply a water-air interface (and therefore dominated by the surface tension of water). Physiologically the lungs contain a substance called **surfactant,** a surface-active material that reduces surface tension. This substance is actually a complex mixture of phospholipids and proteins. The major phospholipid is **dipalmitoyl phosphatidylcholine** (DPPC), and the major proteins have been named **surfactant proteins A, B, C, and D.** DPPC is an essential component of surfactant, acting as a molecule with both hydrophobic and hydrophilic domains, which is thought to be aligned physically at the alveolar surface in such a way as to reduce surface tension. The most abundant surfactant protein is surfactant protein A (SP-A), which is a glycoprotein of molecular weight approximately 28–36 kD. SP-A binds to lipids, calcium, and sugars and works with the other components of surfactant to form an air interface with low surface tension. SP-B and SP-C are smaller proteins (5 and 8 kD) and work with DPPC and SP-A to accelerate the spread of surfactant. SP-D, like SP-A, is a larger glycoprotein (43 kD) made by type II alveolar epithelial cells. Its role in reducing surface tension is not clear.

65. What is the ontogenetic pattern of surfactant proteins in fetal lung?

SP-A: low throughout much of late gestation, but dramatic increase before term.

SP-B and **SP-C:** rise progressively throughout the latter half of gestation.

66. Why is antenatal treatment of fetuses with glucocorticoids beneficial to neonatal cardiopulmonary function?

Glucocorticoids accelerate the terminal maturation of the fetal lung, including stimulation of the endogenous production of surfactant proteins and stimulation of the incorporation of choline into phosphatidyl choline. Pulmonary compliance is high in premature infants, often too high to allow sufficient spontaneous ventilation of the lungs for neonatal survival. For this reason, treatment of women at risk for premature labor and delivery with synthetic glucocorticoid (usually dexamethasone or betamethasone) reduces the risk of perinatal death secondary to respiratory distress.

FETAL GROWTH AND METABOLISM

67. What factors are responsible for fetal growth?

Fetal growth is independent of maternal hormones such as GH, thyroid hormone, and insulin, and also appears to be independent of fetal GH. Fetal growth appears to be only indirectly related to fetal insulin but may depend on production of insulin-like growth factors (IGFs) in fetal tissues and liver. In small-for-gestational-age babies, IGF-1 levels are reduced, suggesting that this hormone may be important for growth at term. Fetal growth also depends on maternal supply of substrates and is reduced when uteroplacental blood flow is reduced or placental growth is compromised.

68. List the substrates for fetal energy supply.

Major substrates

- Glucose
- Lactate

Possible substrates

- Triglycerides
- Fatty acids
- Glycerol
- Ketoacids

69. How does glucose reach the fetus?

Glucose is supplied to the fetus primarily through transplacental transport. The fetus has relatively little gluconeogenic capacity and therefore does not produce much glucose on its own. Just before birth, the enzymes of gluconeogenesis and glycogen synthesis are induced by cortisol, resulting in an increase in glycogen storage as well as hepatic glucose production near the time of birth. Before this time, fetal glucose concentrations depend primarily on placental transfer of glucose from the mother; the flux of glucose across the placenta is directly related to maternal plasma glucose concentration, uterine glucose uptake, and the ratio of maternal to fetal glucose concentrations. Normally a large percentage (about 80%) of glucose uptake from the uteroplacental circulation is metabolized by the placenta; however, when fetal glucose concentrations fall, this percentage drops allowing for relatively greater transfer of glucose to fetal plasma. During periods of rapid fetal growth, the glucose transport across the placenta increases owing to both an increase in transport capacity and an increase in the ratio of maternal to fetal glucose concentrations, which is caused by increased fetal glucose utilization with growth.

70. How do amino acids reach the fetus?

Transport of amino acids into the fetus occurs by a transporter-mediated, energy-dependent process. The placenta contains transport proteins on the brush-border membrane of the villus, which is the interface with maternal blood. As for many other amino acid transporters, these are dependent on Na^+, K^+-ATPase for energy. Some amino acids are also produced in the fetus; serine and glutamate appear to be primarily produced by the fetal liver (from glycine and glutamine) rather than transported across the placenta.

71. What happens when fetuses do not grow normally?

Stunting of the fetus is described as **intrauterine growth retardation.** Such fetuses are termed **small for gestational age.** Although the causes of fetal growth retardation probably are many, the mechanism most likely relates to an insufficient supply of nutrients to the growing fetus. The causes of growth retardation in human fetuses are not well understood and remain an important area of research. However, both epidemiologic data and results of studies in animals suggest that poor maternal nutrition, reduced placental perfusion, chronic fetal hypoxia, and increased maternal corticosteroid concentrations (above the normal increase in cortisol in pregnancy) can all result in intrauterine growth retardation.

BIBLIOGRAPHY

1. Faber JJ, Thorburn KL: Placental Physiology. New York, Raven Press, 1983.
2. Knobil E, Neill JD (eds): The Physiology of Reproduction, 2nd ed. Philadelphia, Lippincott-Raven, 1994.
3. Thorburn GD, Harding R (eds): Textbook of Fetal Physiology. Oxford, Oxford University Press, 1994.

13. EXERCISE PHYSIOLOGY

Paula E. Papanek, Ph.D., MPT

1. What is skeletal muscle?

Whole skeletal muscle, such as the biceps, which is observable and palpable, is really several kinds of tissue. Each muscle comprises long, thin, cylindrical muscle fibers or cells that extend its entire length. As such, these cells can be very long. Each multinucleated muscle cell or fiber is surrounded by and connected to parallel muscle cells by a layer of connective tissue called the **endomysium**. These fibers are then grouped in bundles held together by another layer of connective tissue called the **perimysium**. This encased group or bundle of fibers is called a **fascicle**. Groups of fascicles, bundles of fibers each with associated blood vessels and nerve tissue, collectively are held in close approximation by another layer of connective tissue called the **epimysium**. The epimysium-surrounded fascicles, which run the entire length of skeletal muscle, are then completely surrounded by an important connective tissue called **fascia**. For greater detail, see Chapter 1, Cells, Nerves, and Muscles.

2. What is the role of fascia in skeletal muscle?

Fascia is a tough, dense, and strong connective tissue that covers the entire muscle and then extends beyond the muscle itself to become the fibrous tendon. The fascia is a fusion of all three internal connective tissue layers of skeletal muscle. Fascia separates muscles from one another, permits frictionless motion, and forms the tendon with which muscle is connected to bone. It is often an overlooked component of muscle physiology. Many believe that normal fascial movement is required for free, unrestricted movement of muscle and thus of joints.

3. How is skeletal muscle force measured?

Although terms such as *strength* and *power* are often used to describe force-generating capabilities of skeletal muscle, they are really incorrect. A contracting skeletal muscle produces a force that acts parallel to the muscle fibers; thus it is a linear force. Only an isolated skeletal muscle generates tension that is measurable as a force. In the body, muscles produce movement by rotation of a bone in a plane that is perpendicular to the joint's axis of rotation. The magnitude of the rotation is expressed as a torque. Appropriate measures of strength in the body then are torques with units of foot-pounds (ft-lb) or Newton-meters (N-m).

4. How does skeletal muscle contraction result in movement?

Repetitive cross-bridge cycling with sarcomere shortening pulls the ends of the muscle toward the middle. The strong connective fascial sheath, which unites skeletal muscle via the tendons to the bones, transmits the force to the bones. To produce movement, the muscle's linear force pulls on a bone and causes rotation in a perpendicular plane to the joint's axis. Because muscle typically crosses at least one joint, the segment that is most free will move, resulting in rotational movement at the joint.

5. How does skeletal muscle contract or shorten?

The ability of muscle to contract is a function of microstructural components—specifically, an interaction of the contractile proteins actin and myosin that occurs under the appropriate conditions (the presence of intracellular calcium ions and energy). The availability of energy for contraction comes from the hydrolysis of adenosine triphosphate (ATP), and calcium is released from the sarcoplasmic reticulum (SR) when stimulated by depolarization. The linkage of a neural impulse generated in the central nervous system with a distant skeletal muscle contraction is called **excitation-contraction coupling**.

6. How much does a muscle shorten during a single cross-bridge cycle or power stroke?

If all the cross-bridges in a single muscle were to go through one cycle simultaneously, a muscle would shorten by only 1% of its resting length. The fact that many muscles are capable of shortening up to 60% of their resting length demonstrates that cross-bridge cycling must occur repeatedly, each time with myosin grabbing a new actin site and pulling for extensive shortening and force to be generated.

7. Where does the energy for skeletal muscle contraction come from?

The breakdown of ATP is achieved by the enzyme myosin ATPase located on the globular head. When hydrolyzed, ATP releases the energy to the myosin head and adenosine diphosphate (ADP) + P_i is formed. The energized myosin head performs the power stroke. The reaction is as follows:

$$ATP \leftrightarrow ADP + P_i + energy$$

8. How much ATP does the body store?

Essentially, the body stores enough ATP for only a few seconds' worth of activity. After that, ATP must be resynthesized from ADP + P_i. ATP is a large, heavy molecule. If the body stored enough ATP for a single day's use, it is estimated that even a sedentary person would have to increase body weight by 75%.

9. Where does the ATP come from?

Muscle fibers contain three major pathways to resynthesize ATP: (1) creatine phosphate (CP) system, (2) glycolysis, and (3) aerobic oxidation of nutrients to produce carbon dioxide and water. Each system has different capacities, characteristics, and lag time to produce ATP. Therefore, they are used to meet different ATP demands.

10. Which food is used by which pathway?

Only carbohydrates can be used in glycolysis. Almost all digestible carbohydrates can be converted into glucose or stored as glycogen. Glycogen and glucose are metabolized by glycogenolysis and glycolysis. Any food source that is converted into acetyl-coenzyme A (CoA) is metabolized via the Krebs cycle and oxidative phosphorylation. Specifically, fat is broken down into glycerol, which, through a two-step process, becomes pyruvate and fatty acids. Fatty acids are oxidized through beta oxidation to acetyl-CoA. Beta oxidation occurs in the mitochondria. Proteins are broken down into amino acids and, after deamination (removal of NH_3), can be converted to pyruvate or acetyl-CoA or enter the Krebs cycle. None of the steps in the Krebs cycle or beta oxidation directly uses oxygen, but without the electron transport chain (ETC), a shortage of electron acceptors (nicotinamide adenine dinucleotide [NAD], reduced flavin adenine dinucleotide [FADH]) results, slowing and ultimately inhibiting the metabolism.

11. Which system produces ATP the fastest?

The **CP system** is the most rapid resynthesis system available in humans because it involves only a single enzymatic step. Basically, a high-energy phosphate is transferred from CP directly to rephosphorylate ADP to make ATP. However, there appears to be a finite level of CP stored in cells, and thus its ability to resynthesize ATP is limited. Because this system does not require the presence of oxygen to produce ATP, it is considered an anaerobic source of ATP.

CP ADP + Pi Myosin contraction

X-Bridge cycling

Cr + Pi ATP energized relaxation

myosin

Creatine phosphate–ATP production link in energizing the myosin head to permit cross-bridge cycling (contraction and relaxation).

12. What type of activities does CP and stored ATP fuel?

Collectively, the CP system combined with stored ATP is used for short-term, high-intensity bursts of activity lasting about 10–12 seconds. It is located right at the myosin heads, the site of use. The CP and ATP systems are used for rapid movements such as rapid lifting, high jumping, a 10-yard sprint, getting up from the couch quickly, moving quickly when in danger of being stung by a bee, or jumping out of the way of a moving truck when crossing a street.

13. Can the effectiveness of the CP system be increased?

The CP system responds to training, and recent studies have demonstrated that consuming creatine monohydrate, an ergogenic aid, appears to increase anaerobic performance. Studies are ongoing to determine how much creatine must be taken, for which activities it is beneficial, when it should be taken, and the side effects or toxicity, if any.

14. Where does the energy come from when physical activity lasts longer than 10–12 seconds or is of lesser intensity?

Glycolysis produces ATP anaerobically (without the use of oxygen). Glycolysis occurs within the cytoplasm of skeletal muscle and involves the breakdown of carbohydrate to pyruvate or lactate with the net energy yield of 2 ATP (3 ATP if started with glycogen). Glycolysis produces ATP quickly but is slower than the CP system. Glycolysis alone can support activity lasting several minutes in duration. For moderate-intensity, long-duration activities, carbohydrate and fat produce large quantities of ATP via complete oxidation (Krebs cycle), beta oxidation (fats), and ETC.

15. How are the energy-producing systems controlled?

Both glycolysis and the Krebs cycle are controlled by hormonal and local regulation of the rate-limiting step or by enzyme regulation. Similarly, the ETC also is regulated by the (ADP + P_i)/ATP ratio. Similar to most regulated enzymes, energy-producing systems are subjected to end-product inhibition. For example, increased concentrations of pyruvate inhibit the regulated step in glycolysis and the key enzyme **phosphofructokinase**. In general, increased concentrations of ADP and P_i stimulate metabolism, whereas high concentrations of ATP inhibit further production of ATP. Some of the key enzymes are regulated by hormones such as epinephrine, norepinephrine, glucagons, insulin, and cortisol.

16. Is the end-product of glycolysis pyruvate or lactate?

When glycolysis is slow and the acceptance of reduced NAD (NADH) by the mitochondria is adequate, **pyruvate** is the end product of glycolysis. Pyruvate is converted into acetyl-CoA (a step requiring NAD) and undergoes complete combustion via the Krebs cycle and ETC. When the mitochondria are unable to accept the pyruvate or provide regenerated electron acceptors (NAD or FADH), pyruvate is converted to **lactate**. The conversion of pyruvate to lactate decreases pyruvate concentration, prevents end-product inhibition, and permits glycolysis to continue.

17. When is lactate produced?

Lactate is produced when mitochondrial function is inadequate to accept pyruvate or produce sufficient electron acceptors. This happens when enzymatic activity in the mitochondria is low, when oxygen supply is insufficient, or when glycolysis is rapid. In general, lactate production is increased during hypoxia, ischemia, and hemorrhage; after carbohydrate ingestion; when muscle glycogen concentrations are high; and during exercise hyperthermia.

18. What else can happen to pyruvate?

During exercise or when caloric intake is insufficient, pyruvate can be converted into the nonessential amino acid **alanine**. Alanine is produced by skeletal muscle and can be converted by the liver into new glucose. This is commonly called the **alanine cycle**. In this case, pyruvate is converted to lactate, and the lactate is transported in the blood to the liver and reconverted to pyruvate and then to alanine. The alanine is then converted to glucose for subsequent release.

19. Compare and contrast the energy pathways in terms of their use in physical activity.

In reality, these pathways interact to provide the needed energy for all activity. However, the contribution of anaerobic sources predominates during high-intensity, short-duration activity, whereas aerobic sources dominate in activities lasting more than 5 minutes. This difference is summarized in the following table.

	ANAEROBIC METABOLISM	AEROBIC METABOLISM
Type of activity	Short, explosive	Longer time (>2 min)
Intensity of activity	High	Low to moderate
Example of event	Shot put, 100-m run	≥ 1500-m run
Major system	ATP-CP, glycolysis	Krebs, ETC
Stimulators	ADP, AMP, P_i	ADP, NAD, P_i
Inhibitors	ATP	ATP, NADH
Type of response	Rapid and immediate	Slower but prolonged

20. How do anaerobic and aerobic metabolism interact?

The intensity and duration of activity dictate the pathways for regeneration of ATP and the metabolic and systemic events contributing to fatigue.

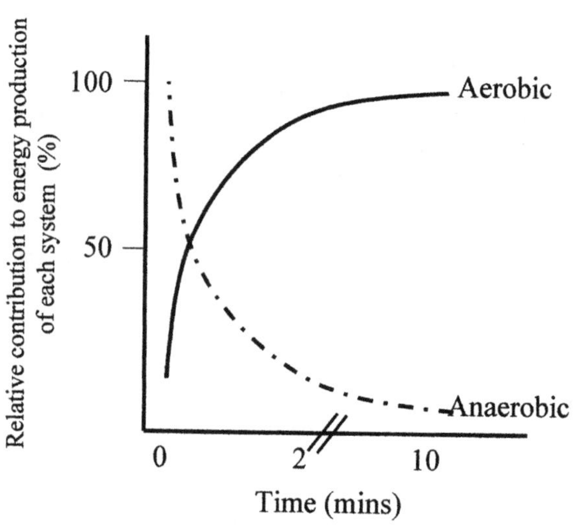

Relative contribution of aerobic and anaerobic metabolism to total energy production as a function of exercise time. Increasing exercise time results in a dominance of aerobic metabolism.

21. Do all skeletal muscles use the same source of ATP and produce the same force?

No. Skeletal muscle comprises different types of muscle cells with different nerve morphology and physiology. This results in different conduction velocities, contractile velocities, force-generating capacity, and metabolic capacities. Basically, when categorized by contractile velocity, the two major subtypes of skeletal muscle are **slow-twitch or type I** and **fast-twitch or type II**. The fast-twitch category is further subdivided based on metabolic capacity. The fast-twitch subdivisions include the following:

- Type IIa (fast-twitch fatigue-resistant) fibers have moderate capacities for both glycolytic and oxidative metabolism.
- Type IIb (fast-twitch fatigable) fibers are large-diameter fibers, produce more force, and have a high glycolytic capacity.

- Type IIab (fast-twitch intermediate) fibers

22. What are FOG, SO, and FG?

Histochemical profiles of skeletal muscle fibers that correspond to fast-twitch oxidative-glycolytic (FOG), slow-twitch oxidative (SO), and fast-twitch glycolytic (FG).

23. How do the response time and fatigue curves for the three main fiber types differ?

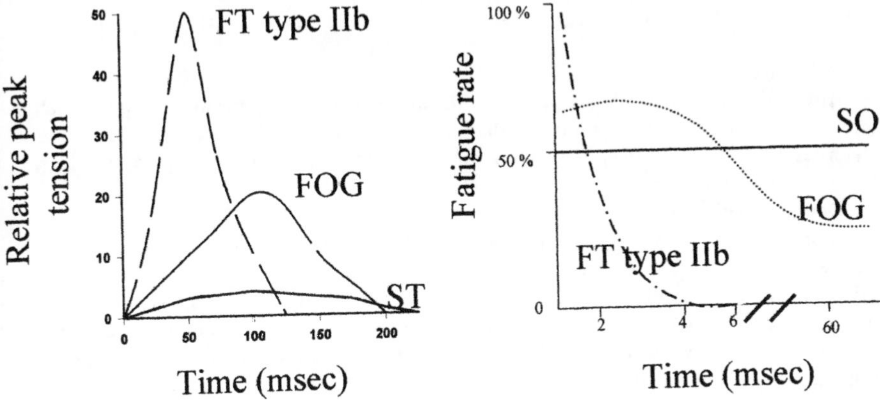

Schematic representation of relative peak tension and fatigue rate of fast-twitch (FT type IIb), fast-twitch oxidative-glycolytic (FOG), and slow-twitch (SO) fibers in human skeletal muscle.

24. Which fiber type is used when?

Slow-twitch fibers have a low threshold and are the first to be recruited during incremental exercise. They have a slow maximal shortening velocity. This is followed by a progressive increase in **FOG** and **FG** recruitment.

25. List the biochemical differences among fiber types.

	SLOW-TWITCH (TYPE I)	FAST-TWITCH (TYPE IIa)	FAST-TWITCH GLYCOLYTIC (TYPE IIb)
Glycogen content	Moderate	Moderate-high	Moderate-high
Capillary density	High	High	Low
Myoglobin content	High	High	Low
ATPase activity	Low	High	High
Mitochondrial density	High	High	Low
Oxidative capacity	High	Moderate high	Low
Color	Red	Intermediate	White
Predominant energy system	Aerobic	Combination	Anaerobic

26. How does skeletal muscle contraction result in physical activity or exercise?

The control of motor function is a complex integration of many parts of the central and peripheral nervous systems. Each plays an important role in the coordinated movement patterns of daily living and in high-skill activities such as sports. The major components of motor function include:

- Motor cortex (stores rough drafts of planned activities)
- Subcortical areas (prime drive for conscious movement)
- Cerebellum and basal ganglia (for precise temporal and spatial execution)
- Thalamus (relay center)

- Spinal neurons (conduction system)
- Skeletal muscle motor end plates (reception and signal conversion)
- Muscle receptors (signal reception and transmission)
- Proprioceptors (for error correction)

When all systems are functioning appropriately, the **motor cortex** with input and modification from **subcortical areas** and the **cerebellum** initiates and modifies (via **proprioception** and visual information) neural output in terms of frequency and intensity to selected muscles for contraction and thus movement. In addition, the central nervous system controls the neuroendocrine responses, which facilitate the supply of substrates for energy metabolism.

27. Define exercise.

Any physical activity that has an energy demand above resting metabolic rate and that disturbs homeostasis. It is the result of alternating contraction and relaxation of skeletal muscles, which results in the movement of a joint or series of joints through its range of motion.

28. Define exercise physiology.

A branch of physiology that specifically deals with the integration and function of the body during exercise and how exercise alters the structure and function of the body. This includes acute responses to exercise as well as the health benefits associated with exercise training. This is done at the various levels: whole body, organ systems, organs, cellular level, and subcellular level. Interest in exercise physiology has spawned many subdisciplines of exercise physiology, including biomechanics, strength and conditioning, and clinical exercise physiology, including sports medicine.

29. How does exercise differ from physical fitness?

Physical fitness is often defined as sufficient physical structure, function, and capacity to perform and respond favorably to whatever specific task an individual person requires. Exercise is any physical activity. Physical fitness is a term that has its origin in physical education. In the 1950s, the physical fitness movement gained momentum when endorsed by President Eisenhower. This endorsement was fueled by three pieces of information: (1) an alarming number of military draftees failed their induction exams, many with physical defects; (2) autopsies of young soldiers killed in the Korean war showed significant coronary artery disease; and (3) U.S. children performed poorly on a minimal muscular fitness test when compared with European children of similar ages. This information prompted President Eisenhower to create the President's Council on Youth Fitness. During President Kennedy's term, the name was changed to the President's Council on Physical Fitness in efforts to promote school fitness or physical education classes of all ages and to develop a "fit society." Today, we speak of physical fitness in terms of general health as well as the protection from many preventable diseases.

30. What is Healthy People 2020?

Healthy People 2020, previously called Healthy People 2000, is a U.S. Department of Health and Human Services' initiative that spells out specific health objectives. Initially, the target year was 2000, but, because the objectives were not met by that year, the name was changed to reflect the new target goal of 2020. The objectives are designed to improve the health and well-being of all Americans and deal with issues such as fitness, body composition, mental health, tobacco and alcohol use, and nutrition.

31. Name a specific goal of Healthy People 2020 in terms of physical fitness.

To increase the proportion of people 18 years old and older who engage in physical activity regularly, preferably daily for at least 30 or more minutes, to develop and maintain the cardiorespiratory system.

32. Why is physical fitness important from a public health standpoint?

The three leading causes of death in the United States are diseases of the heart and blood vessels, cancer, and chronic obstructive pulmonary disease. For each of these degenerative diseases, epidemiologists have identified major risk factors and separated them into three categories: inherited or biologic, environmental, and behavioral. Because nothing can be done currently in terms of modification of inherited risk factors (age, gender, race, and susceptibility), health care providers and researchers have focused on environmental and behavioral risk factors. A major behavioral risk factor for each of the three major diseases is inactivity or a lack of regular exercise.

33. What are the behavioral risk factors for degenerative disease?

Smoking	Alcohol consumption
Inactivity	Overuse of medication
Poor nutrition	Pressure to succeed

34. Why is inactivity a risk factor for many chronic diseases?

There is an inverse relationship between physical activity and premature cardiovascular mortality and all-cause mortality. That is, a sedentary lifestyle increases the incidence of these diseases.

35. How does regular exercise decrease morbidity and mortality?

Regular exercise or training has both **direct effects** on organ systems and **indirect effects,** all of which contribute to the health benefits of exercise.

DIRECT EFFECTS	INDIRECT EFFECTS
Stronger, more efficient heart muscle	Better stress management
Lower blood pressure	Improved immune system
Better insulin sensitivity and glucose control	
Improved body composition	
Lower-low-density lipoprotein concentration	
Higher high-density lipoprotein concentration	

In general, the higher the activity level or level of cardiorespiratory fitness, the lower the mortality and the longer the life span.

36. What is homeostasis?

The maintenance of a constant or **optimal** internal and cellular environment that is compatible with cell life in the face of external and internal influences. Homeostasis is achieved through the integration of multiple compensatory or regulatory systems making continual adjustments. Homeostasis is a dynamic constancy and not an absolute constancy. A dynamically constant internal environment is necessary for optimal cell function.

37. What are the components of a homeostatic control system?

- A **receptor,** which is excited by a stimulus
- An **integrating center,** which processes the information for comparison to its set-point and determines the appropriate response
- The **effector,** which, in response to a signal from the integrating center, responds to correct the disturbance
- The **evoked responses,** which return the internal environment back to normal

The restoration of the internal environment decreases the initiating stimulus and as such is called a **negative feedback control system**.

38. List examples of negative feedback homeostatic control systems involved in adapting to exercise.

Although numerous systems are involved in maintaining homeostasis during exercise, three major systems are vital to exercise:

1. Arterial blood pressure and blood volume regulation, including the baroreceptors
2. Regulation of blood glucose
3. Temperature regulation

39. Why is exercise described as a great challenge to homeostasis?

Physical activity or muscular exercise is the repetitive contraction of groups of skeletal muscle that permits movement about a joint or series of joints. Physical activity or contraction of skeletal muscles of any kind changes the internal environment at a variety of levels and, as such, is a broad homeostatic challenge. For example, during exercise:

- Glucose utilization can be increased twentyfold.
- Skeletal muscle pH drops dramatically.
- Six to 10 lb of water can be lost from the system as sweat.
- Temperature can increase to 106°F.
- Cardiac output can increase from 4.5 L/min to 25 L/min even in untrained adults.

These disturbances must be compensated for to promote cell survival.

40. Why are changes in skeletal muscle associated with whole-body responses to exercise?

Of the approximately 660 skeletal muscles in the human body, more than 400 are under voluntary control. Skeletal muscle constitutes greater than 40% of total body weight and is responsible for three major functions: force production for locomotion and breathing, force production for posture, and heat production during cold exposure. The relative mass of skeletal muscle is indicative of its ability to elicit large changes in homeostasis. The diverse needs of the skeletal muscle are met by multiple systems. For example, because of an increased demand for oxygen, cardiac output or blood flow must increase. Similarly, increases in ventilation and transport of oxygen to the red blood cells by the respiratory system must occur. The acids made by skeletal muscle result in extracellular acidity and are a serious challenge to acid–base homeostasis. Thus, the individual organ systems of the body serve as primary support systems that permit skeletal muscles to perform their functions. Therefore, the whole-body or physiologic responses to exercise function to support skeletal muscle and restore homeostasis.

41. What is ultimately the driving factor for the physiologic changes associated with exercise?

The majority of changes that occur in response to exercise are related to the increased demand for energy to fuel skeletal muscle contraction. For movement of any kind to occur, skeletal muscle must contract or shorten. Skeletal muscle shortening is powered by the hydrolysis of ATP. During exercise, energy utilization can increase from 1.2 kcal/min to 18–30 kcal/min, or a 25-fold increase. These bioenergetic demands dictate physiologic changes in a predictable fashion.

42. What is the difference among exercise, sporting activities, and the physical activities of daily living or work?

From a metabolic point of view, nothing. The ATP demands and whole-body response to sprinting to intercept a pass or sprinting to catch a bus differ only in their magnitude and skill level. Within a single step, the ATP needs of skeletal muscle have increased above rest. The energy or ATP utilization during heavy exercise can increase by 200 times above resting levels. The ability to sustain this or any type of activity is directly linked to the ability of skeletal muscle to produce an equivalent amount of ATP. That is, contractions continue as long as sufficient ATP is produced. If work intensity increases, the amount of ATP required to perform those contractions increases regardless of the motivation for the movement.

43. Does that mean that any activity, even kissing, burns calories?

From a purely metabolic point of view, yes. Kissing is physical activity, and the number of calories has been determined. In fact, the caloric requirements for nearly all activities have been determined and are published in table format in standard exercise physiology textbooks.

44. Graph the relationship between exercise (work) and ATP production.

Increases in work intensity can only be met by a concomitant increase in ATP production. If ATP production does not match work or ATP utilization, work or, in this case, skeletal muscle contraction will cease.

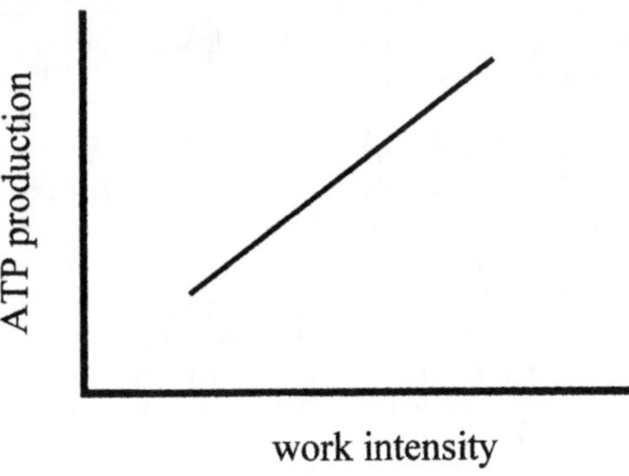

45. Can the ATP demands of exercise be measured?

No. ATP is used at the subcellular level, and aerobic metabolism occurs within the mitochondria and cannot be measured directly. Measuring oxygen consumption at the mouth is a commonly used indirect method for assessing the ATP needs of metabolic work or exercise.

46. What does skeletal muscle require to produce ATP?

A constant supply of substrates (glucose, fatty acids, and oxygen) and an appropriate environment through the removal of waste products (carbon dioxide, acids, adenosine, heat, and potassium).

47. How is oxygen related to exercise?

Because the synthesis of ATP is most efficient under aerobic conditions, the amount of oxygen used or consumed is an indirect measure of ATP synthesis and thus of ATP utilization. Because ATP synthesis cannot be measured, oxygen consumption usually is measured to indicate ATP need. This is best demonstrated in the following figure. The time course of oxygen utilization indicates that oxygen consumption will increase until a new steady state is achieved where oxygen (ATP) demands are met by oxygen (ATP) delivery. *Note that the y-axis is labeled oxygen consumption in liters/min.*

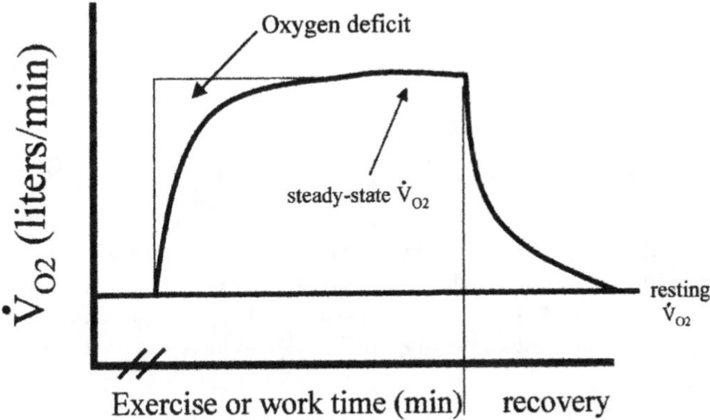

Relationship between exercise or metabolic work and oxygen consumption (L/min). Oxygen consumption and thus ATP production increases until ATP production appropriately balances ATP consumption during work at which a steady state is achieved. Oxygen consumption (ATP production) will be maintained until intensity is changed in either direction.

48. Where does the ATP come from if it takes time for oxygen consumption to increase?

The delay in reaching a new steady state (where oxygen need is met by supply) is often called the **oxygen debt** or **deficit**. Many think that this suggests that the ATP for this work was supplied by anaerobic sources.

49. What is the oxygen debt?

The lag between the onset of metabolic work or exercise and reaching the increase in oxygen consumption; that is, the difference between the oxygen uptake in the first few minutes of exercise and the oxygen needed to provide the necessary ATP for work. ATP needs increase instantaneously, but matching the oxygen needs with an increase in oxygen consumption takes a variable length of time; thus, a deficit is created. Controversy exists about whether the ATP for this work is provided by anaerobic metabolism or by stored sources or is just a lag in measurement. The oxygen debt is decreased with training, suggesting an ability to induce more rapidly the necessary systems to move oxygen more quickly in response to exercise.

50. What is the relationship between oxygen consumption and work when the load is continuously increased?

A progressive increase in workload is called an **incremental workload**. This is like running up a hill and with each step the hill gets just a little steeper, so you run just a little bit faster. If workload is progressively increased, the need for ATP is increased; therefore, the oxygen need is similarly increased until a plateau is reached. The relationship between workload and oxygen consumption is shown in the figure. Oxygen consumption continues to increase so long as oxygen demands are increased to produce ATP to meet the energy needs of the increasing work.

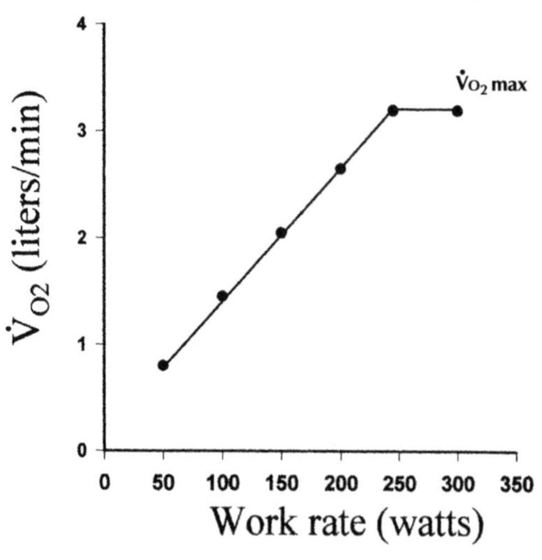

Relationship between oxygen consumption (L/min) and incremental work or ATP needs. Oxygen consumption will increase to match work in a near linear fashion until a maximal level is obtained.

51. Is there a maximal workload or a limit to the capacity to exercise?

Yes. Each individual has a maximal workload or maximal exercise level at which the increased oxygen demand is no longer met with an increase in oxygen consumption. This is defined as **maximal oxygen consumption ($\dot{V}O_2$max)** and is seen as a plateau on the curve in the figure in question 50.

52. What is the significance of $\dot{V}O_2$ max?

Maximal oxygen consumption or $\dot{V}O_2$max represents the maximal capacity to transport and use oxygen during exercise. As such, many consider $\dot{V}O_2$max to be the best indicator of cardiovascular and respiratory fitness. $\dot{V}O_2$ increases in a linear fashion relative to workload or exercise until $\dot{V}O_2max$ is reached. This plateau can be thought of as the physiologic maximum or limit in the ability to transport and deliver oxygen to working muscle. As an index of fitness, $\dot{V}O_2max$ increases with training and decreases with age. Higher values are associated with an increased capacity to perform physical activity or work.

53. What determines $\dot{V}O_2max$?

Oxygen consumption is a function of the cardiovascular system's ability to deliver oxygen specifically to the working muscle, the respiratory system's ability to get oxygen into and carbon dioxide out of the blood, and skeletal muscle's ability to take in and use the oxygen aerobically to produce ATP. Training and genetics influence $\dot{V}O_2max$. This is best described by the Fick equation.

54. What is the Fick equation?

$$\dot{V}O_2 = CO \times (aO_2 - \bar{v}O_2)$$

where $\dot{V}O_2$ is O_2 consumption in mL of O_2/min; CO is cardiac output in L/min; $aO_2 - \bar{v}O_2$ is the difference in arterial and mixed venous O_2 contents in mL of O_2/L.

This equation states that the ability to consume oxygen is a function of the ability of the cardiovascular and respiratory systems to deliver oxygen-enriched blood in combination with the ability of skeletal muscle to extract and utilize oxygen.

55. What is the role of the cardiovascular system during exercise?

According to Fick's equation, the cardiovascular system functions to deliver oxygen and substrates to the specific working muscle for use, to deliver hormones to their target site to facilitate substrate availability, and to remove metabolic wastes from the muscle, including heat. The circulatory system serves as the conduit for transport and exchange of oxygen and waste products, whereas the heart serves as the driving pump to meet such needs.

56. What are the cardiovascular responses to acute exercise?

Two major adjustments occur during exercise to meet oxygen demands.

1. Cardiac output must be increased. This increase is achieved by increasing heart rate and stroke volume

2. Blood flow must be redistributed specifically away from relatively inactive tissue to the working muscle while maintaining appropriate blood flow and pressure to critical organs such as the brain.

57. What controls the cardiovascular responses to exercise?

The cardiovascular centers in the medulla are the primary extrinsic controllers of heart rate and stroke volume. Input to these centers is via the baroreceptor reflex. A dramatic increase in the sympathetic nervous system output both neurally and from the adrenal medulla gland results in increased concentrations of circulating catecholamine, both epinephrine and norepinephrine, during exercise to increase heart rate and stroke volume. Furthermore, intrinsic mechanisms such as the Frank-Starling law of the heart facilitate stroke volume in response to increased venous return. Other factors that influence cardiovascular function include venous return and blood volume, which are influenced by body size, training, and external environmental temperatures.

58. How is venous return increased during exercise?

- Skeletal muscle pump
- Increased cardiac output
- Greater negative pressure in the thoracic cavity as a function of increased ventilation

59. How much can cardiac output increase during exercise?

Resting cardiac output is on average 5 L/min with an average heart rate of 72 bpm and stroke volume of approximately 70 mL per beat. In endurance-trained individuals, maximal cardiac output measures exceed 34 L/min for men (70 kg) and exceed 23 L/min for women (50 kg). Consider that this is equal to seventeen 2-L bottles of soda or just over 9 gallons of blood being pumped through an organ the size of one's fist every minute.

60. What is the relationship among heart rate, stroke volume, mean arterial pressure, and cardiac output with oxygen consumption or workload?

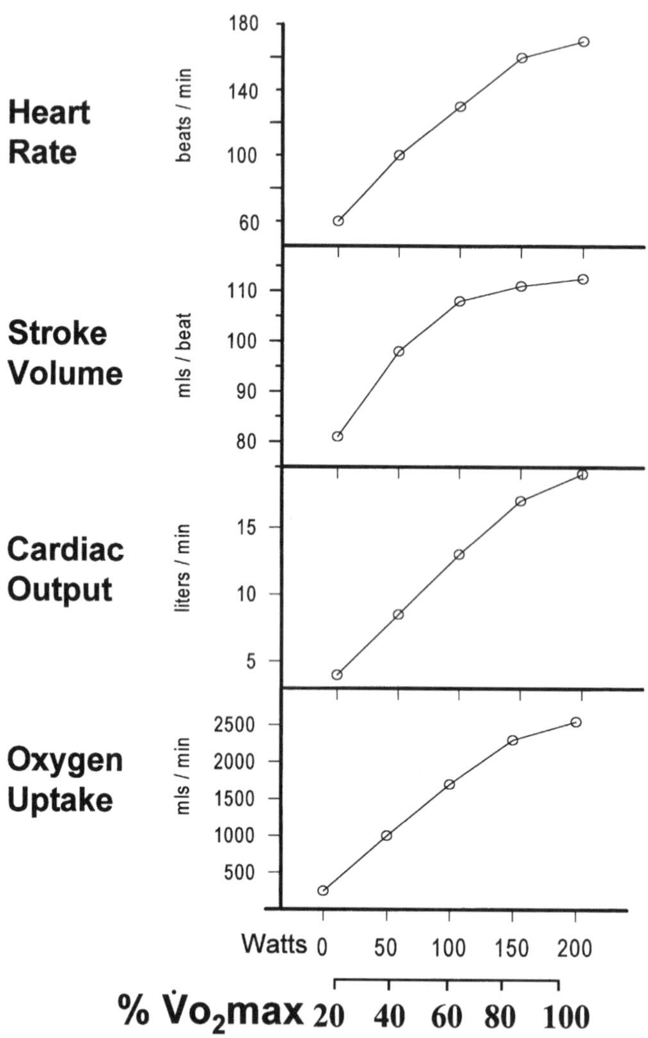

Cardiovascular responses to incremental exercise or work.

61. What is the maximal heart rate?

Commonly, maximal heart rate is considered to be 220 bpm. At heart rates higher than 220 bpm, filling time is decreased, and stroke volume and thus cardiac output are compromised.

62. How are exercise heart rate maximums calculated for use in determining exercise intensity?

Generally, one of two formulas is used to calculate exercise heart rate maximum: the age formula or the Karvonen formula.

- The **age formula** is simply 220 minus your age. For example, a 46-year-old man's maximal heart rate is 220 − 46 = 174 bpm.
- The **Karvonen formula** is explained in question 133.

Neither of these formulas puts a physiologic limit on heart rate, and heart rates can exceed calculated values. Heart rate maximums are used more for safety during exercise.

63. Is there a difference in cardiac output between men and women?

If you measure straight cardiac output in terms of liters per minute, men have a higher cardiac output. In general, men are larger, which means they have a bigger heart, a greater stroke volume, larger blood volume, and higher hematocrit and hemoglobin concentration. Each of these factors contributes to a greater stroke volume and thus cardiac output and oxygen consumption. When data are normalized per gram of lean body mass, the gender differences are significantly diminished. That is, women have a lower cardiac output, but they have less lean muscle mass and smaller body mass as well.

64. What is the role of the microcirculation of skeletal muscle during exercise?

The capillaries of skeletal muscle intertwine with the individual fibers and form an intricate tortuous network with extensive capillary-to-fiber (cell) contact. The tortuosity of the network enhances the transit time of the blood in the muscle. Collectively, this facilitates diffusion of oxygen and nutrients. The microcirculatory system is controlled by autoregulation and local controllers, and capillary density responds to training.

65. How is blood flow selectively distributed to skeletal muscle when sympathetic or vasoconstrictor tone is high?

At rest, the microcirculation of skeletal muscle is vasoconstricted or has a high resistance to blood flow, a function of sympathetic stimulation. With the initiation of exercise, it is hypothesized that a selective withdrawal of sympathetic tone to skeletal muscle results in a relative vasodilation. The prime determinant of skeletal muscle blood flow is intrinsic, that is, inherent within the muscle itself. During exercise, oxygen tension and pH decrease; the concentration of carbon dioxide, extracellular potassium, adenosine, and local temperature all increase, and each acts as a direct local vasodilator. These local factors are directly linked to contraction and metabolism; therefore, the greater the demand, the greater the vasodilation. Collectively, local factors vasodilate the microcirculatory system of skeletal muscle and result in a decrease in resistance and an increase in blood flow. The high sympathetic tone vasoconstricts nonmetabolically active tissue, which effectively facilitates the selective redistribution of blood flow to the area of least resistance (i.e., the dilated capillaries of active skeletal muscle).

66. How does blood flow to skeletal muscle change with exercise?

Because of the high tone in the microcirculation at **rest,** skeletal muscle gets only 15–20% of the total cardiac output at rest. Using the average cardiac output of 5 L/min, blood flow would be less than 1 L/min to all skeletal muscle. During heavy work or **exercise,** cardiac output can increase well above 20 L/min. If an average cardiac output of 25 L/min is coupled with vasodilation in skeletal muscle, 80–85% of the blood flow will be distributed to the muscle. This would be equivalent to more than 20 L of blood delivered to working skeletal muscle per minute.

67. What is the relationship between blood pressure and incremental exercise?

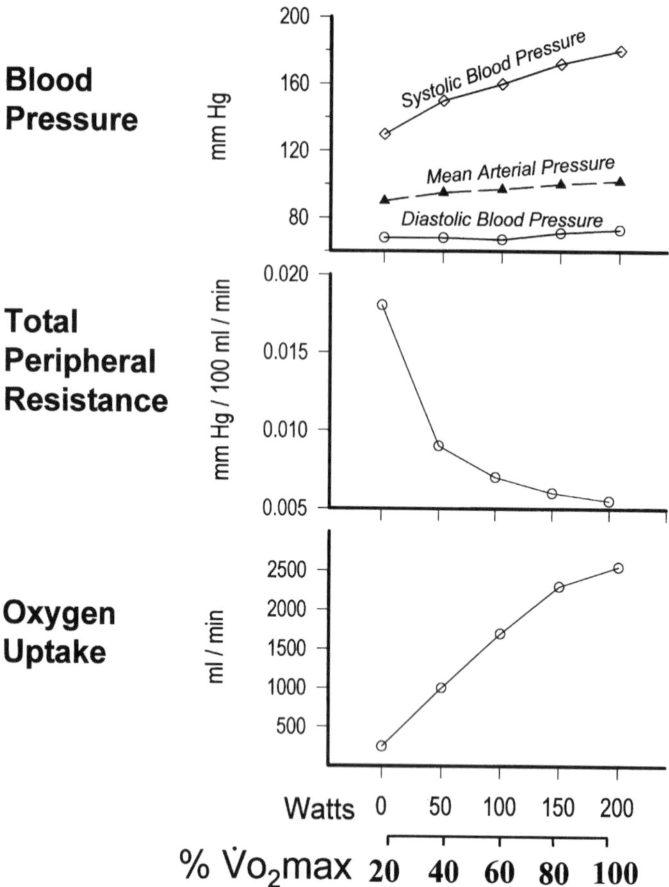

Blood pressure, total peripheral resistance, and oxygen uptake responses to incremental exercise or work. Note that mean arterial pressure changes very little despite large increases in work and decreases in total peripheral resistance.

68. How does blood pressure change during aerobic exercise?

During exercise, systolic blood pressure increases as a function of pumping more blood through the system per minute. The degree of the response is related to the type and intensity of exercise. Diastolic blood pressure is an index of total peripheral resistance and is the sum of all of the resistance beds. During exercise, many of the microcirculatory beds are vasoconstricted. Skeletal muscle, which represents a large circulatory bed, vasodilates. As a result, diastolic blood pressure either decreases or stays the same during exercise. In fact, an increase in diastolic blood pressure is an abnormal response to exercise and a reason to terminate a graded exercise tolerance test.

69. Besides the redistribution of blood flow, what else facilitates oxygen delivery during exercise?

According to Fick's equation, $\dot{V}O_2$ is the product of oxygen delivery (cardiac output) and oxygen extraction ($aO_2 - \bar{v}O_2$). At rest, oxygen extraction of skeletal muscle is relatively low (approximately 5 mL of oxygen is removed per 100 mL of blood). During exercise, when oxygen need is significantly increased, oxygen extraction increases nearly linearly with work rate to a maximal value of approximately 160 mL O_2 per L of blood. This equates to an extraction of 85% of the oxygen delivered in the presence of an increase in blood flow. (See figure.)

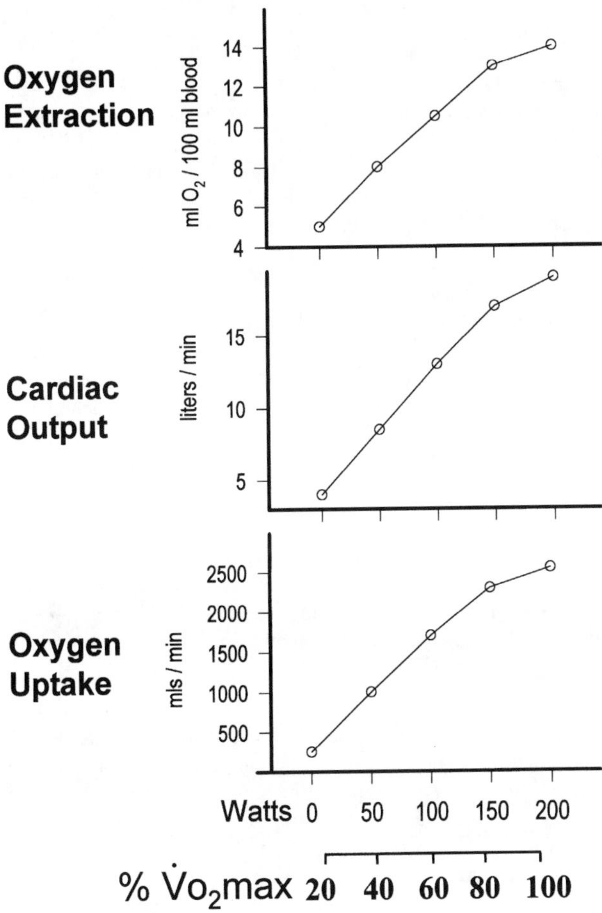

Oxygen extraction by skeletal muscle, cardiac output, and oxygen uptake responses to incremental exercise or work.

70. List the direct influences on oxygen extraction.

- Skeletal muscle blood flow
- Mitochondrial density
- Capillary density
- Training
- Arterial oxygen content
- Muscle mass
- Fiber type
- Pulmonary function

71. What are additional, indirect influences on oxygen extraction?

Exercise conditions including barometric pressure (altitude) and air pollution can indirectly influence extraction by affecting pulmonary function and the partial pressure of oxygen in the inspired air.

72. What determines oxygen content of blood?

The oxygen-carrying capacity (CaO_2) is 20 mL of oxygen per 100 mL of blood. CaO_2 is a function of hemoglobin and the percent arterial saturation (SaO_2). In women, hemoglobin is generally lower, which contributes to the lower $\dot{V}O_2$max reported in women. Hemoglobin concentration is increased with endurance training, which contributes to the training-induced increases in $\dot{V}O_2$max.

73. What determines SaO_2 during exercise?

Hemoglobin is contained in the body's 4–6 billion red blood cells. Each hemoglobin can carry four molecules of oxygen when fully saturated. In healthy individuals, saturation is determined primarily by the partial pressure of oxygen in either the tissue or blood and the affinity between oxygen and hemoglobin. For a complete discussion of hemoglobin saturation and changes with exercise, see Chapter 5, Respiratory Physiology.

74. How is oxygen delivery increased during exercise?

The increase in aerobic metabolism and skeletal muscle contraction results in the increase of metabolic and contractile wastes. These include but are not limited to increases in PCO_2, 2,3-diphosphoglycerate (2,3-DPG), hydrogen ion concentration, and temperature. Each of these shifts the oxyhemoglobin saturation curve to the right. This is a local phenomenon, which increases the oxygen extraction in face of an increased blood flow to match oxygen demands of the increased metabolism.

75. What is the function of the respiratory system during exercise?

The respiratory system's primary function is to enable **gas exchange** between the body and the environment. In addition, the respiratory system plays an important role in maintaining **acid–base homeostasis,** particularly during exercise. The effective exchange of oxygen into the circulation requires an appropriate matching of pulmonary blood flow with ventilation.

76. Are the ventilatory responses the same for all types of acute exercise?

No. During **submaximal constant work,** ventilation increases dramatically with the onset of exercise. This is followed by a more gradual increase in minute ventilation or the amount of air moved per minute. In contrast, during **incremental exercise,** minute ventilation increases in a near-linear fashion with workload or oxygen consumption up to 50–75% of $\dot{V}O_2$max. When $\dot{V}O_2$ is greater than 75% of $\dot{V}O_2$max, minute ventilation increases in a more exponential pattern. At rest, minute ventilation in a 70-kg man is approximately 7.5 L/min. During **maximal exercise,** minute ventilation can increase to 120–175 L/min.

77. How is minute ventilation changed during exercise?

Minute ventilation is the product of the amount of air moved per breath and the frequency of breathing. During exercise, respiratory rate can increase from resting values of 12–15 breaths per minute (bpm) to 40–50 bpm. Tidal volume, or the volume of air per breath, can increase from resting values of 0.5 L to greater than 3.0 L/min.

$$\text{Minute ventilation} = \text{tidal volume (L)} \times \text{bpm}$$

78. How are the ventilatory responses to exercise controlled?

Both the frequency (rate) and depth (tidal volume) of ventilation are controlled by motor neuron output from the respiratory control centers located in the medulla oblongata. The respiratory control center receives input from central and peripheral chemoreceptors, which are sensitive to changes in pH and arterial PO_2 and PCO_2. Exercise-induced decreases in pH and PO_2 and increases in P_{CO_2} each tend to increase minute ventilation. There is also some experimental evidence to suggest that afferent neural impulses originating in the motor cortex to drive skeletal muscle activity may spill over and assist in the drive of ventilation.

79. Summarize the changes in ventilation during incremental exercise

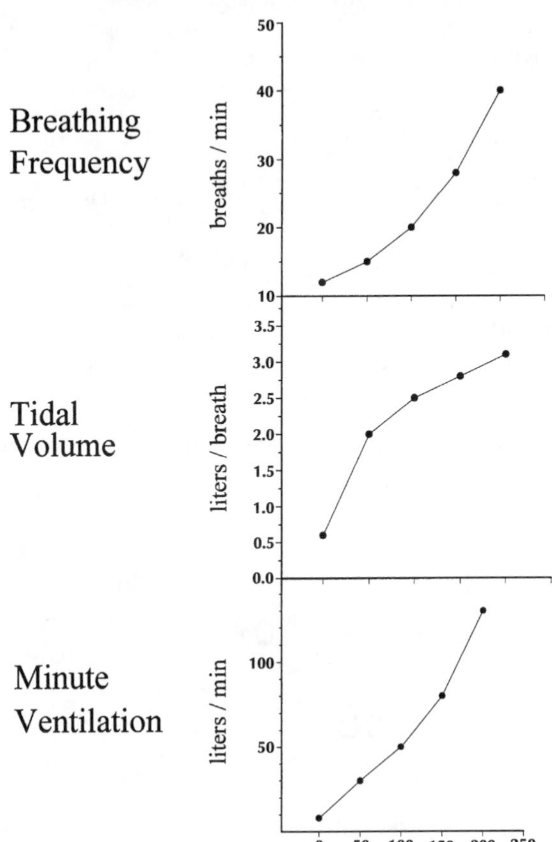

Respiratory responses to incremental work or exercise including breathing frequency, tidal volume, and minute ventilation.

80. What signals the respiratory control center to change ventilation?

In addition to chemoreceptor input, the respiratory control centers receive afferent information from peripheral receptors, including muscle spindles, Golgi tendon organs, and joint pressure receptors. Others have suggested that skeletal muscles have special chemoreceptors, which may respond to potassium and hydrogen ion concentrations with direct input to the respiratory centers. Finally, mechanoreceptors in the heart send afferent information relative to increases in cardiac output. These mechanoreceptors may also play an important role in providing afferent information to control respiration after the initiation of exercise.

81. Which dominates ventilatory control during exercise: chemoreceptors or neural input?

There is no clear agreement about which factors are the major regulators of breathing during exercise. Controversy also exists regarding the controllers during different types of exercise (submaximal versus heavy). There is evidence to suggest regulation only by neural input; there is evidence to suggest regulation only by humoral input; and, finally, there is some evidence to support regulation by a combination of humoral and neural controllers. It is likely that ventilation is regulated by an interaction between these two types of information. Under this scenario, the primary drive to breathe during exercise would be mediated neurally, and precise adjustments to match ventilation would be provided by humoral input regarding the specific changes in PCO_2.

82. What happens to arterial blood pH during exercise?

One important and potentially dangerous by-product of exercise metabolism is an increased production of hydrogen ions or free acids from skeletal muscle. The increase in acid concentration and corresponding decrease in pH is a significant threat to homeostasis. Skeletal muscle pH can drop to 7.2. Uncompensated, the drop in pH threatens enzyme kinetics and compromises the production of ATP.

83. What is the role of the respiratory system in acid–base balance during exercise?

Under normal conditions, excess H^+ is buffered by the bicarbonate system. During exercise, when acid is produced from the production of lactate, the bicarbonate formed is converted to carbon dioxide and water via carbonic anhydrase. This excess production of carbon dioxide increases the PCO_2 and further drives the increase in minute ventilation. Thus, exercise-induced metabolic acidosis is accompanied by increases in PCO_2 and ventilation. Blowing off the excess carbon dioxide provides an effective method to compensate for the exercise-induced metabolic acidosis.

84. Show how these multiple systems are linked to support exercise.

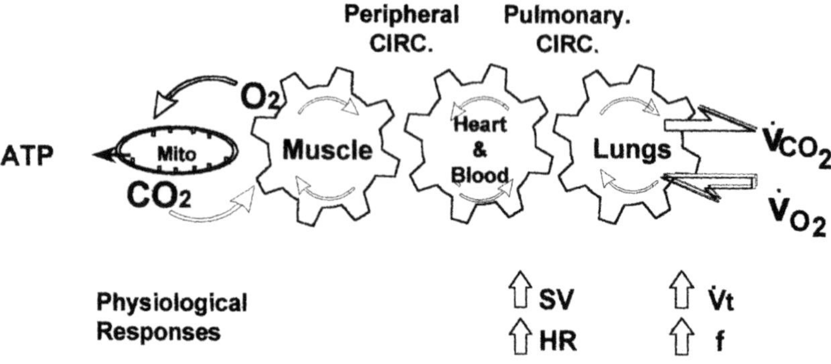

Interdependency of the respiratory, cardiovascular, and microcirculatory systems to deliver oxygen and remove metabolic wastes to produce ATP by the mitochondria. Each system must function optimally to meet the needs of working skeletal muscle. The weakest system will always be the rate-limiting system.

85. What are the endocrine responses to acute exercise?

HORMONE	CHANGE DURING EXERCISE	ENERGY FUNCTION	GROWTH FUNCTION	OTHER EXERCISE FUNCTIONS
Growth hormone	Increase	FFA mobilization, gluconeogenesis, decreases glucose uptake	Stimulates protein synthesis	
Epinephrine	Increase	Glycogenolysis, FFA mobilization		Increases heart rate, stroke volume, and TPR

(*Table continued on following page.*)

HORMONE	CHANGE DURING EXERCISE	ENERGY FUNCTION	GROWTH FUNCTION	OTHER EXERCISE FUNCTIONS
Thyroxine tri-iodothyronine	Increase	Mobilizes fuels	Stimulates growth	
Cortisol	Increase with heavy	Mobilizes fuel substrates (FHA, protein), increases gluconeogenesis		Breaks down skeletal muscle
Aldosterone	Increase			Saves sodium and aids in fluid homeostasis
Vasopressin	Increase when ≥50% $\dot{V}O_2$max			Decreases water loss by kidney, aids fluid homeostasis, increases TRP
Insulin	Decrease	Uptake of glucose, amino acids, and FHA into tissues		
Glucagon	Increase	Glucose and FFA mobilization and gluconeogenesis		
Endorphins	Increase when ≥20% $\dot{V}O_2$-max			Blocks pain

FFA = free fatty acid; TPR = total peripheral resistance.

86. Does respiration limit exercise performance?

Although the pulmonary system can limit physical performance in some disease states, ventilation generally is not considered a limiting factor in healthy adults during prolonged submaximal exercise. The diaphragm has two to three times more oxidative capacity and capillary density than other skeletal muscle, uses glycogen sparingly, and has a high resistance to fatigue. The diaphragm favors oxidation of fat over carbohydrate, making it less dependent on glycogen and carbohydrate supply. In normal healthy individuals, even at maximal exercise, the blood exiting the lungs remains nearly saturated, demonstrating the capacity of the system.

87. Can the pulmonary system ever limit exercise?

Yes. Any pathology in the pulmonary system can compromise performance by decreasing SaO_2 or increasing the work of breathing. Pathology includes damage from environmental pollutants, asthma, or other respiratory diseases.

88. Can the pulmonary system limit exercise in elite athletes?

Pulmonary ventilation may be limiting for elite athletes or highly trained individuals performing prolonged heavy work, such as a marathon. At these levels, the competition between respiratory and skeletal muscles for blood flow and oxygen may be a factor.

89. Does the cardiovascular system limit exercise?

One theory about what limits exercise capacity is known as the **central theory.** It holds that exercise is limited when sufficient oxygen cannot be delivered to skeletal muscle, which is a function of the cardiovascular system. Fick's equation demonstrates the important role of the cardiovascular system in maintaining oxygen consumption. A cardiovascular limitation is hypothesized because once stroke volume maximum is reached, increases in cardiac output can occur only with higher heart rates. At heart rates over 200 bpm, the filling time is compromised, so stroke volume actually decreases. Thus, there is a difficult balance between high enough heart rates and sufficient filling time. Because minute ventilation and respiratory rates can be increased even at $\dot{V}O_2$max when heart rate maximum has been reached, the cardiovascular system is generally considered the limiting factor. In addition, as core temperature increases secondary to heat production by skeletal muscle, the need to deliver blood to the cutaneous circulatory bed to facilitate sweating and heat loss comes into direct competition for blood flow to skeletal muscle.

90. What is the anaerobic threshold?

The term **anaerobic threshold** was first used in the mid-1960s to describe the sudden increase in blood lactate that occurs at high workloads. This was interpreted as an increased lactate production most likely due to local hypoxia (low blood oxygen partial pressures) or ischemia (low blood flows). When oxygen is lacking, pyruvate is converted into lactate. As a result, the production of lactate was interpreted as evidence that there was a lack of oxygen in contracting skeletal muscle. This is controversial. Today, most prefer the term **lactate threshold** to describe the time during which lactate appearance in the blood in no longer linearly related to the workload.

91. What is the lactate threshold?

In the figure below, there is an interesting relationship among the onset of lactate in the blood, the drop in arterial pH, and the change in minute ventilation during exercise. The exercise intensity at which a systematic increase in blood lactate levels occurs is called the **lactate threshold**. Although still being investigated, most would agree that skeletal muscle continually produces lactate during exercise. However, as seen in the figure, blood lactate concentration does not increase until much higher exercise intensities are reached.

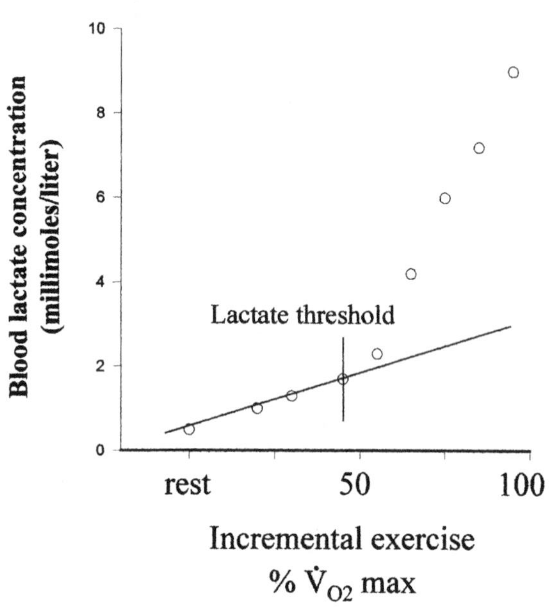

Blood lactate concentration as a function of incremental exercise. Lactate is continually being produced and released into the systemic circulation. Lactate threshold represents the workload where blood lactate concentration begins to increase in a nonlinear fashion.

92. What causes the sudden increase in blood lactate?

There are several theories:

- Decreased removal of lactate from the circulation
- Increased recruitment of fast-twitch glycolytic fibers, which produce more lactate
- Imbalance between glycolysis and mitochondrial respiration
- Tissue hypoxia or ischemia
- Altered ratio of $NADH/NAD^+$

93. Does muscle become hypoxic during exercise?

Although technically impossible to measure directly, to date, there is no experimental evidence to demonstrate hypoxia within skeletal muscle during incremental exercise. Estimates of the $NADH/NAD^+$ ratio even at high workloads suggest that sufficient oxygen is available to permit the ETC regeneration of electron acceptors. Thus, there is no evidence that skeletal muscle is hypoxic, so it is unlikely that hypoxia contributes to the lactate threshold.

94. Why is the lactate threshold important?

The lactate threshold for any given individual is relatively reproducible for a given exercise. Research indicates that the exercise intensity at lactate threshold is the maximal intensity of exercise that can be maintained at a steady state. This means that the higher the lactate threshold, the higher the intensity that can be sustained during endurance exercise. Simply put, given the same $\dot{V}O_2$max, you could run at 70% of your maximal effort instead of being able to run at only 50% of your maximal effort.

95. How is lactate threshold determined?

Typically, an incremental exercise test is performed in which an arterial catheter is inserted for serial blood sampling. The workload is increased incrementally until maximal capacity is reached. Lactate levels are measured from small samples of blood taken every couple of minutes. Blood lactate concentrations are plotted against workload, and the break point from linearity is determined.

96. Can lactate threshold be determined without an arterial catheter?

No. However, there is often a close association between the lactate threshold and a breakpoint in minute ventilation. This close association has been extensively studied. Some believe the lactate threshold can be estimated from gas exchange data collected during indirect gas colorimetry. In this case, at the lactate threshold and change in arterial pH, there very often is a ventilatory breakpoint or a disproportionate increase in ventilation relative to the change in workload. This breakpoint is called the **ventilatory threshold**. Ventilatory threshold is a crude (at best), noninvasive estimate of lactate threshold.

97. Is lactate production detrimental?

No. Many people used to think lactate production was responsible for muscle fatigue and delayed-onset muscle soreness; this is now known to be incorrect. Lactate is an important substrate for cardiac muscle energy production and is an important intermediate step in gluconeogenesis. In addition, the production of lactate from pyruvate regenerates NAD^+ and permits glycolysis to continue during high demands for ATP. Furthermore, the conversion of pyruvate to lactate when pyruvate production exceeds entry into the mitochondria for metabolism eliminates end-product inhibition of the key glycolytic enzymes. This facilitates energy metabolism. Lactate also can be converted by the liver back to pyruvate and as part of the Cori cycle synthesis of new glucose.

98. What is the ventilatory threshold?

The exercise intensity at which there is a deviation in linearity in minute ventilation simultaneously with an increase in ventilatory equivalents for oxygen ($\dot{V}_E/\dot{V}O_2$). This nonlinear point has traditionally been thought to occur secondary to the metabolic (lactate) acidosis (drop in pH and increase in PCO_2) occurring in relationship to the lactate threshold. Both pH and PCO_2 drive the increase in ventilation.

99. Are the ventilatory threshold and lactate threshold the same?

No. Although some have suggested that ventilatory threshold and lactate threshold are the same and can be used interchangeably, several studies suggest this is incorrect. Differences between lactate threshold and ventilatory threshold as large as 8% of $\dot{V}O_2$max have been reported.

100. Can ventilatory threshold and lactate threshold change?

Yes. Both lactate threshold and ventilatory threshold respond to training (i.e., shift to the right). The thresholds have practical implications both in sport performance and in designing exercise training programs for endurance athletes. Because fatigue is associated with high levels of lactate, exercising just below lactate threshold is important. With training, the shift in threshold permits working at a higher percentage of maximum without lactate build-up in the circulation.

101. What is fatigue?

The inability to continue exercise at a desired or given intensity. Often, **fatigue** and **performance limitation** are incorrectly used interchangeably. Fatigue is really a process and should be defined by the failing system for a specific type of exercise. For example, muscular fatigue during resistance-type exercise is characterized by the inability to sustain a generated force, despite an appropriate effort. Performance limitation is generally considered to focus on what limits $\dot{V}O_2$max.

102. Describe the two major theories regarding sites of fatigue.

1. **Central fatigue.** The central nervous system is primarily responsible for fatigue by either a reduction in the number of motor units firing or a decrease in the frequency of motor unit firing. There is limited evidence in support of this theory.
2. **Peripheral fatigue.** Peripheral fatigue occurs as the result of neural, mechanical, or energetic system failures. The peripheral theory supports the conclusion that fatigue is the result of failure at the cellular level to provide ATP secondary to disrupted homeostasis.

103. List the potential mediators of skeletal muscle fatigue during prolonged exercise.

- Metabolic acidosis
- Decreases in glycogen
- Electrolyte imbalances
- Dehydration
- Hypoglycemia
- Damage to skeletal muscle
- Changes in muscle membrane excitability
- Inability to supply ATP adequately
- Mechanical failure owing to high H^+ concentration
- Failure of temperature regulatory systems resulting in hyperthermia

104. Define DOMS.

Delayed-**o**nset **m**uscle **s**oreness (DOMS) is a common overuse injury that appears 24–48 hours after strenuous exercise (delayed). Although originally thought to be due to lactate, this is clearly not the case. Current evidence for the mechanisms for DOMS indicates that excessive mechanical force results in skeletal muscle and connective tissue damage or injury. Associated with the cell damage or injury is a classic inflammatory response, including an increase in cell mediators such as histamine, kinins, and likely prostaglandins; increased macrophage, mast cell, and lysosomal activities; edema formation; and an increase in local temperature. Each of these stimulates sensory nerve endings and results in pain.

105. What limits $\dot{V}O_2$max?

Currently there are two theories to explain $\dot{V}O_2$max limitations:

1. The **central limitation theory** focuses on the central nervous system and the systemic circulation as limiters. This includes changes in blood volume, arousal, cardiac function, and oxygen transport. Central theory proponents believe that sufficient oxygen-enriched blood cannot be transported to the skeletal muscle without compromising systemic blood pressure and blood flow to essential organ systems, particularly the brain or temperature regulatory beds such as cutaneous microcirculation.
2. In contrast, the **peripheral limitation theory** has focused on factors occurring in the skeletal muscle itself. These factors include structural and functional elements, such as capillary density, mitochondrial density, oxygen extraction capabilities, and oxygen utilization capability of the mitochondria.

106. List the functional limitations for different types of exercise.

EXERCISE	FUNCTIONAL LIMITATION AND MECHANISM
Intense <30 s	Energy depletion (CrP and ATP)
Intense 0.5–10 min	Energy depletion (CrP and ATP), acidosis, accumulation of waste products, electrochemical disturbance
Low intensity <90 min	Hyperthermia, muscle damage
Low intensity >90 min	Low muscle glycogen, hypoglycemia, muscle damage, low liver glycogen, dehydration, hyperthermia, electrochemical disturbance, central nervous system and cardiovascular disturbance

CrP = creatinine phosphate.

107. What limits all-out anaerobic performance?

During high-intensity exercise lasting less than 180 seconds, contractions are dominated by a very high percentage of type IIb fibers (> 70%). Type IIb fibers have a high glycolytic capacity, which means ATP needs are met primarily by anaerobic glycolysis and the creatine phosphate system. The primary result is a large production of lactate with resulting muscle acidosis and spillover to systemic acidosis. The elevated H^+ concentration interferes with metabolism or the mechanics of contraction by interfering with troponin's ability to bind calcium. Collectively, these limit the exercise time.

108. Describe the skeletal muscle adaptations to endurance exercise training.

Skeletal muscle responds to endurance training with characteristic adaptations designed to increase the tolerance to the metabolic challenge. Although the change in cross-sectional area is minimal, muscle fibers change their biochemical or metabolic features to facilitate this type of activity. Changes in skeletal muscle include:

- Hypertrophy of slow-twitch fibers
- Increased myoglobin content
- Increase in mitochondrial density and size
- Increase in glut 4 transporters
- Increase in oxidative enzyme content
- Increase in capillary density, which increases the autoregulatory capacity of the muscle itself

These changes not only result in an increased capillary-to-fiber ratio, which promotes oxygen delivery, but also permit a more rapid redistribution of blood to working muscle after endurance training. Collectively, these changes facilitate the delivery, extraction, and utilization of oxygen and thus increase ATP production for skeletal muscle contraction and delay the onset of metabolic acidosis.

109. Does endurance training burn more fat?

Yes, with aerobic conditioning, the activities of the enzymes involved in beta oxidation and those involved in liberating free fatty acids into the circulation are increased. This permits a greater utilization of fat as a fuel or substrate (burn more fat) and spares carbohydrate (glycogen) stores. Therefore, a greater percentage of fat is burned at intensities below the lactate threshold.

110. What are the cardiovascular adaptations to aerobic training?

In addition to the skeletal muscle changes noted above, aerobic training induces adaptations in the cardiovascular and respiratory systems. Specifically, $\dot{V}O_2max$ is increased because more oxygen can be delivered and consumed. The cardiovascular adaptations include:

- Cardiac hypertrophy
- Increased stroke volume at rest and during submaximal and maximal workloads
- Greater ejection fraction
- Greater end-diastolic volume
- Lower heart rate
- Faster heart rate recovery
- Increase in cardiac output
- Increases in blood volume and plasma volume
- Slight increase in red blood cell numbers

111. Why does aerobic training decrease the incidence of heart attacks?

Although the long-term benefits of aerobic training are multifactorial, a major factor in lowering the risk of myocardial ischemia is exercise-induced bradycardia. Myocardial oxygen consumption is best estimated by the **double product,** which is heart rate × systolic blood pressure. Because heart rate is lower at rest and during all levels of exercise or physical activity, the heart is less likely to exceed its oxygen delivery capacity. Thus, endurance exercise training results in a lower oxygen demand of the heart for a given cardiac output, avoiding the damaging effects of ischemia.

112. What are the respiratory adaptations to aerobic training?

Without appropriate adaptations in the respiratory system, adaptations in the cardiovascular system would be meaningless. The specific adaptations are designed to maximize the efficiency of oxygen delivery. Specific adaptations include:

- Slight increase in maximal tidal volume
- Decreases in respiratory rate at rest and during submaximal exercise and an increase at maximal levels
- Increase in maximal minute ventilation
- Increase in oxygen diffusion in the alveoli during maximal exercise (unchanged at rest and during submaximal exercise)
- Improved ventilation/perfusion ratio, permitting optimal O_2 uptake from the alveoli into the pulmonary capillaries

113. Does oxygen extraction change with aerobic training?

Although the content of arterial oxygen does not change with training, the venous content is lower. That is, the skeletal muscle extracts more, so the $aO_2 - \bar{v}O_2$ is increased with training. This is a function of the skeletal muscle changes from endurance training, including increases in capillary density and myoglobin content. The net effect is to extract more of the delivered oxygen into the skeletal muscle for use by mitochondria for ATP production.

114. What happens to the lactate threshold with aerobic training?

The lactate threshold shifts to the right, so it will occur at a higher workload. Thus, the **onset** of lactate will occur at a higher percentage of a greater $\dot{V}O_2max$. This appears to be the result of an enhanced clearance of lactate by muscle and a shift toward fatty acid metabolism (produce less lactate). In addition, there is not only a delayed onset, but also an increased tolerance to the acidosis that occurs with training.

115. Describe the mechanisms of skeletal muscle adaptations to resistance training.

Skeletal muscle adaptations to resistance training are partially mediated by adaptations within skeletal muscle and partially associated with changes in the neural motor system. The initial or rapid increases in strength are primarily a function of the neural motor system and learning—that is, a greater ability to recruit motor units. The skeletal muscle adaptations require protein synthesis via transduction, translation, and synthesis, all of which require more time.

116. What are the neural adaptations to resistance training?

- Increase in integrated electromyographic activity, which increases force generation
- Increase in motor unit firing rate, which increases force production and duration of contraction
- Greater ease of motor unit recruitment, so that more motor units are fired simultaneously for greater force production
- Improved motor unit synchronization or coordination, which increases force production and permits a more efficient application of the generated force
- Coordination of antagonists, timing, and inhibition of Golgi tendon organs

117. List the skeletal muscle adaptations to resistance training.

Neural and Skeletal Muscle Tissue Adaptations to Strength Training

	ADAPTATIONS		SIGNIFICANCE
↑	Muscle mass	↑	Muscle strength
↑	Cross-sectional area	↑	Contractile capacity
↑	Type I and II fiber area	↑	Strength
↑	Intracellular glycogen content	↑	Glycolytic capacity
↑	Intramuscular high-energy phosphate pool	↑	Phosphagen metabolism

(Table continued on following page.)

Neural and Skeletal Muscle Tissue Adaptations to Strength Training (cont.)

	ADAPTATIONS		SIGNIFICANCE
↑	Intramuscular ATP utilization rate	↑	Capacity for maximum contraction
↑	Androgen receptors	↑	Androgen-induced hypertrophy
⇔	Glycolytic enzymes	⇔	Adequate
↓	Capillary density (weightlifters); ↑ in bodybuilders	↓ or ↑	Diffusion capacity
↑	Rate of motor unit activation	↑	Rate of force development
↑	Integrated electromyographic activity	↑	Force production
↑	Coordination of antagonist and muscle groups	↑	Effectiveness of force application
↑	Motor unit synchronization	↑	Force; ↑ efficiency in application of force
↑	Time high-threshold motor units can be activated	↑	Length of time maximal force can be maintained
↑	Inhibition of Golgi tendon organs	↓	Inhibition of maximal muscle contraction

↑ = increased, ↓ = decreased, ⇔ = no change.

118. How is muscle size related to force production?

Force production is directly proportional to the cross-sectional area of the muscle. In response to training, particularly resistance training, skeletal muscle hypertrophies, resulting in an increased cross-sectional area and a concomitant increase in force production.

119. What is the force–velocity relationship?

A **force–velocity curve** is created when the rate of shortening (velocity) is plotted against the force developed. During an isotonic contraction, the muscle changes length. Muscle is capable of shortening at different velocities depending on the load and intrinsic properties. During a shortening or **concentric** contraction, increasing the load results in a decrease in the shortening velocity. That is, when the load is light, the velocity of shortening is fast. When the load is maximal, velocity is zero, and the load does not move. In terms of eccentric or lengthening contraction, note that the force for any given eccentric contraction is greater than the maximal concentric force by 50–100%. That is, skeletal muscle can generate more eccentric force at any velocity than concentric force. These high eccentric forces are the primary reason for exercise-induced muscle injury, which is prevalent after exercise with an eccentric bias.

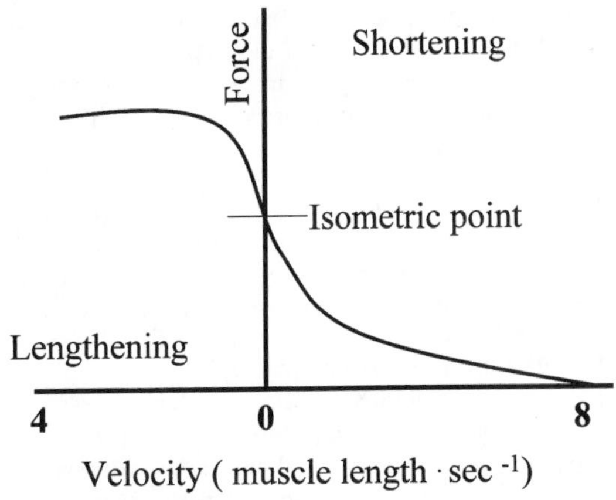

Relationship between velocity or shortening and force-generating capacity of human skeletal muscle.

120. What is the length–tension relationship?

The amount of tension that a muscle is capable of generating for a given threshold stimulus is critically dependent on its initial resting length relative to its optimal length. Optimal length is defined as the fiber length at which maximal force is generated and where optimal actin–myosin overlap exists. It is an inverted U-shaped curve. Because the optimal length is the site of optimal force-generating capabilities and is at the peak of the U, changes in fiber length in either direction compromise force.

121. Does fiber type influence performance?

No one knows for sure. Descriptive studies of elite athletes suggest that muscle fiber composition differs for different sports. For example, elite sprinters have 55–75% fast-twitch fibers, whereas elite distance runners have 60–90% slow-twitch fibers. Although this difference suggests that fiber type may be important in sport performance, the studies report a large variability within athletes of a given sport. Clearly, fiber composition is just one component to performance, and one cannot eliminate the complex physiologic interactions of the other systems or ignore the role of training, personality, and psychological components.

122. How does skeletal muscle mass increase?

No one knows for certain. No receptors, signal transducers, or integrating centers have been identified that are responsible for skeletal muscle size. Skeletal muscle is approximately 20% protein and 60–70% water. In humans, skeletal muscle **hypertrophy,** an increase in fiber size, is thought to be the dominant response to training versus an increase in fiber numbers (**hyperplasia**). The increase in fiber size is the result of an increase in protein synthesis. All protein synthesis is regulated by gene expression and is influenced by the cellular environment. Both recruitment and load are known to stimulate muscle DNA translation and thus protein synthesis. Exercise training, nutrition, humoral factors, overall health, and gender are all capable of modifying the protein synthesis in response to the same signal. These factors can either facilitate or inhibit protein synthesis.

123. Other than exercise, what else causes skeletal muscle hypertrophy?

Any work that is an overload stimulates protein synthesis. Furthermore, growth hormone and androgens (endogenous and synthetic) stimulate protein synthesis, as does appropriate nutrition. Research is currently under way to investigate ergogenic aids for their hypertrophic potential. This is not only important in terms of sports and exercise, but also clinically relevant in terms of aging and many patient populations that experience muscle wasting secondary to disease.

124. Why do training adaptations occur?

The major objective of the cellular and organ system adaptations is to facilitate the response to specific tasks or challenges associated with exercise. Because each type of exercise disturbs homeostatic balance in a specific way, the adaptations are designed to respond more quickly to that specific signal and restore homeostasis more quickly. For example, as a result of the increased cardiac output demands, the heart hypertrophies to perform the increased work but at a lower oxygen cost. This and other adaptations have as side benefits a decrease in morbidity and mortality from all causes.

125. How much exercise is required for a training adaptation to occur?

Any amount of exercise that is an overload to the current system will induce adaptations. Specific adaptations depend on the frequency, duration, and intensity of exercise as well as rest intervals. Adaptations occur in response to planned and appropriate overload.

126. What is the overload principle?

An exercise must specifically overload the capacity of the target to evoke a training adaptation and enhance physiologic function. That is, adaptations occur only when a specific system has been required to do more work than it normally performs. If the overload principle is followed, the exercise intensity, duration, and frequency must be manipulated continually to continue to induce adaptations. Adaptations are appropriate to the specific stimulus.

127. What is the principle of task specificity?

Training adaptations respond to the specific initiating stimuli. If one trains the arms, then the arms respond, and the legs show no training adaptations. Similarly, training to shoot free throws is done by shooting free throws, not by swimming. By definition, the principle of **task specificity** means that specific exercise elicits specific adaptations creating specific training effects or changes in performance. Those systems not stimulated show minimal if any adaptations; this includes the biochemical, neural, and mechanical aspects of exercise. Furthermore, the adaptations are specific to the intensity of the stimuli. Walking for 30 minutes per day results in adaptations to walking with many associated health benefits, but it will not make you a good sprinter or able to complete a marathon.

128. What is the reversibility principle?

Simply stated, **use it or lose it**. Detraining occurs rapidly. If a sufficient stimulus is not provided, the training improvements are rapidly lost. Significant losses can be measured within 1–2 weeks, and bed rest can decrease $\dot{V}O_2$max by 25%, increase resting heart rate, and reduce maximal cardiac output in just 20 days. The central point is that the training benefits are only transient and rapidly reversible unless sufficient stimuli (exercise) are provided to prevent it. Research suggests that training benefits show signs of reversal within 3 days. Therefore, to sustain the adaptations or prevent their loss, exercise should be performed every 48–72 hours. In support of this, studies have demonstrated the effectiveness of 3 days per week frequency vs. 1–2 days per week in terms of retaining cardiovascular training effects.

129. How much exercise is needed to get a beneficial effect in terms of cardiovascular disease?

Healthy People 2020 recommends 30–45 minutes of aerobic exercise 3–5 times per week. Originally, it was thought that this exercise needed to be continuous and of an intensity over 65% of $\dot{V}O_2$max. However, it is now recognized that a cumulative total of 30–45 minutes, that is, the total minutes throughout the day, is sufficient to reap important health benefits, including decreases in cardiovascular mortality. Furthermore, studies have reported the effectiveness of low-risk exercises (low injury rate) such as walking in improving health.

130. What type of exercise or machine is best for cardiovascular disease prevention?

According to the American College of Sports Medicine, in selecting the mode of exercise, any exercise that involves the use of large muscle groups over prolonged periods and is rhythmic and aerobic in nature results in the greatest improvements in $\dot{V}O_2$max and reduction in cardiovascular disease risk. Examples include:

Walking
Cross-country skiing
Machine-based stair climbing
Swimming
Cycling
Rowing
Rope skipping
Endurance activity

Key in the selection of the mode of exercise is selecting one that is enjoyable, affordable, and readily available for participation and ideally has a limited risk of injury. For all ages, **walking** has continually proved to be one of the best exercises for cardiovascular disease prevention.

131. What factors influence training adaptations?

Initial level of fitness
Intensity of training
Frequency of training
Duration of training
Genetics

132. How is training intensity determined?

- Calories per minute
- Absolute workload (watts)
- Relative workload (% of $\dot{V}O_2$max)
- Workload relative to lactate threshold
- Workload at a particular heart rate or a percentage of maximal heart rate
- Multiples of METs
- Rating of perceived exertion

Percentages of **heart rate maximums** and **ratings of perceived exertion** are the most common techniques used for fitness and include a percentage of age-adjusted heart rate maximum (HR_{max} = 220 – age), the Karvonen formula, or the Borg scale of perceived effort.

133. What is the Karvonen formula?

This formula determines exercise intensity based on age-adjusted heart rate maximum but takes into consideration resting heart rate (an index of initial fitness level). To calculate: Subtract standing heart rate (HR) from age-adjusted heart rate maximum (HR_{max}) to obtain heart rate reserve. Calculate intensity range by multiplying high and low ranges by heart rate reserve. To each range value, add back the resting heart rate to obtain target training heart rates.

To calculate the target heart rate for exercise in the range of 50–85% maximum:

$$\text{Target HR range} = [(HR_{max} - HR_{rest}) \times 0.50] + HR_{rest} \text{ and}$$
$$[(HR_{max} - HR_{rest}) \times 0.85] + HR_{rest}$$

134. What is resting metabolic rate?

The amount of oxygen consumed to provide ATP for the metabolic processes occurring at rest. For men it is 3.7 ml O_2/body weight in kg/min. For women it is 3.2 ml O_2/body weight in kg/min. Resting metabolic rate (RMR) differs from basal metabolic rate (BMR). The requirements for measuring RMR are much less stringent and often include the thermic effect of food, whereas BMR can be measured only following a minimum of a 12-hour fast and refraining from performing any physical activity for several hours prior to the test. Typically, BMR is measured after an overnight stay in a special facility. RMR is a good estimate of BMR and can be measured 3 hours after a light meal or exercise. Lean body mass has the greatest effect on increasing either RMR or BMR.

135. Are METs a baseball team?

No, a MET is a unit of metabolic work. MET stands for **metabolic equivalent**. Average resting metabolic rate for men and women is 3.5 mL of oxygen uptake per kilogram of body weight per minute, which means that 3.5 mL O_2/kg body weight/min are burned or metabolized to make ATP while just resting. This is equal to approximately 1.2 kcal/min.

136. How are METs used to quantify work?

By knowing the energy cost of different types of activity and converting them to their requirement for oxygen, one can use multiples of METs to define intensity. Thus, 1 MET is resting activity, 2 METs is work above rest, and 10 METs requires 10 times more oxygen than at rest and is thus harder. METs have been worked out for many activities. METs are commonly used to express exercise intensity and for exercise prescriptions because they are easy to understand and remember for many people. Low intensity is 3–4 METs, moderate is 6–8 METs, and vigorous exercise increases metabolic rate above 10 METs.

137. Define calorie.

The quantity of heat required to raise the temperature of 1 kg of water 1°C. It is most appropriately called a kilogram calorie or a **kilocalorie (kcal)**. As such, a quantity of food containing 250 kcal contains sufficient energy to increase the temperature of 250 kg of water 1°C. Thus, kilocalorie is a unit of expressing energy. Humans are inefficient in converting kilocalories to ATP, and they lose 40–60% of the energy as heat. Energy consumption may be measured by measuring heat loss or, more conveniently, by measuring oxygen uptake. This is because oxygen is required in the combustion of food. Measuring oxygen consumption allows us to calculate the energy cost (kilocalories) of different activities.

138. How can you determine the calories burned by measuring oxygen consumption?

Oxygen is consumed in the combustion of food to release energy for activity. The more oxygen consumed, the more energy used. Each liter of oxygen burned is 5 kcal. Therefore, if resting oxygen is 3.5 mL of oxygen/kg/min for a 70-kg man, then at rest he burns the following:

$$3.5 \text{ mL} \times 70 \text{ kg} = 245 \text{ mL } O_2/1000 = 0.245 \text{ L } O_2$$

$$0.245 \text{ L } O_2 \times 5 \text{ kcal/L} = 1.225 \text{ kcal/min at rest}$$

This equals 74 kcal/hr (1.225 × 60 min/hr) or 1764 kcal in a single day just for resting metabolism.

139. How many calories do you burn when you exercise?

It depends on the type of exercise, the intensity, and, in some instances, the body weight. For example, if a 70-kg man performs 30 minutes of aerobic exercise at an intensity level of 8 METs, he is burning the following:

$$3.5 \times 8 \times 70 = 1960/1000 = 1.9 \text{ L } O_2 \times 5 \text{ kcal/L} = 9.8 \text{ kcal/min} \times 30 = \text{total of } 294 \text{ kcal}$$

BIBLIOGRAPHY

1. Brooks GA, Fahey TD, White TP: Exercise Physiology: Human Bioenergetics and Its Application, 2nd ed. Mountain View, CA, Mayfield Publishing Company, 2000.
2. Durstine JL, King AC, Painter PL, et al (eds): American College of Sports Medicine Resource Manual for Exercise Testing and Prescriptions. Baltimore, Williams & Wilkins, 1998.
3. Powers SK, Howley ET (eds): Exercise Physiology: Theory and Application to Fitness and Performance, 4th ed. New York, McGraw-Hill, 2001.
4. Rowell LB, Shepherd JT: Exercise: Regulation and Integration of Multiple Systems. In Handbook of Physiology. New York, Oxford University Press, 1996.

14. TEMPERATURE REGULATION

Paula E. Papanek, Ph.D., MPT

1. Is there a normal body temperature?

Internal or core temperature remains nearly constant despite exposure to wide ranges in environmental or external temperature. Typically, the average normal body temperature is 98.6°F (37°C), with ranges in temperature from 97° to 99°F (36.1–37.2°C). That is, core temperature is controlled within ± 1°F (± 0.6°C).

2. Why is body temperature so tightly regulated?

Similar to oxygen tension and intracellular and blood pH, changes in extracellular temperature can have a profound effect on cellular function. Many enzymes required for cellular survival function optimally within a narrow temperature range. Therefore, maintaining appropriate temperature is vital for homeostasis.

3. What is the source of internal heat?

Heat production is a byproduct of all metabolism. On average, 40–60% of the energy from hydrolysis of adenosine triphosphate (ATP) is lost as heat. Thus, heat production and internal temperature are a function of energy utilization or metabolic activity. Anything that increases cellular metabolism (increases in thyroid hormone, epinephrine, or norepinephrine; increased basal metabolic rate; or exercise) increases heat production.

4. What is thermal balance?

The balance between the heat-producing (heat gain) systems and the heat-loss systems. At rest, radiation and convection to the air are the primary heat-loss systems if the environment is cooler and dryer than skin temperature. During exercise or when core temperature is elevated, evaporation from sweating becomes the predominant heat-loss mechanism.

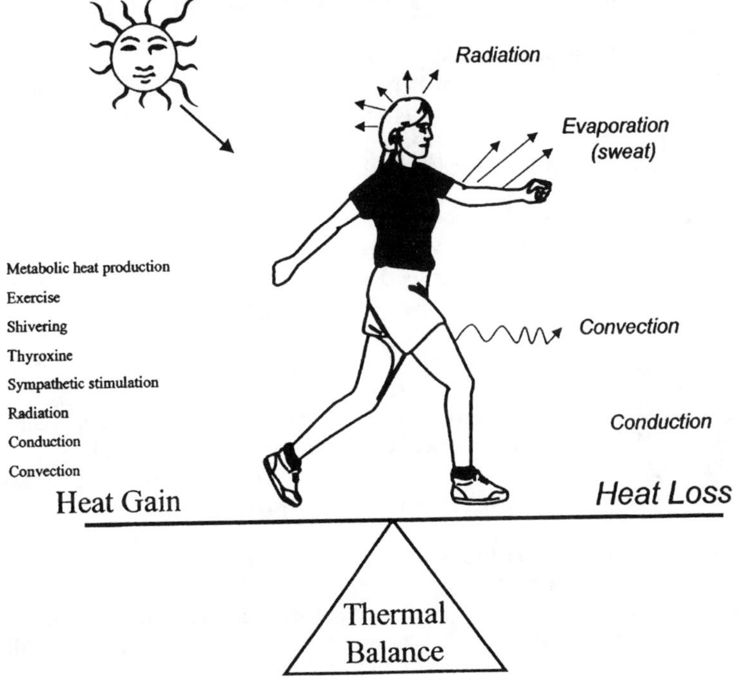

5. What are the upper limits of extreme heat that humans can tolerate?

Heat tolerance depends almost entirely on whether the heat is dry or wet.

- When the heat is completely **dry** and evaporation is effective, humans can tolerate external temperatures of **150°F (65.6°C)** for several hours.
- If the air is **100% saturated** or **humidified,** core temperature begins to rise whenever the environmental temperature is above 94°F (34.4°C).

The upper limits of tolerable core temperature are often recorded during exercise and range up to 104°F (40°C), with the low end of normal range of 95.5–96.5°F (35.3–35.8°C) recorded in the early morning or during cold weather.

6. How does the body keep core temperature constant?

Body temperature is controlled by balancing heat production with heat loss. When heat loss equals heat production, **homeostasis,** or balance, is achieved. When either is out of equilibrium, body temperature either increases or decreases.

7. What are the medical terms for elevated and decreased body temperature?

Hyperthermia is excessively high body temperature, and **hypothermia** is low body temperature.

8. Is there a critical body temperature?

When body temperature rises **above 106–110°F (41.1–43.3°C), heat stroke** develops. These core temperatures are extreme and require external intervention targeted to decrease body heat or survival is doubtful. If body temperature falls **below 94°F (34.4°C),** the ability to regulate core temperature is lost.

9. Define heat stroke.

A self-perpetuating condition that occurs because the hypothalamus has become excessively heated, greatly diminishing its heat-regulating capacity. It is often defined as the state where core temperature is elevated such that central nervous system is damaged.

10. List the signs and symptoms of heat stroke.

Headache
Dizziness progressing to delirium
Cessation of sweating
Confusion
Abdominal distress or nausea
Rapid, strong pulse rate
Variable blood pressure
Unconsciousness
Hot, dry skin

11. What are the consequences of heat stroke?

If body temperature is not quickly decreased, **circulatory shock (hypotension)** ensues. In addition, the hyperpyrexia directly damages neurons. The brain can tolerate only a few moments of excessive temperatures. High temperature also damages the kidneys, liver, and other organs, which also contributes to mortality.

12. What is the treatment for heat stroke?

Heat stroke is a medical emergency or crisis, and emergency medical treatment should be sought immediately. If efforts to decrease core temperature are not successful, mortality is high. Any method available must be used to assist in cooling to prevent cellular damage, including dousing the patient with water or applying ice or cold towels.

13. What increases the risk for heat stroke?

By far, the biggest risk factor for heat stroke is a past medical history of heat stroke. For reasons unknown, once someone has had an episode of heat stroke, they are at a greater risk of developing heat stroke again. Anyone with a history of heat stroke therefore requires additional attention and monitoring.

14. Is heat exhaustion another name for heat stroke?

No. They are different but related pathophysiologic states. **Heat exhaustion** is often a precursor to heat stroke.

15. List the signs and symptoms of heat exhaustion.

Profuse sweating
Fatigue
Excessive thirst
Excessive weakness
Pale, cool skin

16. What is the treatment for heat exhaustion?

Stop all activity and treat heat exhaustion with fluid replacement and any method available to cool the body. Untreated, heat exhaustion is likely to progress to heat stroke.

17. What are the mechanisms for heat loss?

- **Conduction** is the direct transfer of heat from the body to other objects—for example, lying on cool pavement.
- **Radiation** is the loss of heat through electromagnetic waves emitted from the body.
- **Convection** is the loss of heat into the air and removed by convection currents. Conduction and convection are effective whenever the body is in contact with cool water or air.
- **Evaporation** is the loss of heat from the body surface as sweat is vaporized and evaporated.

Independent of physiologic mechanisms for heat loss are **behavioral responses** directed at temperature regulation. These behavioral responses are dictated by the psychic perception of being overheated and result in environmental adjustments, such as removing clothing, seeking cooler locations, or drinking cool beverages. These behaviors occur both consciously and subconsciously.

18. What method of heat loss is the predominate system at rest?

- Radiation—60% of heat loss
- Evaporation (both respiratory and sweating)—22%
- Conduction to the air—15%

Radiation and conduction are ineffective when external air temperature is greater than skin temperature. In this case, the primary heat loss system is **evaporation** via **sweating**.

19. Where is temperature sensed?

The **hypothalamus** traditionally has been regarded as the primary thermosensitive site within the central nervous system. Thermoregulatory sites also may exist within the spinal cord, skeletal muscle, and splanchnic organs. Although the role of these accessory sites is still under investigation, it is clear that multiple sites sense changes in temperature dictated by their accessibility either to the heat produced by the body or to their proximity to the external surface. These thermosensitive sites include:

Rectum
Tympanic membrane
Esophagus
Right atrium

Temperatures at these sites may differ by a tenth of a degree depending on blood flow and regional heat production. The areas with the highest perfusion (hypothalamus) respond more quickly to changes in heat production than those with low blood flow (e.g., rectum).

20. Are there temperature receptors?

Thermoreceptors for warmth or heat are predominately unmyelinated C fibers but also include small myelinated A delta fibers. These fibers are tonically active.

21. Are there temperature receptors for cold?

Yes. Cold information is relayed indirectly by a decrease in the rate of neuronal discharge from the warm receptors and directly by cold receptors. Cutaneous cold receptors are innervated by small myelinated A delta fibers and C fibers. By the time core temperature has decreased a few tenths below normal, the warm fibers have been completely shut off. Additional cold information is, therefore, detected by specific cold receptors located in the skin, abdomen, spinal cord, and likely within other internal structures.

22. What type of receptors are warm and cold receptors?

Both warm and cold receptors are tonically active and belong to the type of sensors that encode information proportionally to the magnitude of the stimulus intensity and rate of change. That is, the receptors are capable of providing information to the thermoregulatory centers regarding not only the current temperature, but also the speed at which the temperature is changing. This warning or anticipatory information provides greater safety in maintaining core temperature. Neither the cold nor the warm receptors respond to mechanical stimuli. When stimulated, the receptors respond with an increase in firing rate.

23. How sensitive are these receptors?

The cutaneous receptors are capable of responding to small changes in temperature (0.005°C). The thermoreceptors appear to have a specific temperature range in which they are active. Collectively, the receptors provide an entire range of temperature sensing.

24. Why are cold and heat sometimes painful?

Information sensed by the cutaneous thermoreceptors is carried by the same A delta and C fibers that carry pain afferent information. This likely explains why extremes in temperature that result in high afferent activity are sensed as burning pain.

25. What are the primary thermal afferent pathways?

With the exclusion of facial and inguinal/scrotal areas, which have separate afferent pathways and processing nuclei, the majority of thermal A delta and C fiber afferents terminate in the superficial laminae of the dorsal horn. The ascending pathways pass up the anterolateral quadrant of the cord on the contralateral side of the appropriate receptive field. There is preliminary evidence that the afferent pathway is the spinothalamic tract. Temperature-responsive neurons in the nucleus raphe magnus and medial-dorsal raphe nuclei appear to receive information regarding warmth, whereas the pontine reticular formations react to cutaneous cooling. Information is not only relayed, but also processed by these nuclei as it is relayed to the midbrain raphe nuclei and reticular formation and finally diverges on the sensory thalamic nuclei and the hypothalamic thermoregulatory area.

26. Where are the temperature regulation centers?

Input from central and peripheral thermoreceptors converge in the temperature-regulating centers located in the **anterior hypothalamus** and **preoptic area**. These areas are responsible primarily for promoting heat loss, whereas separate and distinct heat-producing areas are located bilaterally in the **posterior hypothalamus**.

27. What is the hypothalamic thermostat?

The overall heat-controlling center of the hypothalamus. Signals from the posterior hypothalamus, the preoptic area, and the periphery converge to dictate the effector response and control core temperature.

28. How does the hypothalamic thermostat work?

When the hypothalamic thermostat detects that temperature is too hot or cold, either heat loss or heat production responses are initiated. The system response is analogous to a thermostat with effectors of both a furnace and air conditioner (see figure).

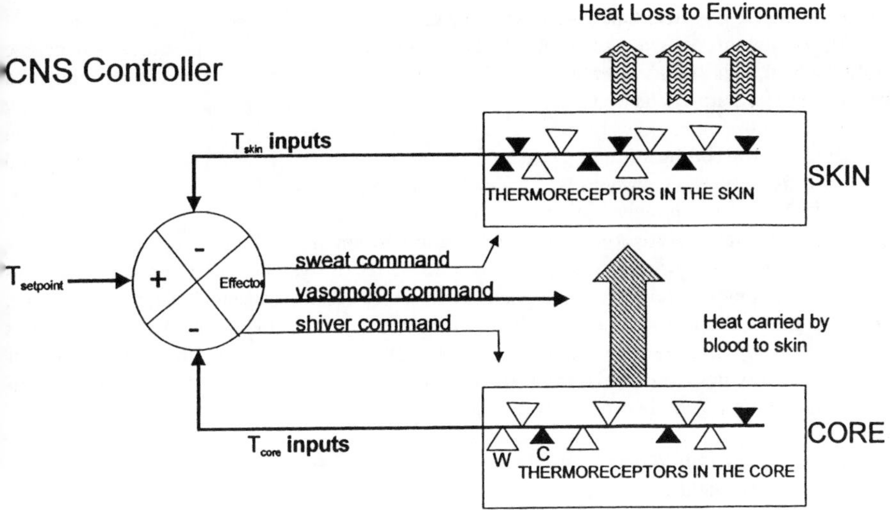

Thermoreceptors are located throughout the body, but the dominant input for temperature regulation is obtained from receptors located in the skin and core. Input from both cold (C) and warm (W) receptors is processed by the central nervous system (CNS) controller and compared with the temperature setpoint ($T_{setpoint}$) of the hypothalamus. The controller makes adjustments (effector limb) as necessary by either stimulation or inhibition of sweating, shivering, and vasomotor responses.

29. What three physiologic effectors are invoked in response to an increase in core temperature?

1. Massive vasodilation of the cutaneous circulation, a vasomotor response
2. Sweating
3. Inhibition of all heat production mechanisms

30. What is the role of the cutaneous circulation in temperature regulation?

The rate of blood flow through the cutaneous circulation can be increased to 30% of cardiac output. This high redistribution of blood flow results in up to an eightfold increase in heat conduction from the core to the skin surface when fully dilated.

31. How are changes in cutaneous circulation controlled?

Heat conduction is controlled via alteration in **arterial vascular resistance**. In response to an increased core temperature, the sympathetic nervous system output to the cutaneous circulation is inhibited, resulting in decreased vasoconstriction and increased blood flow.

32. Explain the mechanisms of sweating.

Stimulation of the anterior hypothalamic-preoptic area results in a robust increase in sweating via an increase in autonomic output. Sweating is initiated when the core temperature is increased above 98.6°F (37°C). Sweat glands are innervated by sympathetic cholinergic nerves. Sweat glands also can be stimulated by elevated concentrations of epinephrine and norepinephrine, which modulate the sweating responses to exercise.

33. How much can a person sweat?

The amount depends on the rate of sweat production and whether the person is heat acclimated. In general, a nonacclimated person can sweat up to 1 L/hr, whereas the acclimated individual can lose up to 3 L/hr. Some individuals can lose several pounds of water weight during a single bout of exercise in the heat.

34. How effective is sweating in temperature regulation?

The evaporation of sweat can remove 10 times more body heat than is produced under basal conditions. In addition, acclimated individuals lose less salt in their sweat, which contributes to better fluid and thermal homeostasis.

35. Describe the composition of sweat.

Sweat is formed by sweat glands, which release the primary secretion with a composition similar to plasma (without proteins). As the sweat travels up the sweat duct, significant proportions of the sodium and chloride are absorbed. The final composition of sweat under resting conditions is 5 mEq/L for both sodium and chloride. At these low rates of sweating, most of the water is also absorbed resulting in a relatively high concentration of other constituents, including lactic acid, urea, and potassium. During exercise or in response to strong sympathetic stimulations, sweat formation is greatly increased, and reabsorption is less effective. As a result, the concentration of sodium and chloride is increased up to 50–60 mEq/L in a nonacclimated person. Large amounts of water, sodium, and chloride can be lost through this important heat-loss system.

36. What are the physiologic adaptations to heat?

- Lower threshold for sweating, which prevents an early increase in core temperature
- Increased sweat rate, which provides a greater evaporative heat loss and lower core temperature
- Increase in plasma volume for better blood pressure control, a lower heart rate, maintenance of stroke volume, and maintenance of sweat rates

37. What three physiologic mechanisms preserve core temperature in response to cold?

1. Massive skin vasoconstriction mediated by stimulation of the posterior hypothalamus
2. Sympathetic-mediated piloerection, which traps air and effectively creates an air insulator
3. Increase in heat production

38. Name the heat production systems.

- Shivering is stimulated by increased activity of anterior motor neuronal activity, which can raise heat production fourfold to fivefold.
- Chemical- or sympathetic-mediated increase in cellular metabolism or heat production occurs via stimulation of brown fat.
- The anterior hypothalamus-preoptic area stimulates production of thyrotropin-releasing hormone, which stimulates thyroid-stimulating hormone release from the pituitary, resulting in an increase in thyroxine secretion. Thyroxine induces an increase in cellular metabolism.

39. What is brown fat?

Brown fat is thermogenic fat. It is typically located surrounding internal organs and the aorta. In animals, brown fat is capable of providing a 500-fold increase in heat production. In adult humans, brown fat stores are limited, and heat production increases only 10–15%. Infants have a greater amount of brown fat and effectively use chemical thermogenesis. In the neonate, this is a key factor in maintaining normal body temperature.

40. Define fever.

An increase in body core temperature of one to several degrees caused by an illness or toxin.

41. List the causes of fever.

Bacterial disease
Brain tumors
Environmental conditions

42. How do bacteria cause fever?

Bacteria liberate toxins, which cause white cells to release pyrogens and reset the hypothalamus.

43. How do pyrogens reset the hypothalamus?

Pyrogens act both directly and indirectly through endotoxins on the hypothalamic thermostat. Basically, phagocytized bacteria release interleukin-1, otherwise known as **leukocyte pyrogen**. On reaching the hypothalamus, interleukin-1 causes an increase in body temperature within 5–10 minutes, thus producing a fever. Interleukin-1 produces fever via the formation of prostaglandin E_2, which resets the hypothalamic thermostat. Body temperature remains elevated as long as the new higher set-point is maintained by the pyrogens.

44. Why does aspirin decrease a fever but not change normal body temperature?

Aspirin inhibits the cyclooxygenase enzymes and decreases the formation of prostaglandins from arachidonic acid. Because prostaglandins mediate fever, aspirin effectively decreases a febrile response. Conversely, prostaglandins are not involved in normal temperature regulation, so aspirin has no effect.

45. Should fevers be treated?

There is sufficient evidence to suggest that fever is a natural defense response to bacterial infection or toxins. In response to pyrogens, core temperature is increased to a new set-point. This elevated temperature is detrimental to bacteria. Once the bacteria are destroyed by the elevated temperature, pyrogen production and thus interleukin-1 and prostaglandin E_2 production are decreased, and normal body temperature is restored by vasodilation and sweating.

This chapter is dedicated to the memory of my mentor and friend, Dr. Melvin J. Fregly.

BIBLIOGRAPHY

1. Fregly MJ, Blatteis CM (eds): Handbook of Physiology. New York, Oxford University Press, 1996.
2. Guyton AC, Hall JE (eds): Textbook of Medical Physiology, 9th ed. Philadelphia, W.B. Saunders, 2000.

15. PHYSIOLOGY OF AGING

Paula E. Papanek, Ph.D., MPT

1. What is aging (senescence)?

Although subjective, accepted classifications include:

Old age: 65–75 years of age
Very old age: 75–85 years
Oldest old age: > 85 years

In physiology, aging is often defined as the accumulation of negative or deleterious alterations in the physiologic processes and their external manifestations or functional presentations that begin after conception and occur until death—or the process of growing old regardless of chronologic age. Another definition is the sum of all changes, including physiologic, psychological, and metabolic, that occur in an organism with the passage of time and increase the probability of death. It is a state of decreased ability to maintain homeostasis.

2. Why are the elderly the fastest growing segment of the population?

The elderly population is growing for several reasons. Life expectancy is increasing; the birth rate in the 1950 and 1960s (the Baby Boomers) was high; and the birth rate is decreasing because of a trend in the 1980s and 1990s toward smaller families. The over-65 age group is growing at a nearly exponential rate.

3. What is the average life span?

The life span of someone born in 1990 is 25 years longer than someone born in 1900. A woman who lives to age 65 years can expect to live, on average, 19 more years and a man an additional 15 years. Thus, once one gets past 65, the average life span is 84 years for women and 80 years for men. Major factors affecting longevity include genetics, gender, ethnicity, social class, physical environment, obesity, and lifestyle choices.

4. Why do gender differences exist in longevity?

Women over 65 outnumber men 3 to 2. After the age of 85, women outnumber men 5 to 2. These differences have been attributed to environmental and genetic causes. Environmental causes include less life stress, which contributes to cardiovascular disease, and lower rates of cigarette smoking (although women are quickly catching up). Genetic causes include the protective effects of estrogen, especially in the cardiovascular system, and protection against oxidative damage resulting in fewer mitochondrial DNA mutations and deletions.

5. Do all physiologic aging processes occur at the same rate?

There is significant heterogeneity in the aging process. There is a range or variability even within a given organ system or person. For example, the pulmonary system may age faster in one person, but functionally, this person may experience little or no change in another system. Further, aging changes are typically more prevalent in some systems as opposed to others. This explains why one 65-year-old individual may be relatively healthy while another is frail and failing. Chronologic age is simply age in number of years, whereas physiologic age is the age relative to functional capacity.

6. What is lipofuscin and what does lipofuscin have to do with aging?

Lipofuscin is a complex pigment that is thought to result from end-stage lipid peroxidation probably by the oxidation of fat with free radical reactants. The exact composition of lipofuscin depends on the tissue of origin and thus varies from cell to cell. It appears to accumulate in cells with the highest metabolic activity. Because lipofuscin accumulates in tissue with aging, it is hypothesized to interfere with cellular processes and function. For example, the accumulation of lipofuscin in the skin is responsible for the age spots typical in older adults. Lipofuscin accumulation also has been demonstrated in aging brains. Direct deleterious effects of lipofuscin have yet to be documented, and its role in the aging process is still hypothetical.

7. What are ceroid and amyloid?

Both of these pigments are either by-products of metabolism or have been shown to accumulate in aging and diseased tissue. Ceroid is a by-product of cell membrane peroxidation, and amyloid contains several protein products. Amyloid accumulates in the vascular system with age, and levels of amyloid are high in the brains of people with Alzheimer's disease.

8. What is apoptosis?

Apoptosis is a type of programmed cell death. It is used by both vertebrates and invertebrates to actively remove unwanted, unneeded, or unused cells. Apoptosis is thought to be controlled by local hormones and growth factors.

9. Is there a single test to determine functional age in a person or organ system?

Geriatric assessment requires a combination of many diagnostic tests including physiologic, psychological, physical competence, and ambulatory skills. These tests would be performed in addition to tests used to ascertain specific organ function such as a renal clearance test to determine renal function and a Berg balance test to determine static and dynamic balance.

10. List the diseases that are primarily limited to the elderly.

Osteoporosis
Osteoarthritis
Adenocarcinoma
Prostatic adenocarcinoma
Temporal arteritis
Polymyalgia rheumatica

11. What diseases are often associated with aging?

Type 2 diabetes mellitus (T2DM), Parkinson's disease, Alzheimer's disease, cancers, emphysema, and essential hypertension. Note, however, that hypertension is now being observed in younger adults with increasing frequency.

12. How does the central nervous system (CNS) change with aging?

There is a progressive loss of brain weight. Other changes include a decrease in size and number of brain cells in all locations, decreased metabolic activity, decreased blood flow, and decreased conduction velocity of peripheral nerves. It appears that the loss is greatest in terms of gray matter.

13. What nervous system impairments are a normal part of aging?

Normal aging, in the absence of disease, is not associated with major impairments of neurologic function. Changes in CNS function are attributed to disease and pathology. However, chronic and severe abnormalities do develop in 30% of adults over the age of 80. The major categories of CNS dysfunction include changes in cognition; changes in sensory systems; and changes in ability to execute actions. Delirium, dementia, and changes in judgment, comprehension, and memory are all examples of cognitive changes (major safety issues for the elderly).

14. List the changes that occur in the aging eye.

- **Presbyopia:** loss of accommodation power, especially near objects
- **Myopia:** nearsightedness
- **Hyperopia:** farsightedness
- **Cornea:** increased thickness, decreased curvature, reduced epithelial regeneration, decreased lens elasticity
- **Anterior chamber:** decreased volume and flow of aqueous humor

- **Iris:** decreased dilator muscle cell number and activity (decreased ability to dilate)
- **Retina:** loss of rods, some loss of cones, reduced cone pigment, decreased light sensitivity, reduced color vision
- **Visual field:** decrease in the size
- **Cataracts:** chemical changes in the lens composition producing opacity do occur more frequently in the elderly, but this is this is considered an eye disease

15. How prevalent are eye diseases in people aged 75–85 years?

Cataracts: 46%
Macular degeneration: 28%
Glaucoma: 7.2%
Blindness: 2.5%

16. Are there any aging-associated changes in the ear?

Presbycusis is the decreased ability to hear sounds, especially sounds with a high frequency. Bilateral presbycusis typically occurs in aging as a consequence of changes in the inner ear and central auditory pathway. Loss of hair cells and supporting cells of the basal coil of the cochlea results in a loss of the hearing sensitivity for high-frequency pure tones. Nerve loss in the central auditory pathway results in a decrease in hearing sensitivity in the low-frequency region.

17. List the somatosensory changes with aging.

- Decreased tactile sensitivity
- Decreased sensitivity to vibration (high-frequency stimulation)
- Decreased two-point discrimination sensitivity (touch acuity)
- Decreased stereognosis (ability to identify an object based solely on tactile manipulation)
- Decreased density of cutaneous mechanoreceptors mediating fine touch and vibration

18. Describe the type of changes in olfaction with aging.

Hyposmia (decline in olfactory ability) and anosmia (a complete loss of olfactory ability) occur regularly in the elderly. Changes that occur include a decreased sensitivity or increased threshold to odor plus a decreased ability to identify odors (good and bad). The mechanism for these changes is not well delineated. However, there is a decrease in the number of bipolar sensory neurons located in the olfactory mucosa and a loss of neurons in the higher nerve centers responsible for smell. It is likely that the change in odor sensitivity is a consequence of aging-related decreases in the CNS.

19. Does taste sensation change with aging?

If smell or olfaction has changed, taste and appetite are significantly compromised. However, relatively few changes specifically occur in taste sensation that are solely attributed to the aging process. There appears to be small changes in taste sensitivity and discrimination, particularly between intensities of the same food or chemical, and some changes in flavor identification particularly when in a mixture.

20. Do we need more or less sleep as we age?

Actually, we sleep less as we age. Infants sleep 16 hours/day. With puberty and through most adulthood, we sleep 8 hours/day. In the late adult stage, we sleep 6 hours/day. In the elderly, sleep in often more fragmented with a reduction in stage IV or slow-wave sleep and REM (rapid eye movement) sleep.

21. What changes occur in the skin with aging?

It is nearly impossible to separate out the effects of aging from the cumulative effects of repetitive trauma on the skin. Constant exposure to the environment, temperature extremes, trauma, and ultraviolet radiation have consequences on the skin. With repetitive trauma and aging, the skin heals and grows slower, is less elastic, and is more prone to injury. The skin is a less-effective barrier to infections, and within the skin, there is atrophy of the sweat glands, pressure and touch sensors, and hair follicles. The skin appears dry, atrophic, scaling, and hairless. In addition, the number of capillaries decreases. Collectively, the skin is less able to assist in thermoregulation as the sweating response and blood flow are diminished. The skin loses structural support, and the remaining capillaries are more easily damaged, which explains the easy bruising in this population.

22. What changes occur in the vestibular system?

The vestibular system provides spatial orientation information, along with proprioception and visual systems. Sensory receptors in the otoliths and semicircular canals degenerate with aging and contribute to the decrease in vestibular sensitivity. If proprioception, vision, and vestibular systems are all functioning, then vestibular changes alone are likely insignificant. However, there appears to be a decreased ability of the vestibular system to correct and maintain balance when it is the sole source of sensory information, for example, when vision is compromised. These changes contribute to the increased risk of falls.

23. List the major cardiovascular changes with aging.

Heart

- Decreased maximal heart rate
- Increased resting heart rate*
- Decreased cardiac reserve (max-rest)
- Decreased stroke volume*
- Increased myocardial work and oxygen consumption
- Decreased resting and exercise cardiac output
- Decrease in left ventricular compliance
- Decreased ejection fraction
- Slight left ventricular wall hypertrophy without change in chamber sizes
- Calcification of the valves
- Fat layer added to pericardium
- Myocardial/pericardial stiffness
- Coronary arteriosclerosis

Vascular

- Increased total peripheral resistance
- Atherosclerosis
- Decreased elasticity
- Decreased aortic compliance
- Rarefaction (decrease in capillary density)

Neural

- Blunted or decreased sensitivity of the baroreceptor reflex
- Decreased adrenergic responsiveness
- Selective decrease in inotropic, chronotropic, and vasodilating responses to β-adrenergic stimulation

Blood

- Decreased total body water
- Decreased blood volume
- Increase in blood cholesterol, low-density lipoprotein (LDL)

*An equal number of authors suggest that these do not change at rest but are altered in response to stressors.

24. List the changes in cardiovascular regulatory hormones that occur with aging.

NO CHANGE	DECREASE	INCREASE
Angiotensinogen	Plasma renin activity	Norepinephrine
ANF	Aldosterone	
AVP (or decrease)	Angiotensin II	
	AVP/ADH	

ANF = atrial natriuretic factor or peptide; AVP = arginine vasopressin.

25. Are the cardiovascular changes really attributable to aging or disease?

Atherosclerosis is a degenerative disease of the vascular wall that results in a thickening of the wall and a loss of distensibility. Consequences of atherosclerosis and arteriosclerosis include changes in total peripheral resistance (TPR) that may increase myocardial work, decrease stroke volume, and decrease cardiac output. Therefore, many of the changes seen are attributed to disease as opposed to the aging process per se.

26. Does the electrocardiogram (ECG) change with age?

There are no ECG changes linked directly to aging. However, ECG can detect disease processes that are more common in the elderly, including ischemic heart disease.

27. What cardiac changes are directly attributed to aging?

No significant cardiac cellular abnormalities are attributed solely to aging. A decrease in the number of pacemaker cells has been noted in the sinoatrial (SA) node, such that by age 75, there are only about 10% as many cells as in a younger adult and an increase in lipofuscin accumulation in the cells. Although the increase in lipofuscin alters the color of the heart, there are presently no known consequences of this change. In the absence of disease, the SA node functions normally.

28. Does cardiac output always decline with age?

In physically fit older persons, without underlying cardiovascular disease, there is no decline in cardiac output. This suggests that the decrease in cardiac output is not directly attributed to aging, but rather to cardiovascular disease. In healthy adults, age-induced cardiac hypertrophy, fat layer in the pericardium, decline in baroreceptor sensitivity, increased total cholesterol and LDL, and increase in blood pressure do not occur regularly. That is, many of the age associated changes in the cardiovascular system (see question 23) are related to inactivity, obesity, and other diseases rather than the aging process.

29. Describe the changes in blood cells with aging.

The erythrocytes show a variety of changes, including smaller size, changes in permeability (increase intracellular sodium and decreased potassium), decreased activity of several enzymes including glucose-6-phosphate dehydrogenase, increased fragility, less elasticity as evidenced by a decrease in reversible deformity, and increased agglutinability. However, the erythrocyte cycle or age, hematocrit, red blood cell (RBC) count, and hemoglobin remain unchanged in healthy adults through at least age 65. Bone marrow is reduced, which decreases the rate of repletion (slower) in response to hemorrhage or destruction, but ultimately RBC count is restored to normal. Erythrocyte sedimentation rate (ESR) increases with age. 2,3,-Diphosphoglycerate (2,3-DPG) levels are lower in adults ages 65–74 and decline even further by 85 years. Platelet concentration is unchanged, but there are some changes in immunity that may be related to changes in T- and B-cell mediated processes.

30. What are the age-related changes in the kidney?

The traditional thought was that renal function as assessed by creatinine clearance decreased by 1 mL/min per year after the age of 40. However, there is great heterogeneity in the change in renal function with aging. Aging per se does not seriously compromise renal function in the absence of disease, particularly in terms of hypertension. The major age-related anatomic and physiologic changes in the kidney include:

- Progressive but gradual decline in total kidney weight with the greatest decrease occurring in the renal cortex
- Progressive but gradual decrease in the total number of glomeruli
- Decreased urine concentrating ability
- Decreased urine diluting ability
- Decreased ability to respond adequately to either a water load or dehydration
- Alteration in control of antidiuretic hormone (ADH) or AVP secretion
- Progressive decline in effective renal plasma flow
- Progressive decline (controversial) in glomerular filtration rate (GFR)
- Decreased bladder capacity

31. Does water and electrolyte balance change because of aging kidneys?

In healthy, normal older adults, the kidney is capable of maintaining water and electrolyte balance. There is no change in either water and electrolyte distribution or a change in acid–base balance in basal conditions. However, the aging kidney does not respond as robustly to either dehydration or water stimuli. The changes in total body water that do occur in the elderly are more related to changes in body composition, not renal function.

32. Are there changes in the urinary tract with aging?

Incontinence is the involuntary loss of urine of sufficient amount or frequency to be a social or health problem. Incontinence is a major problem for the elderly, particularly for women, and conservative estimates suggested that over 30% of community-living elderly women are incontinent. The greater prevalence in women occurs because of changes in the lower urinary tract and pelvic floor musculature. Incontinence increases the risk of infections and chronic wounds in this population.

33. Is incontinence inevitable?

No. Incontinence is not a normal response to aging, and often it is treatable. Patients with incontinence need to be referred for appropriate treatment. However, several age-related changes may contribute to the increased incidence.

34. List the changes that contribute to an increase risk of incontinence with aging.

Females	***Males***
Estrogen deficiency	Prostate size
Weak pelvic floor and bladder outlet	Impaired urinary flow
Decreased urethral muscle tone	Urinary retention
Atrophic vaginitis	Detrusor instability

35. How is the prostate affected by aging?

After about 40 years of age, the prostate begins to change. These changes include atrophy of the smooth muscle with subsequent replacement of the muscle cells with collagen and proliferation of fibrous tissue within the prostate. After age 60, the cells of the prostate continue to atrophy in a more uniform pattern. However, despite the atrophy of these cells, other parts undergo hyperplasia. Unlike almost all other organs, which decrease in size, the prostate can double its size with aging.

36. What is benign prostatic hypertrophy (BPH)?

BPH is really more of a hyperplasia (increase in cell number) than hypertrophy. It is characterized by increases in the noncancerous cells in the inner portion of the gland. Because of its location, the increasing size of the prostate (could double) results in obstruction of the urethra and urine outflow from the bladder.

37. What about changes in fluid balance with aging?

Typically, aging is associated with a loss of skeletal muscle, which is replaced by fat. Lean tissue has a significantly higher water content than fat. Consequently, there is a loss of total body water relative to mass. This makes it more difficult to regulate body temperature, especially in response to a thermal challenge. Further, a decreased urine concentrating ability with aging increases the risk for dehydration.

38. List the reasons why the elderly are at greater risk for dehydration.

- Decreased urine concentrating ability
- Decreased antidiuretic hormone (ADH) or AVP response to increased osmolality
- Decreased total body water
- Decreased angiotensin-II–stimulated thirst and salt intake in response to dehydration

39. Why is there greater incidence of edema with aging?

A decrease in plasma protein concentration occurs with aging. This lowers osmotic pressure in the capillaries and predisposes the elderly to edema formation based on the Starling equilibrium. Further, any change in renal function secondary to disease (more common in the elderly) increases the risk of edema formation.

40. Which physiologic changes may explain the increase in drug toxicity in the elderly?

- Decline in renal function associated with disease
- Decreased total body water
- Increased body fat percentage altering drug distribution
- Altered hepatic clearance associated with disease

41. What is responsible for the change in pulmonary efficiency in aging?

Changes can be grouped into five broad categories: changes in (1) **mechanical properties,** (2) **flow,** (3) **volume,** (4) **gas exchange,** and (5) **lung defense**. For example, changes may occur both in the lung and within the chest wall that increase the work of breathing and decrease PaO_2, altering ventilation.

42. List the changes in the lung that are typical of aging.

- Enlarged alveolar ducts
- Thinning and separation of the alveolar membrane
- Thickening of the supporting membranes between alveoli and capillaries
- Increased mucous gland activity
- Increased alveolar compliance
- Decreased capillary numbers (rarefaction)
- Decreased ventilation/perfusion matching
- Decreased tissue extensibility (alveolar wall)
- Early airway closure
- Decreased lung elastic recoil

43. List the common mechanical changes in the respiratory system that typically occur with aging.

- Increased costovertebral stiffness
- Increased rigidity of the chest wall
- Decreased chest wall compliance
- Increased anterior–posterior diameter
- Atrophy of respiratory muscles
- Decreased strength of intercostal muscles

Functionally, these changes result in an increase in minute ventilation requiring an increase in the work of breathing, increased oxygen demand by the respiratory muscles, and greater respiratory muscle fatigue

44. Which lung volumes and flows change with aging?

REDUCED	INCREASED
Vital capacity	Residual volume
Total lung capacity	Physiologic dead space
Inspiratory reserve capacity	
Maximal ventilatory volume	
Maximal expiratory flow	
FEV_1	
All flow rates in general	

FEV_1 = forced expiratory volume in 1 second.

45. How does oxygen flux change with aging?

- Reduced diffusing capacity
- Lower resting arterial oxygen tension
- Increased alveolar-arterial oxygen gradient ($P_AO_2 - P_aO_2$) suggesting increased $\dot{V}/\dot{Q}$ mismatch
- Decreased alveolar surface area
- Decreased pulmonary blood volume
- Decreased 2,3-DPG (shift oxyhemoglobin curve to the left)

46. List the changes in the lung defense system.

- Decreased cilia number
- Decreased strength of remaining cilia
- Decreased effectiveness of alveolar macrophages
- Decreased effectiveness of mucus escalator
- Decreased cough reflex
- Decreased cough effectiveness due to changes in chest wall mechanics
- Decreased gag reflex, which increases risk of aspiration

47. When does the aging process begin in the respiratory system?

The respiratory system appears to be mature by age 20, and pulmonary function begins to decline by age 25.

48. Are the respiratory changes age-related or related to disease or lifestyle?

Both environmental and lifestyle factors have major effects on respiratory changes typical of aging. Lifestyle habits such as smoking and lack of physical exercise are most notable for accelerating these changes. It is nearly impossible to separate the direct effect of aging from lifestyle and disease including occupational and environmental inhalants. Environmental factors, living in an urban as opposed to rural area, industrial exposures, frequency of infections, and exposure to toxic free radicals accelerates the aging changes. A major environmental factor is exposure to secondary cigarette smoke.

49. Can the aging respiratory system meet minimal or basal needs?

In the absence of pathology, both the lungs and heart can meet the needs for delivery of oxygen at rest. However, the reserve capacities are diminished. In the presence of a challenge, or when combined with disease, the oxygen delivering capacity may be exceeded.

50. What age-related changes occur in skeletal muscle?

There is a loss of about 30% of strength from 50 to 70 years of age and an additional 30% after age 70. Additional changes include:

- Sarcopenia
- Loss of mitochondria
- Decreased tendon strength
- Decreased skeletal muscle elasticity
- Loss of heterogeneous fiber type pattern
- Rarefaction (loss of blood vessels)
- Decreased oxygen extraction
- Decreased respiratory enzyme activity
- Decreased force-production capability

51. What is sarcopenia and why does it occur?

Sarcopenia is the process of age-related loss of muscle mass. The etiology is probably multifactorial. Sarcopenia is associated with both a change in the size of the individual muscle fibers and a decrease in the total number of cells. Current hypotheses include:

- Decreased activity (sedentary lifestyle)
- An altered hormonal milieu (decreased testosterone, estradiol, and growth hormone levels)
- Reduced protein synthesis

- Poor nutrition, particularly low protein intake
- Decreases in neural activation patterns resulting in a decreased release of growth factors

52. What are the consequences of sarcopenia?

A loss of skeletal muscle cross-sectional area or loss of muscle mass is directly related to a loss of force-producing capability (a smaller muscle is weaker). Sarcopenia contributes to the weakness in the elderly population. In addition, lean tissue is more metabolically active that fat. The loss of lean tissue equals a decrease in basal metabolic rate, which results in an increase in body fat.

53. Are there changes in connective tissue with aging?

Collagen becomes stiffer and weaker as it increases in density with aging. Changes in blood flow result in a decreased ability to provide nutrients and remove waste products, which is essential for healthy collagen. Cross-linkage develops between elastin fibers, and water and elasticity are lost. Consequently, the connective tissue becomes more rigid and frays easier. Depending on the site of change, this can result in fragile tendons or the presence of increased cross-linkage, restrictions that can limit mobility.

54. What specific changes happen to cartilage?

Hyaline cartilage becomes dehydrated and stiffer and wears thin in areas of weight bearing, such as hips and knees. The production of chondroitin sulfate is decreased which decreases the osmotic attraction force and the ability to maintain hydration. The dehydration is associated with a decreased ability to absorb and distribute forces across a bone surface. Consequently, joint forces may become concentrated and represent an overload, resulting in tears or injury to the joint cartilage. These injuries (even microtraumas) stimulate an inflammatory response that may further accelerate joint pathology. In addition, there is a decrease in secretion of the naturally occurring lubricant by chondroblasts, resulting in a decreased efficiency of lubrication and acceleration of joint pathology.

55. Does maximal oxygen consumption decrease with aging?

Changes in oxygen extraction by the lungs and a decrease in cardiac output result in a decreased maximal oxygen consumption. It is estimated that, after the age of 50, maximal oxygen consumption declines about 0.45 mL/kg/min each year. Exercise training may help to maintain cardiac output, prevent the loss of pulmonary function, and thus help maintain maximal oxygen consumption.

56. What changes occur in body composition with aging?

The most dramatic and obvious change is an increase in fat and the loss of lean body mass with age. Average body fat for a male in his 20s is 18%, whereas it is 38% for a male in his 60s.

57. What is the one percent rule?

The one percent rule describes the loss of skeletal muscle mass after the mid 20s at about 1% per year and the loss of bone mineral density of about 1% per year after the peak in the late 20s. Skeletal muscle mass is replaced by fat, and bone density progressively decreases. This continues until menopause or andropause, at which time both processes are accelerated.

58. Can the muscle of elderly adults increase in size and function with exercise?

High-intensity resistance or strength training (an intensity greater than 60% of maximal lifting capacity) results in increases in both size and force-production capacity of skeletal muscle. The increases in size and force production in the inactive adults ages 60–72 are equal or better than gains measured for younger adults. This strongly suggests that the losses in skeletal muscle function are more a consequence of lifestyle than the pathology of aging. Although many health benefits are associated with aerobic or endurance exercise such as walking, jogging, biking, or swimming, these types of exercise involve a high number of repetitions with little resistance. They do not induce muscle hypertrophy. It is clear that the appropriate signal for skeletal muscle hypertrophy is high-intensity resistance training.

59. What is osteoporosis and why does it happen earlier in women?

Osteoporosis is the gradual and progressive deossification of bone resulting in decreased strength, increased risk of fractures, changes in stature and posture, and pain. The imbalance between resorption (osteoclast) and deposition (osteoblast) to favor resorption results in a decrease in bone mineral density and a concomitant increase in fracture risk. Because the gonadal steroids play an important role in calcium and bone homeostasis, they have important effects on bone strength. In women, menopause occurs at an earlier age than andropause. The absence of estrogen accelerates bone resorption and thus the osteoporosis. Bone loss of 1% per year begins at age 30 or so for women but not until age 50 in men. Women have a lower bone mineral density (BMD) to begin with, and they begin to lose it nearly two decades sooner. More than 25 million Americans have been diagnosed with osteoporosis. Women are more than four times more likely to be affected than men, which demonstrates the important role of estrogen.

60. Are osteoporosis and osteopenia the same?

They are two different levels of the same process. According to the World Health Organization, normal BMD is not more than 1 standard deviation below young adult mean. **Osteopenia** is defined as a BMD between 1 and 2.5 standard deviations below young adult mean, and **osteoporosis** is defined as a BMD greater than 2.5 standard deviations below young adult mean and the presence of fragility fractures.

61. Is osteoporosis a normal consequence of aging in women?

No. Osteoporosis is a disease and is not an inevitable consequence of aging.

62. What determines BMD?

BMD is the consequence of many factors including:

- **Nutrition**. Ensure appropriate vitamin D and calcium intake, limiting caffeine and other diuretic-inducing foods and foods high in sodium phosphate such as carbonated beverages.
- **Genetics**. The BMD of your parents and grandparents is important, as is ethnicity.
- **Smoking**. Another big negative of smoking is that it arrests bone formation and stimulates resorption and also decreases healing in bone.
- **Alcohol**. Excessive intake decreases BMD.
- **Hormones**. Estrogen and testosterone play important permissive roles in bone growth, and parathyroid hormone and calcitonin directly alter bone homeostasis.
- **Drugs**. Steroids, in particular glucocorticoids, accelerate bone loss as does hyperthyroidism.
- **Physical activity**. Physical activity stimulates osteoblastic activity, which increases BMD.

Each of these plays a role in determining the net effect or balance between osteoclast and osteoblast activity and ultimately determines whether more bone is being resorbed or deposited.

63. What role does estrogen play in BMD?

Estrogen plays an important role in determining and sustaining peak BMD. In the absence of estrogen, the pattern of bone resorption exceeds deposition. During menopause or the premature withdrawal of estrogen, bone resorption is dramatically accelerated such that bone density can decline at a rate of 6–8% during the first year. These patterns are nearly identical for men in terms of testosterone dependence. Unlike women, however, peak BMD is greater and the decrease in testosterone occurs later in life. Also, testosterone is often normal in elderly men, and frank hypogonadism is not inevitable.

64. Does a past history of low estrogen affect BMD later in life?

Yes. Studies now suggest that disrupted menses, either amenorrhea or oligomenorrhea, is associated with an increase risk of hip fractures in elderly women. There is clear evidence that normal estrogen levels are important for a lifetime of healthy bones.

65. Describe the impact of osteoporosis on the elderly?

Osteoporosis accounts for 87% of fractures and 65% of accidental deaths in the elderly. Hip fractures as a consequence of osteoporosis and falls accounts for over 300,000 hospitalizations per year and 40% of nursing home admissions. In addition, the incidence of falls increases with age. Osteoporosis results in > 175,000 femur fractures and > 500,000 vertebral fractures annually. The mortality rate from hip fractures is very high.

66. What is menopause?

The permanent loss of menstruation and of ovarian follicular activity. Median ages for menopause are 49–51 years of age. Typically, menopause is preceded by a 12-month time period known as **perimenopause** in which the menstrual cycle is irregular.

67. Does perimenopause last only 12 months?

Women wish it were so. There are case reports where perimenopausal symptoms began in patients as early as their mid 30s and lasted until menopause in their 50s.

68. List the symptoms of menopause.

AUTONOMIC NERVOUS SYSTEM IMBALANCE	PSYCHOGENIC	SYSTEMIC CONSEQUENCES
Hot flashes	Headaches	Vaginitis
Perspiration	Insomnia	Accelerated atherosclerosis/thrombosis
Palpitations	Mood changes	Skin atrophy
Angina pectoris	Irritability	Breast atrophy
Fatigue	Depression	Osteoporosis
	Nervousness	Degenerative arthropathy
	Apprehension	Hirsutism
	Anxiety	Obesity

69. How is each organ system affected by menopause?

ORGAN OR SYSTEM	EB	MAJOR CHANGES
Vulva		Decrease in pubic hair, atrophy of labia majora and vulva skin
Vagina		Atrophy, loss of elasticity, alkalization, increase in bacterial infections
	+	Vaginal dryness and possible painful intercourse
Cervix		Atrophy, decreased mucus production
Uterus		Atrophy
Oviducts	+	Shortened, decrease in diameter, becomes fibrotic
Ovary		Atrophy, becomes fibrotic, blood vessels sclerose
		Decreased primordial and graafian follicles
Skin		Loss of water and elasticity; thins; accumulates age spots; loss of sebaceous and sweat glands; increased sensitivity to temperature, humidity, and trauma
Bladder and urethra		Atrophy of urethra, increased cystitis, urinary atrophy, dysuria, and noninflammatory urethritis. Incontinence
Cardiovascular system		Increase in hemoglobin and total cholesterol, LDL. Higher incidence of cardiovascular disease
Skeletal system	+	Osteoporosis

EB + = ameliorated in part or totally with estrogen replacement therapy.

70. What reproductive changes occur in men with aging?

Reproductive function in men generally is not affected by aging. That is, men well into their 80s have reproduced, with sperm found in the ejaculate of about 50% of men in their 80–90s. However, there maybe a marked decrease in libido.

71. What cause the decreased libido in men?

Although this is clearly multifactorial, the decrease in free testosterone seems to be a major mechanism.

72. What changes in sexual function occur in men?

In men, aging is associated with a decrease in erotic responsiveness, speed and duration of erection, amount of preejaculate mucus secretion, nocturnal erections, and capacity for multiple climaxes. This is associated with a decrease in libido and an age-related decline in sexual function. This is really erectile not ejaculatory dysfunction. Impotence is not just a problem for aging men. One percent of men age 25 are impotent, more than 7% are by age 50, and 55% experience erectile dysfunction by age 75. Much of this has been changed by drugs such as sildenafil (Viagra) that improve blood flow in the penis.

73. Do men have a menopause?

Menopause is the absence of menstruation, which men do not have to lose, but there may be a male equivalent. Total testosterone levels do decline slightly in men, but not until much later, and they remain within the normal range. This has often been called **andropause**. However, free testosterone (biologically active) decreases with aging primarily due to a change in the binding characteristics of sex hormone–binding globulin (SHBG). This results in andropause.

74. Which hormones decrease with aging?

Estrogen, free testosterone, adrenal production of dehydroepiandrosterone (DHEA), and DHEA-sulfate, growth hormone activity, and insulin-like growth factor (IGF) axis.

75. List two important clinical changes in the endocrine system that occurs more frequently with aging.

1. Impaired glucose tolerance and undiagnosed diabetes mellitus
2. Age-related hypothyroidism (decline in thyroid-stimulating hormone [TSH] and thyroxine [T_4])

76. Why is there an increase in glucose intolerance with aging?

Obesity, increases in abdominal fat mass, insulin resistance, poor diet, physical inactivity, decreased lean body mass, and a relative decrease in insulin secretion all contribute to changes in glucose metabolism. Proper exercise and diet in combination with a weight loss program or the maintenance of normal body weight and lean body weight are the best prevention.

77. Are the gastrointestinal changes that are common in the elderly pathologic or related to aging?

Proper nutrition and health start at the mouth. The loss of dentition and decreases in salivation compromise chewing and swallowing. Collectively, these may alter food choices and place a person at risk of malnutrition. However, no known changes in bowel function are solely attributable to aging. Rather, aging is associated with an increased risk of ulcers, dysphagia, constipation, cholelithiasis, and cancers of the stomach, pancreas, and large intestine.

78. What is physical frailty?

Frailty is defined as a state of reduced physiologic reserves. Frailty is associated with increased susceptibility to disability. A variety of clinical conditions are correlated with frailty, including fractures, falls, loss of independence, generalized weakness, impaired mobility, and decreased endurance. Loss of muscle strength or weakness is a major determinant of frailty, and it may be caused either by the actual aging of the muscle or by disuse atrophy. Among nondisabled, community-dwelling and independent adults, the single entity with the greatest predictability of frailty is lower-extremity function. That is, reduced leg strength or cross-sectional area is the greatest predictor of frailty.

79. Compare and contrast aging with the long-term benefits of an exercise training program.

ORGAN OR SYSTEM	AGING EFFECT	BENEFIT OF EXERCISE
Cardiovascular		
Maximal oxygen consumption	Decreased	Increased
Cardiac output	Decreased	Increased
Blood pressure	Increased	Decreased
Total peripheral resistance	Increased	Decreased
Total cholesterol	Increased	?
Triglycerides	Increased	Decreased
LDL	Increased	?
HDL	Decreased	Increased
Immune system	Decreased	Increased
Muscles		
Strength	Decreased	Increased
Endurance	Decreased	Increased
Flexibility	Decreased	Increased
Body composition		
Bone	Decreased	Increased
Lean body mass	Decreased	Increased
Fat mass	Increased	Decreased
Metabolic systems		
Basal metabolic rate	Decreased	Increased
Temperature regulation (heat loss)	Decreased	Increased
Cognitive function		
Anxiety	Increased	Decreased
Depression	Increased	Decreased
Cognitive function	Decreased	Increased

LDL = low-density lipoprotein; HDL = high-density lipoprotein.

BIBLIOGRAPHY

1. Hampton JK, Craven RF, Heitkemper MM: The Biology of Human Aging, 2nd ed. DuBuque, IA, WCB Publishers, 1997.
2. Lamberts SW, Van Den Beld AW, Vander Lely AJ: The endocrinology of aging. Science 278(5337): 419–424, 1997.
3. Lewis CB, Bottomley JM: Geriatric Physical Therapy: A Clinical Approach. Norwalk, CT, Appleton & Lange, 1994.
4. National Center for Chronic Disease Prevention and Health Promotion: Chronic Disease Notes and Reports. Vol. 12, No. 3. Bethesda, MD, National Center for Chronic Disease Prevention and Health Promotion, 1999.
5. Shephard RJ: Aging and exercise. In Fahey TD (ed): Encyclopedia of Sports Medicine and Science. Internet Society for Sport Science: http://sportsci.org. Accessed March 7, 1998.
6. Timiras PS (ed): Physiological Basis of Aging and Geriatrics, 2nd ed. Boca Raton, FL, CRC Press, 1994.

FINAL EXAM: CELLS, NERVES, AND MUSCLES

Choose the single best answer to each of the following questions or incomplete statements. Answer key at end.

1. **Which of the following substances are components of the plasma membrane?**
   a. phospholipids
   b. receptor proteins
   c. cholesterol
   d. carbohydrates
   e. all of the above

2. **Which of these statements is true regarding the cellular fluid compartments?**
   a. The concentration of intracellular potassium is higher than the concentration of extracellular potassium.
   b. The concentration of intracellular sodium is higher than the concentration of extracellular sodium.
   c. The osmolarity of the intracellular fluid is higher than the osmolarity of the extracellular fluid.
   d. The concentration of intracellular glucose is higher than the concentration of extracellular glucose.
   e. There are no proteins in the intracellular fluid compartment.

3. **Which of these substances can readily diffuse across the cell membrane?**
   a. glucose
   b. amino acids
   c. carbon dioxide
   d. sodium ions
   e. hydrogen ions

4. **Substances with high diffusion coefficients:**
   a. are more soluble in water than in lipid
   b. require specialized transport proteins to cross the cell membrane
   c. include large polar molecules
   d. usually cross the cell membrane by simple diffusion
   e. include sodium and potassium ions

5. **The rate of simple diffusion of an uncharged solute across the cell membrane is *inversely* proportional to:**
   a. the membrane area
   b. the concentration gradient of the solute across the membrane
   c. the diffusion coefficient of the solute
   d. the thickness of the cell membrane
   e. the number of receptor proteins in the cell membrane

6. **Which of the following events occurs during osmosis?**
   a. Water molecules are pumped across the cell membrane by active transport.
   b. Water molecules diffuse across the cell membrane from a region of low solute concentration to a region of high solute concentration.
   c. Water molecules move across the cell membrane by facilitated diffusion.

d. The fluid volume on both sides of the membrane remains the same.
e. The fluid osmolarity on both sides of the membrane is unchanged.

7. **Which of the following processes directly requires metabolic energy (ATP)?**
   a. facilitated diffusion
   b. simple diffusion of uncharged solutes
   c. movement of ions through membrane ion channels
   d. primary active transport
   e. secondary active transport

8. **Which of these events is rate limiting and saturable?**
   a. simple diffusion of uncharged solutes
   b. movement of ions through membrane ion channels
   c. the movement of oxygen molecules across cell membranes
   d. facilitated diffusion
   e. osmosis

9. **Which of these statements is true regarding the movement of glucose across the cell membrane?**
   a. Glucose is a large polar molecule that requires a specialized transport protein to cross the cell membrane.
   b. The movement of glucose across the cell membrane directly requires ATP.
   c. The movement of glucose across the cell membrane is directly proportional to its concentration gradient across the membrane.
   d. Glucose can cross the cell membrane by passive diffusion or active transport.
   e. Glucose is transported from the inside to the outside of the cell.

10. **The Na^+ K^+ pump:**
   a. participates in a countertransport process
   b. directly requires ATP
   c. exchanges three intracellular Na^+ ions for two extracellular K^+ ions
   d. is an electrogenic exchange mechanism that generates a net negative intracellular charge
   e. does all of the above

11. **Which of the following does *not* describe the process of secondary active transport?**
   a. directly requires ATP
   b. derives energy secondarily from the sodium concentration difference across the cell membrane
   c. participates in the absorption of sugars and amino acids in the gastrointestinal tract
   d. may represent either cotransport or countertransport processes
   e. is a rate-limiting, saturable process

12. **Pharmacologic block of the Na^+ K^+ pump in cardiac muscle cells by digitalis glycosides results in:**
   a. a net increase in the intracellular sodium concentration
   b. a reduced electrochemical gradient for Na^+ influx across the cell membrane
   c. a reduced activity of the sodium-calcium exchanger
   d. an increased force of contraction in the heart secondary to an enhanced intracellular Ca^{2+} concentration
   e. all of the above

13. **What is the main difference between voltage-gated and ligand-gated ion channels?**
   a. Voltage-gated ion channels are located in cardiac cell membranes, whereas ligand-gated ion channels are located in neuronal cell membranes.

b. Only voltage-gated ion channels can be studied by patch-clamp techniques.
c. Voltage-gated ion channels are activated by changes in membrane potential, whereas ligand-gated ion channels are activated by the binding of a chemical messenger.
d. Only ligand-gated ion channels are found in the resting conformational state.
e. Only ligand-gated ion channels contain an α-subunit protein.

14. Which of the following statements is true regarding the resting membrane potential of a cell?
a. The resting membrane potential value is closer to the K^+ equilibrium potential than to the Na^+ equilibrium potential, because the cell membrane is preferentially permeable to K^+ ions.
b. The resting membrane potential shows a negative value indicating an excess of negative charges at the inside of the cell membrane.
c. The Nernst equation can be used to calculate the equilibrium potential for a single ion species.
d. The Goldman constant-field equation predicts the resting membrane potential value as a function of ion concentrations and membrane permeabilities.
e. All of the above statements are true.

15. Which of the following statements is true of cell excitability in cardiac ventricular cells?
a. An increase in the K^+ permeability of the cell membrane results in depolarization.
b. The K^+ channels activate at more negative membrane potentials than the Na^+ channels.
c. The membrane potential becomes more positive during repolarization.
d. The plateau phase of the action potential is caused by the influx of Ca^{2+} ions through voltage-gated Ca^{2+} channels.
e. The activation of the Na^+, K^+ pump is the main event mediating repolarization.

For questions 16–24, select the correct answer from the four choices below. Each answer can be used more than once.
a. calcium channel
b. sodium channel
c. potassium channel
d. ligand-gated channel

16. Ion flux through this channel may increase several thousand-fold during the neuronal and cardiac action potentials.

17. Ion flux through this channel mediates the repolarization phase of the neuronal action potential.

18. Ion flux through this channel primarily determines the level of resting membrane potential.

19. This ion channel is highly expressed in the cell membranes of neuronal and cardiac cells but not in most smooth muscle cells.

20. This ion channel is *not* directly activated by depolarization.

21. The sustained inactivation of this channel following the action potential is associated with the refractory period.

22. Ion flux through this channel provides the activator ion for neurotransmitter secretion.

23. Drugs that block this channel would be expected to prevent the upstroke of the cardiac and neuronal action potentials.

24. Ion flux through this channel is most closely associated with the upstroke of action potentials and contraction in smooth muscle cells.

Choose the single best answer to each of the following questions or incomplete statements.

25. Which of the following statements is true regarding the propagation of an action potential along a nerve axon?

a. Saltatory conduction is associated with a slowing of action potential propagation.
b. The original action potential propagates for the length of the axon.
c. Multiple sclerosis is associated with increased conduction velocity.
d. Large myelinated nerve fibers conduct faster than small unmyelinated nerve fibers.
e. The propagation of action potentials requires a direct source of ATP.

26. The concentration of neurotransmitter in the synaptic cleft is determined by:

a. the rate of active uptake of the transmitter by the surrounding neurons
b. the amount of transmitter released by the presynaptic nerve terminal
c. the rate of enzymatic breakdown of the transmitter in the synaptic cleft
d. the diffusion rate of the transmitter from the presynaptic nerve terminal to the synaptic cleft
e. all of the above statements

27. Which of the following statements regarding the excitability of postsynaptic neurons is true?

a. Spatial summation of inhibitory postsynaptic potentials would tend to depolarize postsynaptic neurons.
b. Temporal summation of inhibitory postsynaptic potentials would tend to depolarize postsynaptic neurons.
c. A single excitatory postsynaptic potential is generally associated with a prolonged refractory period of the postsynaptic neuron.
d. Spatial and temporal summation may concurrently regulate the level of resting membrane potential of the postsynaptic neuron.
e. A single excitatory postsynaptic potential is generally associated with the firing of an action potential at the postsynaptic neuron.

28. Under normal physiologic conditions, the acetylcholine that participates in skeletal neuromuscular transmission:

a. is stored in the muscle fiber end plate
b. undergoes reuptake by the muscle fiber end plate following neurotransmitter combination with the acetylcholine receptor
c. is first hydrolyzed to acetate and choline, which then undergo reuptake by the muscle fiber end plate
d. opens a channel in the end plate that is permeable to both Na^+ and K^+
e. generates a small end plate potential that can be summated to produce an action potential in the muscle fiber, depending on the frequency of prejunctional motoneuron activity

29. During the cross-bridge cycle for activation and relaxation of contractile force in skeletal muscle:

a. ATP is used to cause the myosin cross-bridge to release from the actin molecule, leading to muscle relaxation

b. Ca^{2+} combines with actin to expose an actin binding site for combination with myosin
c. the actin filament shortens to reduce the length of the sarcomere
d. the myosin filament shortens to reduce the length of the sarcomere
e. Ca^{2+} combines with calmodulin to activate myosin light chain kinase

30. Which of the following events does *not* occur during the cross-bridge cycle for activation and relaxation of contractile force in smooth muscle?
a. The Ca^{2+}-calmodulin complex activates myosin light chain kinase.
b. ATP is used to phosphorylate the myosin light chain and thus increase its affinity for actin.
c. The phosphorylated myosin spontaneously combines with actin.
d. ATP is used to provide chemical bond energy to flex the myosin head and generate contractile force.
e. The thick and thin filaments shorten, causing muscle contraction.

31. Calcium:
a. initiates contraction of striated muscle by binding to regulatory proteins on the thick filament
b. initiates contraction of smooth muscle by direct binding to the thin filament
c. binds to calmodulin to initiate contraction of striated muscle
d. binds to calmodulin to initiate contraction of smooth muscle
e. does none of the above

32. Myosin light chain kinase:
a. is essential for initiating contraction of striated muscle in response to an increase in cytoplasmic Ca^{2+}
b. initiates cross-bridge cycling in smooth muscle by attaching a phosphate to the light chains on the myosin molecule
c. terminates contraction of smooth muscle by removing a phosphate group from the light chains on the myosin molecule
d. is an important regulatory protein in cardiac muscle
e. is none of the above

33. Which of the following statements is true concerning ATP in skeletal muscle contraction?
a. Less ATP is consumed for each cross-bridge cycle during the contraction of a fast twitch skeletal muscle than during cardiac muscle contraction.
b. ATP is necessary for Ca^{2+} release from the sarcoplasmic reticulum during excitation-contraction coupling.
c. ATP is necessary for detachment of cross-bridges during muscle contraction.
d. Increased cycling of cross-bridges reduces ATP consumption.
e. None of the above is true.

34. Functions of myosin ATPase include:
a. pumping Ca^{2+} back into the sarcoplasmic reticulum
b. cross-bridge cycling in skeletal and cardiac muscle
c. decreasing the affinity of the myosin cross-bridge for the active site on the thin filament
d. maintaining the latch state in skeletal muscle
e. none of the above

35. Troponin:
a. blocks the access of the myosin cross-bridge to the active site on the thin filament in skeletal muscle
b. is an essential regulatory protein for excitation-contraction coupling in skeletal and cardiac muscle but not in smooth muscle

c. pumps Ca^{2+} ions back into the sarcoplasmic reticulum in skeletal and cardiac muscle
d. opens the sarcoplasmic reticulum Ca^{2+} channel in skeletal and cardiac muscle
e. does none of the above

36. Which of the following mechanisms participates in the release of Ca^{2+} from the skeletal muscle sarcoplasmic reticulum following generation of a muscle fiber action potential?
a. depolarization of the T-tubule membrane
b. activation of a voltage-sensitive receptor in the T-tubule
c. opening of a ryanodine-sensitive Ca^{2+} channel in the sarcoplasmic reticular membrane
d. release of Ca^{2+} from a sarcoplasmic reticular store in which the ion is bound to calsequestrin
e. all of the above

37. Excitation-contraction coupling in skeletal muscle:
a. is mediated primarily by the influx of Ca^{2+} ions from the extracellular fluid
b. occurs without a change in transmembrane potential
c. is mediated via the sodium calcium exchange mechanism
d. is mediated via an abrupt decrease in the activity of the Ca^{2+} ATPase, which pumps Ca^{2+} ions into the sarcoplasmic reticulum
e. none of the above

38. The transverse tubule system of striated muscle:
a. stores Ca^{2+} for release during excitation-contraction coupling
b. conducts action potentials to the interior of the cell
c. contains calsequestrin to bind Ca^{2+} ions
d. pumps Ca^{2+} ions from the extracellular fluid into the terminal cisterna of the sarcoplasmic reticulum
e. all of the above

39. The most important function of membrane depolarization during excitation-contraction coupling in skeletal muscle is:
a. maintaining metabolic heat production by triggering hydrolysis of ATP
b. triggering the influx of Ca^{2+} ions from the extracellular fluid into the cytoplasm
c. depolarizing the sarcoplasmic reticulum
d. triggering Ca^{2+} release from the sarcoplasmic reticulum
e. none of the above

40. Which of the following statements does *not* describe an isotonic contraction of a skeletal muscle?
a. The muscle does external work if it is lifting a load.
b. The muscle generates a constant contractile force.
c. The shortening velocity is inversely proportional to the load being lifted.
d. The contraction becomes isometric when the maximal contractile force capable of being generated equals the load attached to the muscle.
e. The overall external length, but not the internal sarcomere length, is reduced.

41. Temporal summation in skeletal muscle refers to:
a. the additional contractile force that occurs during a twitch contraction as stimulus voltage is increased
b. the additional contractile force that occurs as stimulus frequency is increased at a constant voltage

c. the multiple action potentials measured with a needle electrode in skeletal muscle that is subjected to repeated stimulation via the motor nerve
d. the decrease in contractile force occurring in a skeletal muscle during prolonged tetanic stimulation
e. none of the above

42. In the length-force relationship for skeletal muscle:
a. maximum passive force is observed at the shortest muscle length
b. maximum active force is observed at the shortest muscle length
c. maximum active force is observed at the longest muscle length
d. passive force and total force can be equal at long muscle lengths
e. none of the above

43. The velocity of contraction of skeletal muscle:
a. increases as the load on the muscle increases
b. is slower than that of smooth muscle
c. is identical for every skeletal muscle
d. is a constant for a given muscle at zero load
e. none of the above

44. Under physiologic conditions, all of the following mechanisms participate in the regulation of skeletal muscle contractile force *except:*
a. the frequency of action potential firing in motoneurons innervating the muscle
b. the recruitment of active motoneurons innervating the muscle
c. the length of the individual muscle fibers in the muscle
d. the number of individual muscle fibers that are activated in the muscle
e. the amount of neurotransmitter released at the neuromuscular junction during each action potential

45. If a skeletal muscle is shortened from its rest length prior to an isotonic contraction:
a. the maximum velocity of contraction increases
b. the binding of Ca^{2+} to troponin decreases
c. the active force generated as the muscle shortens during an isotonic contraction decreases
d. the maximum force that can be generated by the muscle increases
e. none of the above

46. The mechanical properties of skeletal and cardiac muscle are similar in each of the following *except:*
a. the maximal force of contraction increases in both types of muscle as the muscle is stretched toward its optimal resting length
b. the maximum velocity of contraction (V_{max}) is identical in skeletal and cardiac muscle
c. the velocity of contraction increases in both types of muscle as the weight being lifted during an isotonic contraction of the muscle is reduced
d. the velocity of an isotonic contraction of the muscle at a given load is greater as the muscle is stretched toward its optimal length
e. contraction velocities are zero during an isometric contraction of either type of muscle

47. Which of the following statements regarding pacemaker activity in the heart is not true?
a. Pacemaker potentials are spontaneous depolarizations that occur as a result of changes in ionic conductance in specialized cells in the sinoatrial (SA) node.
b. A slowly developing outward K^+ current is the primary cause of the diastolic depolarization.

c. The heart rate can be determined by any or all of the following variables: slope of the diastolic depolarization, value of the threshold potential, and value of resting membrane potential.
d. The atrioventricular (A-V) node and the Purkinje fibers can also exhibit pacemaker activity.
e. Inward Ca^{2+} current contributes to the depolarization of the cell during the pacemaker potential.

48. Differences between fast-response and slow-response action potentials in the heart include:
a. the absence of a rapid depolarization (phase 0) in the slow-response action potential
b. diastolic depolarization during the fast-response action potential
c. a rapid repolarization phase in the fast-response action potential but not in the slow-response action potential
d. a longer plateau phase (phase 2) in the slow-response action potential compared with the fast-response action potential
e. all of the above

49. Calcium initiates contraction of ventricular muscle by binding to:
a. a calcium-activated ATPase
b. actin
c. myosin
d. tropomyosin
e. troponin

50. Differences between smooth and striated muscle include:
a. the lack of a sarcoplasmic reticulum in smooth muscle
b. a similar shortening velocity but a lower V_{max} in striated muscle
c. a characteristic length-tension relationship in striated muscle but not in smooth muscle
d. a lack of tropomyosin in smooth muscle but not in skeletal muscle
e. none of the above

51. Both cardiac and skeletal muscle:
a. have a thin-to-thick filament ratio of 2:1
b. have T-tubules and a sarcoplasmic reticulum
c. require troponin to activate contraction in response to Ca^{2+}
d. have tropomyosin on the thin filament
e. all of the above

52. Which of the following statements is true regarding contractile filaments in smooth muscle?
a. Contractile filaments in smooth muscle are arranged in sarcomeres.
b. The thin-to-thick filament ratio is lower in smooth muscle than in skeletal muscle.
c. Smooth muscle thin filaments are attached to Z disks that are similar to those in skeletal muscle.
d. Smooth muscle contractile proteins generate active force by cross-bridge cycling and the sliding filament mechanism.
e. Thick filaments are attached to the cytoskeleton.

53. Excitation of smooth muscle can occur:
a. by spontaneous alterations of transmembrane potential accompanied by bursts of action potentials
b. with little or no change in transmembrane potential
c. by graded depolarization without action potentials
d. by current spread from adjacent cells
e. by all of the above

For questions 70–71, select the correct answer from the five choices below.

a. tropomyosin
b. vimentin
c. calmodulin
d. troponin
e. desmin

70. Ca^{2+} binding regulatory protein in smooth muscle.

71. Ca^{2+} binding regulatory protein in skeletal muscle.

For questions 72–79, select the best answer from the three choices below. Each answer can be used more than once.

a. skeletal muscle only
b. smooth muscle only
c. skeletal and smooth muscle

72. Dense bodies.

73. Troponin.

74. Caveolae.

75. Myosin light chain kinase.

76. Myosin ATPase.

77. Syncytial gap junction.

78. T-tubules.

79. Latch state.

ANSWER KEY

1. e
2. a
3. c
4. d
5. d
6. b
7. d
8. d
9. a
10. e
11. a
12. e
13. c
14. e
15. d
16. b
17. c
18. c
19. b
20. d
21. b
22. a
23. b
24. a
25. d
26. e
27. d
28. d
29. a
30. e
31. d
32. b
33. c
34. b
35. b
36. e
37. e
38. b
39. d
40. e
41. b
42. d
43. d
44. e
45. e
46. b
47. b
48. a
49. e
50. e
51. e
52. d
53. e
54. b
55. c
56. d
57. e
58. e
59. e
60. c
61. a
62. e
63. c
64. b
65. c
66. e
67. e
68. k
69. i
70. c
71. d
72. b
73. a
74. b
75. b
76. c
77. b
78. a
79. b

FINAL EXAM: CELL SIGNALING

Choose the single best answer to each of the following questions or incomplete statements. Answer key at end.

1. **Activation of G protein–coupled receptors that signal through $G\alpha_s$ result in:**
   a. increased adenylyl cyclase activation and opening of calcium channels
   b. decreased opening of calcium channels
   c. increased PLC activation and increased activation of cGMP phosphodiesterases
   d. decreased adenylyl cyclase activation and closing of potassium channels
   e. decreased PLC activation and decreased activation of cGMP phosphodiesterases

2. **Pertussis toxin alters G-protein signaling by:**
   a. increasing G_i protein affinity for GTP
   b. activating G_i
   c. increasing interaction of ADP-ribosylated G_i with its receptor
   d. decreasing the affinity of G_i for GTP
   e. none of the above

3. **Cholera toxin alters G protein signaling by:**
   a. preventing GTP hydrolysis
   b. blocking the transfer of ADP-ribosylation moieties from NAD^+ to the α subunit of G_s
   c. blocking ligand binding to the extracellular portion of the receptor
   d. blocking all G proteins
   e. lowering cAMP levels

4. **In vascular smooth muscle cells, vasopressin signals via the V_1 receptor leading to which sequence of events?**
   a. activation of adenylyl cyclase resulting in increased cAMP formation and PKA activation
   b. activation of PLC with subsequent increases in DAG and IP_3 levels
   c. G protein–coupled activation (opening) of potassium channels
   d. activation of guanylyl cyclase resulting in increased cGMP formation and PKG activation
   e. closure of membrane-bound calcium channels

5. **Calmodulin is:**
   a. a major target of cytosolic free calcium
   b. a protein containing four calcium ion binding sites
   c. not an enzyme
   d. an activator of CAM kinases, including myosin light chain kinase
   e. all of the above

6. **How do prostaglandins signal?**
   a. stimulation of adenylyl cyclase activity in platelets
   b. stimulation of adenylyl cyclase activity in smooth muscle
   c. inhibition of adenylyl cyclase in adipocytes
   d. inhibition of adenylyl cyclase in epithelial tissues
   e. all of the above

7. **Which statement best characterizes the purinergic receptors?**
   a. The P_1 subgroup is composed of receptors for ATP.
   b. The P_1 subgroup is made up of adenosine receptors.
   c. The P_2 subgroup comprises receptors for adenosine.
   d. Both P_1 and P_2 subgroups are adenosine-binding sites.
   e. None of the above is true.

8. **Which statement best characterizes receptor tyrosine kinases (RTKs)?**
   a. All RTKs, including the insulin receptor, are dimers.
   b. Dephosphorylation of the receptor facilitates initiation of the signaling cascade.
   c. SH2 domains on intracellular proteins bind to the phosphotyrosine residues on the activated RTK.
   d. Adaptor proteins (e.g., Rab2) provide important enzymatic activity in the cascade of RTK signaling.
   e. RTKs are inactivated by further phosphorylation.

9. **RTKs activate the GTP-binding protein Ras. Which statement best describes Ras?**
   a. Ras is a heterotrimeric G protein.
   b. Ras is in its active state when GDP is bound.
   c. Ras activates the mitogen-activated protein kinase cascade.
   d. Ras binds potassium channels, sterically hindering their opening.
   e. None of the above.

10. **Cancer cells have "acquired" the capacity to escape controlled growth by:**
    a. undergoing mutations in genes involved in signaling pathways
    b. undergoing mutations in signaling receptors
    c. transforming into cells with constitutively active signaling pathways
    d. experiencing cell division even in the absence of growth factors
    e. all of the above

11. **Natriuretic peptides:**
    a. are vasoconstrictor peptides that signal via adenylyl cyclase
    b. have receptors that are dimeric proteins
    c. bind receptors that are themselves ion channels
    d. signal via G-protein coupling to PLC
    e. bind receptors that span the lipid bilayer and possess both a kinase and a guanylyl cyclase domain in their cytoplasmic tail

12. **Which of these regulatory molecules are derived from arachidonic acid?**
    a. thromboxanes
    b. leukotrienes
    c. prostacyclins
    d. prostaglandins
    e. all of the above

13. **Which statement best describes the cyclooxygenases (COXs)?**
    a. COX-1 and COX-2 are constitutively expressed enzymes.
    b. COX-1 expression is rapidly increased by endotoxin and is an early response to inflammation.
    c. Aspirin acetylates and inhibits COX-1 and COX-2, blocking the production of prostaglandins and thromboxanes.
    d. Nonsteroidal anti-inflammatory drugs do not affect COX activity.
    e. None of the above is true.

14. Which statement best characterizes the comparison of TGFβ and RTK receptors?
a. Both are serine-threonine kinases.
b. Both are constitutively active.
c. TGFβ receptors exist as monomers, whereas RTKs exist as dimers.
d. Only the RTK signals via transcriptional activation.
e. Both span the plasma membrane only once.

15. Cytokines such as IL-2 and IL-3 signal via the class 1 cytokine receptors by:
a. activation of Janus kinases
b. activation of interferon-stimulatable response elements (ISREs)
c. activation of adenylyl cyclase
d. activation of tyrosine kinases
e. activation of serine-threonine kinases

16. Which of the following two words best complete the following description of lipopolysaccharide (endotoxin) signaling? LPS binds to the ________ receptor, leading to recruitment and activation of a cytoplasmic adapter protein (MyD88) and eventually the release of NFκB from IκB due to ________ of IκB.
a. toll / dephosphorylation
b. toll / phosphorylation
c. interferon / acetylation
d. interferon / deacetylation
e. toll / acetylation

17. GABA and glycine are inhibitory neurotransmitters that bind to ligand-gated ion channels. These channels conduct primarily which of the following?
a. sodium
b. calcium
c. potassium
d. magnesium
e. chloride

18. What is the function of the magnesium ions associated with the NMDA receptor?
a. to facilitate calcium entry
b. to inhibit channel opening
c. to block glycine binding
d. to cause localized depolarization in the absence of glutamate
e. none of the above

19. Cytoplasmic receptors for steroid hormones such as cortisol and progesterone exist in the absence of ligand in association with proteins called:
a. adaptor proteins
b. heat shock proteins
c. protein kinases
d. transcription factors
e. ubiquitins

20. Which of the following diseases is caused by autoantibodies that recognize and stimulate the thyroid hormone receptor?
a. Chagas' disease
b. Hashimoto's disease
c. lupus
d. Graves' disease
e. Addison's disease

21. What kind of antagonist is described by the following statement: "Even in the presence of excess agonist, the maximum response was never observed when this compound was present."?

a. competitive antagonist
b. noncompetitive antagonist
c. partial agonist/antagonist
d. reversible antagonist
e. none of the above

22. Receptor desensitization occurs when:

a. the number of receptors on the cell surface declines
b. internalization of cell surface receptors increases
c. more new receptors are inserted in the membrane
d. the signaling cascade is exhausted
e. none of the above

ANSWER KEY

1. a
2. d
3. a
4. b
5. e
6. e
7. b
8. c
9. c
10. e
11. e
12. e
13. c
14. e
15. a
16. b
17. e
18. b
19. b
20. d
21. b
22. d

FINAL EXAM: PHYSIOLOGIC GENOMICS

Choose the single best answer to each of the following questions or incomplete statements. Answer key at end.

1. **A multifactorial disease:**
   a. is caused by a mutation in a single gene
   b. is not caused by genetic factors
   c. is the rarest form of genetic disease
   d. has both genetic and environmental components

2. **An example of a qualitative trait is:**
   a. hypertension
   b. blood glucose level
   c. blood pressure
   d. weight

3. **Which of the following statements is false regarding inbred rat strains?**
   a. Animals within an inbred strain are genetically distinct.
   b. Brothers and sisters from one extreme of a trait distribution can be bred to generate an inbred strain phenotypically and genotypically enriched for that trait.
   c. Two inbred rat strains can be crossed and subject to a genome scan to identify quantitative trait loci (QTLs).
   d. Generating an inbred strain requires 20 generations of inbreeding.

4. **Which of the following is false regarding genetic markers?**
   a. Genetic markers are used to link a genomic region to a phenotype.
   b. Genetic markers do not need to be polymorphic in a cross to be useful for genetic linkage analysis.
   c. SNPs are the most abundant type of genetic marker.
   d. Both b and c are false.

5. **Congenic rat strains:**
   a. contain a genomic region of interest (e.g., a QTL) from one strain introgressed onto the genome of another strain
   b. can be used to narrow the genomic interval containing a QTL
   c. can be generated from a consomic strain by an F_2 intercross
   d. are all of the above

6. **Knock-out technology:**
   a. is particularly powerful when genes interact to cause a phenotype
   b. is available in the rat
   c. can be used to validate a candidate gene's role in a complex disease
   d. is very similar to ENU mutagenesis in its ability to globally screen for gene effects

7. **Comparative mapping:**
   a. requires complete genomic sequence
   b. is useful for predicting the location of a QTL in one species based on its map location in another species

c. suggests that, in general, two species that are closer to a common ancestor have had a greater amount of genome rearrangements
d. both a and b

ANSWER KEY

1. d
2. a
3. a
4. b
5. d
6. c
7. b

FINAL EXAM: CARDIOVASCULAR PHYSIOLOGY

Choose the single best answer to each of the following questions or incomplete statements. Answer key at end.

1. **The viscosity of blood is greater than that of water mostly because of:**
   a. the high concentration of plasma proteins
   b. the presence of erythrocytes
   c. clotting factors
   d. the fourth power law
   e. plasma skimming

2. **An increase in capillary pressure of 5 mmHg would:**
   a. increase plasma volume by 5%
   b. cause a reabsorption of water from the interstitial space into the capillary
   c. reduce hematocrit by 25%
   d. increase hematocrit by 25%
   e. increase the net outward flux of water from the capillary to the interstitial space

3. **Which of the following statements about the lymphatic system is *not* true?**
   a. Lymph is derived from the interstitial fluid.
   b. Total normal lymph flow through the thoracic duct is about 2–3 liters/day.
   c. Lymph is actively pumped throughout the lymphatic system.
   d. Lymphatic capillaries are impermeable to protein.
   e. Lymphatic drainage of the gastrointestinal tract is a major route for nutrient absorption.

4. **What is the most important means by which substances are transferred between the plasma and the interstitial space?**
   a. diffusion
   b. perfusion
   c. active transport
   d. carrier-mediated transport
   e. facilitated diffusion

5. **Blood flow (Q) through a vessel is determined by which of the following?**
   a. pressure gradient
   b. Laplace's law
   c. vascular volume
   d. parabolic velocity profile
   e. pulse pressure

6. **Which of the following is greater in the veins than in the arteries?**
   a. pressure gradient
   b. Laplace's law
   c. vascular volume
   d. parabolic velocity profile
   e. pulse pressure

7. Hydrostatic pressure measured in the toe when standing as compared with supine is:
   a. higher
   b. lower
   c. not different

8. Pulse pressure in a patient with aortic regurgitation compared with normal is:
   a. higher
   b. lower
   c. not different

For questions 9–11, select the correct answer from the five choices below.
   a. arteries
   b. arterioles
   c. capillaries
   d. venules
   e. veins

9. The major site of vascular resistance in the systemic circulation.

10. Lack smooth muscle in the vessel wall.

11. Have the largest wall to lumen ratio.

Choose the single best answer to each of the following questions.

12. Which of the following describes the relationship between wall tension and vessel radius?
   a. Poiseuille's law
   b. Ohm's law
   c. Starling's law
   d. Laplace's law
   e. Reynolds' law

13. Which of the following are not innervated by sympathetic neurons?
   a. large arteries
   b. arterioles
   c. capillaries
   d. venules
   e. large veins

14. Which of the following stimulates the release of renin from the kidney?
   a. increased circulating angiotensin II (Ang II) concentration
   b. increased renal perfusion pressure
   c. increased arterial blood pressure
   d. reduced sodium intake
   e. volume expansion

For questions 15–18, select the correct answer from the three choices below. Each answer can be used more than once.
   a. increases
   b. decreases
   c. does not change

15. The diameter of an isolated 50-micron arteriole when flow is increased at constant transmural pressure.

16. The active wall tension in an isolated 100-micron arteriole when transmural pressure is elevated at constant flow.

17. The diameter of a 25-micron arteriole when metabolism of the tissue it feeds is increased.

18. The pO_2 of venous blood draining skeletal muscle as oxygen consumption of the muscle is increased from 1 to 5 mL $O_2 \times 3\ min^{-1} \times 3\ gm^{-1}$.

Choose the single best answer to each of the following questions or incomplete statements.

19. The autoregulatory multiplier effect refers to:
   a. the fact that arterial pressure is the product of cardiac output and total peripheral resistance
   b. the increase in resistance that occurs when cardiac output is elevated
   c. renal autoregulatory mechanisms that protect the glomerulus from rises in pressure
   d. the multiplicative effect of myogenic and metabolic autoregulatory mechanisms
   e. the dependence of arterial resistance on the fourth power of vessel radius

20. After the release of a temporary occlusion of an artery supplying skeletal muscle:
   a. blood flow will be transiently increased above the preocclusion level
   b. sympathetic withdrawal will cause dilation of downstream resistance vessels
   c. blood flow will be increased by active hyperemia
   d. the myogenic response will limit the reduction in flow as pressure falls
   e. sympathetic vasodilator fibers play a role in the observed response

21. Which of the following hormones would be most likely to dilate systemic arterioles in a human?
   a. endothelin
   b. vasopressin
   c. norepinephrine
   d. histamine
   e. none of the above

22. Aortic arch baroreceptor afferents travel in:
   a. Hering's nerve
   b. the vagus nerve
   c. the intermediolateral cell column
   d. the glossopharyngeal nerve
   e. the medullopontine nerve

23. Which of the following series of events best describes the response to a sudden primary reduction in renal excretory ability on a normal sodium diet?
   a. sodium retention → increased MCFP → increased AP → increased sodium excretion
   b. increased AP → increased sodium excretion → decreased MCFP → hypotension
   c. sodium and water retention → blood volume expansion → decreased vascular capacity → decreased resistance to venous return → increased cardiac output
   d. increased renin secretion → increased Ang II → arterial constriction → increased arterial pressure

e. increased renal perfusion pressure ⟶ increased GFR ⟶ decreased sodium excretion ⟶ increased afferent arteriolar resistance

24. If a large fistula were suddenly to open between the femoral artery and femoral vein, cardiac output would:
a. increase suddenly because of the reduced peripheral resistance
b. decrease over time because of reductions in blood volume by the kidney
c. not change because metabolic demands of the peripheral tissue have remained constant
d. not be affected by changes in preload because mean circulatory filling pressure is greater than right atrial pressure
e. do none of the above

25. Resistance to venous return is:
a. higher during exercise than at rest
b. equal to the slope of the venous return curve
c. reduced by increasing sympathetic outflow
d. increased by an increase in mean circulatory filling pressure
e. increased by constriction of arterioles

26. The blood-brain barrier:
a. protects the brain from increases in arterial pressure
b. restricts the movement of some hormones from the blood to the brain parenchyma
c. is involved in enhanced metabolic autoregulation in the brain
d. is often compromised in patients with low circulating renin
e. is created by the tight junctional barriers between the neurons and endothelial cells of cerebral capillaries

27. A person with type A blood has:
a. A antigens (agglutinogens)
b. anti-A antibodies (agglutinins)
c. no agglutinins
d. B agglutinogens
e. all of the above

28. Important components of the blood clotting cascade include all of the following *except:*
a. thrombin
b. factor X
c. calcium
d. agglutinins
e. fibrin

29. Anticoagulants can work by :
a. inhibiting vitamin K–induced production of clotting factors
b. breaking up clots that form in the vessels
c. activating antithrombin III
d. a and c
e. all of the above

30. The ECG normally includes wave forms that represent all of the following *except:*
a. atrial depolarization
b. atrial repolarization
c. ventricular depolarization
d. ventricular repolarization
e. all of the above

31. Analysis of the ECG can identify:
- a. poor ventricular contractility
- b. heart failure
- c. conduction blocks at the AV node
- d. decrease in stroke volume
- e. all of the above

32. Activation of the baroreceptor reflex produces:
- a. an increase in parasympathetic drive
- b. a decease in peripheral resistance
- c. a decrease in cardiac contractility
- d. a and c
- e. all of the above

33. Blood flow to cardiac muscle:
- a. is controlled to a large extent by autoregulation
- b. arises directly from the chambers of the heart
- c. is greatest during diastole
- d. only a and c
- e. all of the above

34. Changes in cardiac output can be produced by:
- a. changes in venous return
- b. Starling's law of the heart
- c. changes in afterload
- d. a and c
- e. all of the above

35. Blood flow to individual vascular beds (organs) can be controlled by:
- a. extrinsic mechanisms including increases in sympathetic drive
- b. Starling's law of the heart
- c. intrinsic autoregulatory mechanisms including the myogenic response
- d. a and c
- e. all of the above

36. The refractory period of cardiac muscle:
- a. equals the R-R interval
- b. helps prevent arrhythmias
- c. blocks the effects of increases in venous return
- d. a and c
- e. all of the above

For questions 37–40, use the following values to calculate the answers:

Arterial pressure = 100 mmHg
Venous pressure = 0 mmHg
Capillary pressure = 10 mmHg
Arterial compliance = 1 mL/mmHg
Venous compliance = 20 mL/mmHg
Blood viscosity = 1.05 centipoise (cP)
Aortic luminal diameter = 2.0 cm
Aortic length = 25 cm
Heart rate = 50 beats/minute
Stroke volume = 100 mL

37. **Cardiac output =**
   a. $2\ L \times min^{-1}$
   b. $3\ L \times min^{-1}$
   c. $4\ L \times min^{-1}$
   d. $5\ L \times min^{-1}$
   e. $6\ L \times min^{-1}$

38. **Total peripheral resistance =**
   a. $5\ mmHg \times L^{-1} \times min$
   b. $10\ mmHg \times L^{-1} \times min$
   c. $20\ mmHg \times L^{-1} \times min$
   d. $25\ mmHg \times L^{-1} \times min$
   e. $30\ mmHg \times L^{-1} \times min$

39. **Arterial stressed blood volume =**
   a. 20 mL
   b. 50 mL
   c. 100 mL
   d. 200 mL
   e. 500 mL

40. **Arterial resistance =**
   a. $5\ mmHg \times L^{-1} \times min$
   b. $12\ mmHg \times L^{-1} \times min$
   c. $16\ mmHg \times L^{-1} \times min$
   d. $18\ mmHg \times L^{-1} \times min$
   e. $20\ mmHg \times L^{-1} \times min$

For questions 41 and 42, review the figure below and select the correct answer from the following five choices:
   a. point 1
   b. point 2
   c. point 3
   d. point 4
   e. point 5

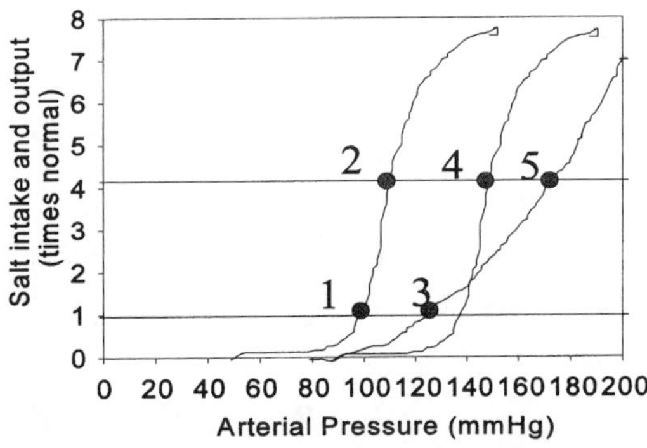

41. **Which point on the graph corresponds to a salt sensitive hypertensive patient on a high-salt diet?**

42. **Which point on the graph corresponds to a patient with one-kidney Goldblatt hypertension?**

Choose the single best answer to each of the following questions or incomplete statements.

43. Chills, vasoconstriction, and shivering best describe which of the following?
   a. sustained fever
   b. hypotension
   c. onset of fever
   d. rapid reduction of the temperature set-point to normal
   e. hyperthyroidism

44. At room temperature, the majority of blood flow to the skin:
   a. acts to meet the temperature regulation needs of the body
   b. travels through arterial shunts
   c. does not enter the capillaries in the dermis
   d. traverses the subdermal venous plexus
   e. does all of the above

45. Which of the following is most likely to occur in anaphylactic shock?
   a. a rise in total peripheral resistance
   b. hypotension and tachycardia
   c. a reduced plasma level of renin
   d. an increased rate of urine production
   e. a decrease in hematocrit

For questions 46 and 47, review the figure below and select the correct answer from the following five choices:
   a. point A
   b. point B
   c. point C
   d. point D
   e. point E

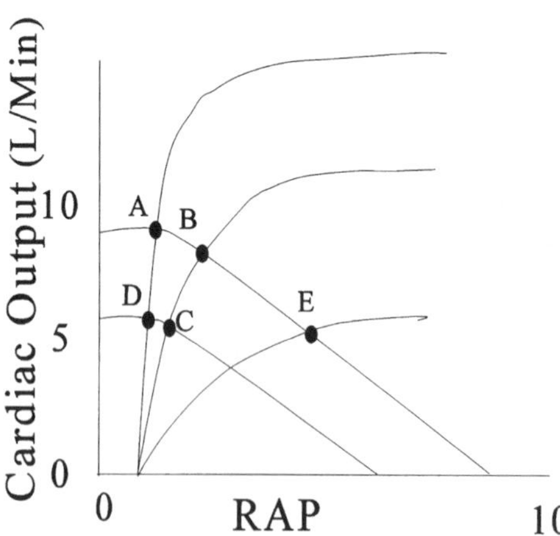

46. Which point on the cardiac function and venous return curves best describes an increase in MCFP alone?

47. Which point on the graph best describes compensated heart failure?

For questions 48–51, select the correct answer from the fifteen choices below.

a. 0.1
b. 0.2
c. 0.3
d. 0.4
e. 1.0
f. 2.0
g. 2.5
h. 4.0
i. 10.0
j. 50.0
k. 80.0
l. 100.0
m. 130.0
n. 150.0
o. 200.0

48. What is the parallel combination of R1 = 10 units, R2 = 10 units, and R3 = 5 units?

49. What is the compliance of a blood vessel in which a change in volume of 20 mL results in a change in pressure 100 mmHg?

50. What is the flow (L/min) in a vascular network with an inflow pressure of 100 mmHg, an outflow pressure of 50, and a resistance of 25 mmHg × 3 min × 3 L^{-1}?

51. What would the heart rate (in beats per minute) be if a person's arterial pressure is 100 mmHg, stroke volume is 80 mL/beat, and cardiac output is 8000 mL/min?

For questions 52–58, select the correct answer from the three choices below.

a. lower
b. higher
c. the same

52. Body temperature set-point compared with actual body temperature when patient is complaining of chills.

53. Plasma angiotensin II concentration in a normal person eating a very low salt diet compared with the concentration in a person eating a high salt diet.

54. Amount of the total blood volume found in the veins compared with the volume found in the capillaries.

55. Total cross-sectional area of the capillaries compared with that of the veins.

56. Active force in a myogenically responsive blood vessel as transmural pressure increases from 75 to 100 mmHg.

57. Activity in the carotid sinus nerve during a 20% reduction of blood volume compared with normal.

58. When blood volume is increased by 20%, cardiac output will also increase. What role does the metabolic autoregulation play in the associated change in total peripheral resistance?

a. Metabolic autoregulation plays no role under these conditions.
b. Total peripheral resistance will decrease because of metabolic autoregulation.
c. Metabolic autoregulation will cause dilation of the veins, resulting in a normalization of cardiac output and total peripheral resistance.
d. Metabolic autoregulation will cause total peripheral resistance to rise, resulting in an increased blood pressure.
e. The metabolic response will be offset by an equal and opposite myogenic response resulting in no change in total peripheral resistance.

Select the most likely diagnosis from the seven choices below for the physical and laboratory findings in questions 59–51.

a. hypertension
b. chronic compensated right heart failure
c. chronic compensated left heart failure
d. acute right heart failure
e. renal failure
f. decompensated chronic left heart failure
g. septic shock

59. 57-year-old male; 5 feet, 9 inches; 214 pounds; arterial blood pressure: 165/90; normal cardiac output; HR: 85.

60. 61-year-old woman; 5 feet, 1 inch; 121 pounds; HR: 160; CO = 3.5 L/min; RAP = 3 mmHg; LAP = 4 mmHg; supine arterial blood pressure: 105/65.

61. 31-year-old male; 6 feet, 1 inch; 195 pounds; recent history of weight gain and exercise intolerance; HR: 80; CO: 5.5 L/min; RAP: 7 mmHg; LAP: 3 mmHg.

ANSWER KEY

1. b
2. e
3. d
4. a
5. a
6. c
7. a
8. a
9. b
10. c
11. b
12. d
13. c
14. d
15. a
16. a
17. a
18. b
19. b
20. a
21. d
22. b
23. a
24. a
25. e
26. b
27. a
28. d
29. d
30. b
31. c
32. e
33. d
34. e
35. d
36. b
37. d
38. c
39. c
40. d
41. e
42. d
43. c
44. e
45. b
46. b
47. e
48. g
49. b
50. f
51. 1
52. b
53. b
54. b
55. b
56. b
57. a
58. d
59. a
60. d
61. b

FINAL EXAM: RESPIRATORY PHYSIOLOGY

Choose the single best answer to each of the following questions or incomplete statements. Answer key at end.

1. **The amount of air remaining in the lungs at end-expiratory level is called the:**
   a. ERV
   b. FRC
   c. RV
   d. V_t
   e. IRV

2. **Determine the ERV from the following information: TLC = 5.80, FRC = 3.20 L, and VC = 4.60 L**
   a. 1.80 L
   b. 2.60 L
   c. 1.40 L
   d. 2.00 L
   e. 1.20 L

3. **What is the hallmark of a restrictive ventilatory impairment?**
   a. decreased VC
   b. increased RV
   c. decreased TLC
   d. decreased ERV

4. **Which of the following does not contribute to hyperinflation?**
   a. decreased pulmonary compliance
   b. airflow obstruction
   c. enlargement of the air spaces
   d. loss of elastic recoil

5. **A patient undergoing a static volume-pressure study had a transpulmonary pressure change of 2.5 cm H_2O following the inspiration of 1000 mL. Determine the static pulmonary compliance.**
   a. 0.02
   b. 0.04
   c. 0.25
   d. 0.40

6. **The widest intrapleural pressure gradient from the top to the bottom of the upright lung:**
   a. is found at RV
   b. is found at TLC
   c. is found at FRC
   d. is found at VC
   e. remains relatively constant

7. **All of the following will result in a decrease in anatomic dead space *except:***
   a. hyperextension of the neck
   b. pneumonectomy
   c. hyperextension of the jaw
   d. tracheostomy

8. **Determine the minute ventilation of a 45-year-old, 57-kg female with a respiratory rate of 12 breaths per minute and a V_t of 400 mL.**
   a. 4.0 L/min
   b. 5.2 L/min
   c. 4.6 L/min
   d. 4.8 L/min
   e. 4.9 L/min

9. **When is alveolar pressure equal to atmospheric pressure?**
   a. at end-inspiratory level
   b. at end-expiratory level
   c. at TLC
   d. at RV
   e. all of the above

10. **Airway resistance is highest at or near:**
   a. TLC
   b. FRC
   c. RV
   d. V_t

11. **Calculate the transpulmonary pressure from the following information: atmospheric pressure = 980 cm H_2O; pleural pressure = 973 cm H_2O; and alveolar pressure = 977 cm H_2O.**
   a. +3
   b. +4
   c. −4
   d. +7
   e. −3

12. **Determine total compliance given the following: lung compliance = 0.3 L/cm H_2O and thoracic compliance = 0.3 L/cm H_2O.**
   a. 0.10
   b. 0.15
   c. 0.30
   d. 0.60

13. **Which of the following relationships describes West's zone 2 of the lung?**
   a. $P_a > P_v > P_A$
   b. $P_v > P_A > P_a$
   c. $P_a > P_A > P_v$
   d. $P_A > P_a > P_v$
   e. $P_v > P_a > P_A$

14. **A coal miner is exposed to 18% oxygen while working. Determine the partial pressure of inspired oxygen if the barometric pressure is 747 mmHg and water vapor is 47 mmHg.**
   a. 126 mmHg
   b. 134 mmHg

c. 143 mmHg
d. 147 mmHg

15. **Increase in the P_{CO_2} that subsequently reduces the affinity of hemoglobin for oxygen is known as the:**
a. Haldane effect
b. Bohr effect
c. Bernoulli effect
d. Pendelluft effect

16. **All of the following will favor reabsorption of fluid into the pulmonary capillaries *except:***
a. decrease in mean capillary pressure
b. decrease in interstitial fluid colloid osmotic pressure
c. increase in interstitial fluid pressure
d. decrease in the capillary filtration coefficient
e. increase in plasma fluid osmotic pressure

17. **Which of the following will stimulate the peripheral chemoreceptors?**
a. decrease in PaO_2
b. decrease in $PaCO_2$
c. increase in arterial pH
d. none of the above

18. **Which of the following will result in the largest increase in minute ventilation?**
a. a decrease in the inspired oxygen from 21% to 18%
b. an increase in inspired carbon dioxide of 4 mmHg
c. decrease in arterial pH from 7.45 to 7.35
d. decrease in the arterial oxygen from 500 mmHg to 150 mmHg
e. increase in arterial pH from 7.10 to 7.30

19. **All of the following mechanisms are involved in high-altitude breathing acclimatization *except:***
a. an increase in alveolar ventilation
b. leftward shift in the oxyhemoglobin dissociation curve
c. increase in the diffusion capacity
d. decreased capillarity
e. an increase in red blood cells and hemoglobin

20. **Calculate the oxygen content of an arterial blood sample with an SaO_2 of 92%; PaO_2 of 75 mmHg; and hemoglobin of 12.0 gm/dL.**
a. 11.27 mL/100 mL
b. 14.89 mL/100 mL
c. 15.02 mL/100 mL
d. 16.08 mL/100 mL

21. **During transient hyperventilation, the RQ will:**
a. increase
b. decrease
c. equal the RER
d. not change

22. **Which of the following determines the rate of gas transfer across the alveolar-capillary membrane?**
a. available surface area
b. membrane thickness

c. solubility coefficient of the gas
d. diffusion coefficient of the gas
e. all of the above

23. A ventilation/perfusion ratio of 0.6 is consistent with:
a. overventilated alveoli
b. low arterial oxygen tension
c. underperfused capillary
d. hyperventilation
e. high arterial oxygen tension

24. Pulmonary vascular resistance is lowest at:
a. FRC
b. TLC
c. end-inspiratory level
d. RV

25. The central chemoreceptors are stimulated by:
a. an increase in $Pa{CO_2}$
b. a decrease in cerebrospinal fluid $P{CO_2}$
c. an increase in cerebrospinal fluid pH
d. a decrease in arterial pH

26. The pulmonary stretch receptors respond to:
a. increases in tidal volume
b. airway hypercarbia
c. hypoinflation
d. smoke and ammonia
e. all of the above

ANSWER KEY

1. b
2. d
3. c
4. a
5. d
6. e
7. c
8. d
9. e
10. c
11. b
12. b
13. c
14. a
15. b
16. e
17. a
18. b
19. d
20. c
21. d
22. e
23. b
24. a
25. a
26. e

FINAL EXAM: RENAL PHYSIOLOGY

Choose the single best answer to each of the following questions or incomplete statements. Answer key at end.

1. **Which of the following statements is true?**
   a. The Na^+, K^+ ATPase pump maintains elevated levels of Na^+ and K^+ in the intracellular fluid.
   b. The intracellular fluid volume is approximately twice that of the extracellular fluid.
   c. By weight, the normal human body is composed of approximately 40% water.
   d. Fluid exchange between the interstitial space and plasma leads to net reabsorption into the systemic capillaries.
   e. None of the above is true.

2. **A 70-kg individual of normal body composition is injected intravenously with 4×10^6 cpm of tritiated water (^3H_2O). Fifteen minutes later a blood sample is taken, and the blood contains 100 cpm/mL ^3H_2O. What is the approximate volume of total body water in this individual?**
   a. 80 liters
   b. 60 liters
   c. 40 liters
   d. 20 liters
   e. cannot be determined

3. **Which of the following best describes the response to a volume load of hypertonic NaCl?**
   a. increased extracellular volume, decreased intracellular volume, increased intracellular osmolality
   b. increased extracellular volume, increased intracellular volume, decreased intracellular osmolality
   c. increased extracellular volume, increased intracellular volume, increased extracellular osmolality
   d. decreased extracellular volume, increased intracellular volume, increased intracellular osmolality
   e. decreased extracellular volume, decreased intracellular volume, increased extracellular osmolality

4. **Which one of the following could lead to hyponatremia?**
   a. inappropriate secretion of antidiuretic hormone
   b. abnormally elevated levels of aldosterone
   c. extreme sweating
   d. nephrogenic diabetes insipidus
   e. abnormally elevated levels of renin

5. **Which of the following sequences of vascular structures could a red blood cell follow when passing through the kidney under normal conditions?**
   a. renal artery → interlobar artery → arcuate artery → glomerular capillaries → peritubular capillaries → efferent arteriole → renal vein
   b. renal artery → interlobar artery → arcuate artery → glomerular capillaries → peritubular capillaries → vasa recta → renal vein

c. renal artery ⟶ arcuate artery ⟶ afferent arteriole ⟶ glomerular capillaries ⟶ efferent arteriole ⟶ vasa recta capillaries ⟶ renal vein
d. renal artery ⟶ interlobular artery ⟶ arcuate artery ⟶ afferent arteriole ⟶ glomerular capillaries ⟶ peritubular capillaries ⟶ renal vein
e. renal artery ⟶ arcuate artery ⟶ glomerular capillaries ⟶ afferent arteriole ⟶ peritubular capillaries ⟶ vasa recta capillaries ⟶ renal vein

6. **What is the net effect (compared with normal conditions) on creatinine clearance in an individual who has just undergone a 50% reduction in renal mass? Assume the individual has come into equilibrium and has not undergone any compensatory hypertrophy of remnant nephrons.**
   a. increased 50%
   b. decreased 50%
   c. not changed
   d. increased 33%
   e. decreased 67%

7. **Which of the following circumstances would lead to an increase in GFR?**
   a. increased colloid osmotic pressure
   b. increased proximal tubule pressure
   c. increased ultrafiltration coefficient
   d. increased tubular flow rate past the macula densa
   e. increased afferent arteriolar resistance

For questions 8–12, determine the answers using the following information:
An individual has a P_{inulin} concentration of 1.2 mg/mL, a urine volume of 120 mL obtained over a 2-hour period, a U_{inulin} concentration of 120 mg/mL, a P_{Na} of 140 mEq/L, a P_{PAH} of 0.1 mg/mL, a U_{PAH} of 50 mg/mL, U_{Na} of 250 mEq/L, and a hematocrit of 40%.

8. **What is this individual's GFR?**
   a. 400 mL/min
   b. 120 mL/min
   c. 100 mL/min
   d. 60 mL/min
   e. 40 mL/min

9. **What is this individual's renal blood flow?**
   a. 1250 mL/min
   b. 833 mL/min
   c. 500 mL/min
   d. 240 mL/min
   e. 167 mL/min

10. **What is the individual's filtration fraction?**
   a. 40%
   b. 30%
   c. 25%
   d. 20%
   e. 12%

11. **What is the individual's fractional sodium excretion?**
   a. 10.0%
   b. 5.0%

c. 1.7%
d. 0.1%
e. 0.01%

12. What is the individual's rate of PAH secretion?
a. 50 mg/min
b. 40 mg/min
c. 30 mg/min
d. 20 mg/min
e. 10 mg/min

Choose the single best answer to each of the following questions.

13. Which of the following will occur following a selective increase in renal efferent arteriolar resistance?
a. Ultrafiltration coefficient will decrease.
b. Afferent arteriolar blood flow will decrease.
c. Efferent arteriolar protein concentration will decrease.
d. Efferent arteriolar hematocrit will decrease.
e. None of the above occurs.

14. What is the approximate hydrostatic pressure in the glomerular capillaries?
a. 100 mmHg
b. 60 mmHg
c. 40 mmHg
d. 20 mmHg
e. 10 mmHg

15. Which of the following will *not* lead to an increase in circulating levels of renin?
a. increased renal sympathetic nerve activity
b. decreased blood pressure
c. increased NaCl delivery to the macula densa
d. hemorrhage
e. none of the above

16. Which of the following statements does not describe the direct effects of angiotensin II?
a. decreased renal blood flow
b. increased proximal tubule sodium reabsorption
c. increased distal tubule sodium reabsorption
d. increased aldosterone release
e. increased renal vascular resistance

17. Which of the following will aid in the excretion of a 1-liter oral load of isotonic saline?
a. inhibition of the renin-angiotensin system
b. decreased renal sympathetic nerve activity
c. dilution of plasma proteins
d. decreased vasopressin levels
e. all of the above

18. Which statement is true regarding the thin descending loop of Henle?
a. This segment is found only in the deep cortical (juxtamedullary) nephrons.
b. Active sodium and chloride reabsorption occurs in this segment.
c. Tubular fluid osmolality decreases from the proximal to distal portions of this segment.

d. ADH-sensitive H_2O absorption occurs in this segment.
e. Passive H_2O reabsorption occurs in this segment.

For questions 19–20, determine the answers using the following information:
An individual excretes 60 mL of urine in 1 hour, has a U_{osm} of 1200 mOsm/kg H_2O, and has a P_{osm} of 300 mOsm/kg H_2O.

19. What is this individual's osmolar clearance rate?
a. 4 mL/min
b. –4 mL/min
c. 3 mL/min
d. –3 mL/min
e. cannot be determined with the data provided

20. What is this individual's free water clearance?
a. 4 mL/min
b. –4 mL/min
c. 3 mL/min
d. –3 mL/min
e. cannot be determined with the data provided

Choose the single best answer to each of the following questions or incomplete statements.

21. Circulating levels of antidiuretic hormone (ADH) will be increased by which of the following?
a. ingestion of 1 liter of isotonic saline
b. ingestion of 1 liter of hypotonic saline
c. ingestion of 1 liter of beer
d. heavy sweating during exercise
e. none of the above

22. Under conditions of dehydration in a normal individual, which of the following tubular segments will contain fluid of the greatest osmolality?
a. proximal tubule
b. distal tubule
c. macula densa
d. thin ascending limb of loop of Henle
e. cortical collecting duct

23. Compared with normal, which of the following would you expect to occur during dehydration?
a. increased water permeability of the collecting duct
b. increased venous pressure
c. elevated levels of atrial natriuretic peptide
d. increased urinary flow rate
e. decreased plasma renin activity

24. Under normal conditions, which tubular segment will contain fluid with the greatest concentration of creatinine?
a. proximal tubule
b. inner medullary thin descending loop of Henle
c. medullary thick ascending loop of Henle

d. distal convoluted tubule
e. inner medullary collecting duct

25. Ammonium is produced from glutamine in which renal tubular segment?
a. proximal tubule
b. inner medullary thin descending loop of Henle
c. medullary thick ascending loop of Henle
d. distal convoluted tubule
e. inner medullary collecting duct

26. Urea permeability is reduced in which segment during water diuresis?
a. proximal tubule
b. inner medullary thin descending loop of Henle
c. medullary thick ascending loop of Henle
d. distal convoluted tubule
e. inner medullary collecting duct

27. Secretion of organic acids and bases occurs in which renal tubular segment?
a. proximal tubule
b. inner medullary thin descending loop of Henle
c. medullary thick ascending loop of Henle
d. distal convoluted tubule
e. inner medullary collecting duct

28. Acid (H^+) is secreted:
a. by cells in the thin descending limb of the loop of Henle
b. by the principal cells of the collecting duct
c. in response to urodilatin
d. by principal cells in the distal tubule
e. by the intercalated cells of the collecting duct

29. Aldosterone-sensitive sodium reabsorption occurs in which renal tubular segment?
a. proximal tubule
b. inner medullary thin descending loop of Henle
c. medullary thick ascending loop of Henle
d. distal convoluted tubule
e. inner medullary collecting duct

30. Potassium excretion:
a. is controlled by angiotensin II and norepinephrine in the proximal tubule
b. is increased when plasma potassium levels are decreased
c. is increased by aldosterone
d. is controlled primarily by renal sympathetic nerves
e. is none of the above

ANSWER KEY

1. b
2. c
3. a
4. a
5. c
6. b
7. c
8. c
9. b
10. d
11. c
12. b
13. b
14. b
15. c
16. c
17. e
18. e
19. a
20. d
21. d
22. d
23. a
24. e
25. a
26. e
27. a
28. e
29. d
30. c

FINAL EXAM: GASTROINTESTINAL PHYSIOLOGY

Choose the single best answer to each of the following questions or incomplete statements. Answer key at end.

1. **Forty minutes after eating a meal of solid foods and liquids, all of which are low in fat, a person is infused with an emulsion of long-chain fatty acids into the duodenum through a catheter. Ten minutes into the infusion:**
   a. antral contractions would be increased in number and amplitude
   b. gastric emptying would be increased
   c. plasma levels of cholecystokinin would be lower
   d. pressures within the orad stomach would be less
   e. the frequency of pyloric contractions would be lower

2. **A catheter with numerous pressure sensors is passed into the esophagus of a patient. Between swallows, normal resting pressures are recorded from the upper esophageal sphincter, the body of the esophagus, and the lower esophageal sphincter. When the patient swallows, the upper esophageal sphincter relaxes and contracts normally, and the upper half of the body of the esophagus contracts normally. However, the lower half of the body of the esophagus does not contract, and the lower esophageal sphincter does not relax. Attempts to elicit a secondary peristaltic contraction by balloon distention of the lower esophagus are unsuccessful. Distention induces contraction of only the muscle directly around the balloon. There is no peristaltic contraction of the lower half of the body of the esophagus, and the lower esophageal sphincter fails to relax. These results indicate a defect in the:**
   a. enteric nervous system
   b. medulla oblongata
   c. smooth muscle of the esophagus
   d. striated muscle of the esophagus
   e. vagus nerve

3. **Administration of a drug that causes an increase in slow wave frequency at all sites of the small intestine would result in an increase in the:**
   a. amplitude of individual jejunal contractions
   b. duration of individual duodenal contractions
   c. maximal frequency at which contractions could occur
   d. rate of occurrence of the migrating motility complex
   e. velocity of propagation of peristaltic contractions

For questions 4–6, select the correct answer from the five choices below. Each answer can be used more than once.

a. gastrin
b. secretin
c. GIP
d. somatostatin
e. CCK

4. **Its release is inhibited by low luminal pH.**

5. **It stimulates biliary HCO_3 secretion.**

6. **It stimulates the release of histamine from enterochromaffin-like (ECL) cells.**

For questions 7–9, choose the correct answer from the five choices below.

a. nitric oxide
b. acetylcholine
c. motilin
d. cholecystokinin
e. secretin

7. **It is a neurotransmitter that causes contraction of intestinal smooth muscle.**

8. **Its release is periodic in a fasting individual.**

9. **It is a neurotransmitter that causes relaxation of the lower esophageal sphincter.**

Choose the single best answer to each of the following incomplete statements.

10. **Sodium taurocholate:**
    a. synthesis in the liver is reduced after ileal resection
    b. is insoluble at pH 6.0
    c. is absorbed by a sodium-coupled secondary active transport mechanism in the ileal mucosa
    d. is a secondary bile salt
    e. forms micelles only at concentrations below the critical micellar concentration

11. **An increase in the incidence of peristaltic contractions over long (> 10 cm) lengths of the small intestine:**
    a. occurs immediately after a meal
    b. is accompanied by increases in slow wave frequency
    c. occurs shortly after the injection of motilin
    d. results in mixing of intestinal contents
    e. occurs shortly after the injection of atropine

12. **The lower esophageal sphincter (LES) differs from the distal body of the esophagus in that:**
    a. intrinsic (enteric) nerves are present in the LES but not in the distal body
    b. the LES is composed of smooth muscle while the distal body is composed of striated muscle
    c. between swallows LES muscle is tonically contracted while distal body muscle is relaxed
    d. nitric oxide contracts LES muscle but relaxes distal body muscle
    e. only the LES receives extrinsic innervation by way of the vagus nerve

For questions 13–15, select the best answer from the four choices below.

a. pepsin only
b. pancreatic lipase only
c. both pepsin and pancreatic lipase
d. neither pepsin nor pancreatic lipase

13. **Activated by brush border enzyme.**

14. **Involved in contact digestion.**

15. **Secreted as a proenzyme.**

For questions 16 and 17, select the best answer from the four choices below.

a. galactose
b. vitamin B_{12}
c. both galactose and vitamin B_{12}
d. neither galactose nor vitamin B_{12}

16. **Enhances Na^+ absorption in the small intestine.**

17. **Malabsorption associated with ileal resection.**

Choose the single best answer to each of the following questions or incomplete statements.

18. **The rate of gastric emptying of a mixed meal of liquids and solids is increased by:**
    a. increases in circulating levels of cholecystokinin
    b. increased contractions of the antrum
    c. increased contractions of the pylorus
    d. relaxation of the orad region of the stomach

19. **Salivary secretion:**
    a. is isotonic at all rates of secretion
    b. is controlled primarily by the hormone secretin
    c. is inhibited by sympathetic nerve stimulation
    d. is directly increased by bradykinin
    e. contains concentrations of K^+ that exceed those in the plasma

20. **Chymotrypsinogen release from pancreatic acinar cells is:**
    a. increased only during the intestinal phase of a meal
    b. reduced by vagotomy
    c. decreased by the addition of a trypsin-inhibitor to the diet
    d. stimulated by dietary glucose
    e. decreased by diversion of the pancreatic duct to the ileum

For questions 21–23, select the correct answer from the five choices below.

a. gastrin
b. VIP
c. GIP
d. CCK
e. somatostatin

21. **Blood levels of this are increased by glucose in the GI lumen.**

22. **Stimulates pancreatic HCO_3^- secretion in the presence of low concentrations of secretin.**

23. **Acts as a neurocrine mediator of smooth muscle relaxation.**

For questions 24–26, select the best answer from the four choices below.

a. internal anal sphincter
b. external anal sphincter

c. both the internal anal sphincter and external anal sphincter
d. neither the internal anal sphincter nor the external anal sphincter

24. Relaxes upon acute distension of the rectum.

25. Contracts in a pattern of rhythmic segmentation.

26. Is under voluntary neural control.

Choose the single best answer to each of the following questions or incomplete statements.

27. Which one of the following statements about gastric HCl secretion is *not* true?
a. Gastric acid secretion is dependent on the fusion of tubulovesicles with the canalicular membrane of parietal cells.
b. Gastric acid secretion is dependent on the local paracrine release of histamine within the gastric mucosa.
c. Administration of a specific inhibitor of H^+, K^+ ATPase will only partially abolish gastric acid secretion.
d. Gastric acid secretion is neurally stimulated during the cephalic phase of a meal.
e. Histamine-induced gastric acid secretion is mediated by increases in parietal cell cAMP levels.

28. Which one of the following physiologic events does *not* occur during the cephalic phase of a meal?
a. The concentration of amylase in the salivary juice increases.
b. The concentration of amylase in the pancreatic juice increases.
c. The gallbladder contracts.
d. Gastric acid secretion increases.
e. Secretin release from intestinal S cells is directly stimulated.

29. Which one of the following statements about bile salts is *not* true?
a. Bile salts play a role in the emulsification of dietary lipids in the intestinal lumen.
b. Bile salts promote the intestinal absorption of lipid-soluble vitamins.
c. Bile salts may be secreted and reabsorbed 3–5 times during a single meal.
d. Bile salts are resistant to bacterial metabolism within the lumen of the GI tract.
e. The concentration of bile salts in the GI lumen increases after the ingestion of a fatty meal.

ANSWER KEY

1. d
2. a
3. c
4. a
5. b
6. a
7. b
8. c
9. a
10. c
11. c
12. c
13. d
14. d
15. a
16. a
17. b
18. b
19. e
20. b
21. c
22. d
23. b
24. a
25. d
26. b
27. c
28. e
29. d

FINAL EXAM: ENDOCRINE PHYSIOLOGY

For questions 1–8, select the chemical nature of the hormone in question from the five choices below. Each answer can be used more than once. Answer key at end.

a. amine/tyrosine derivative
b. polypeptide/protein
c. steroid
d. glycoprotein
e. carbohydrate

1. **Human chorionic somatomammotropin**

2. **Human chorionic gonadotropin**

3. **1,25$(OH)_2$D**

4. **Thyroxine**

5. **Adrenocorticotropic hormone (ACTH)**

6. **Follicle-stimulating hormone (FSH)**

7. **Cortisol**

8. **Epinephrine**

Choose the single best answer to each of the following questions.

9. **Which of the following exerts its action through a cell surface receptor?**
   a. cortisol
   b. 1,25$(OH)_2$D
   c. thyroxine
   d. vasopressin
   e. aldosterone

10. **Which of the following hormones has the slowest metabolic clearance rate (longest half life)?**
    a. oxytocin
    b. growth hormone (GH)
    c. aldosterone
    d. cortisol
    e. thyroxine

For questions 11–14, select the correct answer from the five choices below.

a. stimulates luteinizing hormone (LH) secretion
b. inhibits prolactin secretion
c. inhibits growth hormone
d. stimulates ACTH secretion
e. stimulates GH secretion

11. Somatostatin:

12. Dopamine:

13. Gonadotropin-releasing hormone (GnRH):

14. Corticotropin-releasing hormone (CRH):

Choose the single best answer to following question.

15. Which of the following represents an example of insensitivity to the peripheral action of a hormone?
a. hyperprolactinemia
b. neurogenic diabetes insipidus
c. secondary adrenal insufficiency
d. hypogonadotropic hypogonadism
e. nephrogenic diabetes insipidus

For questions 16–20, select the correct adrenal response to administration of ACTH from the five choices below.

a. exaggerated increase in progesterone with no change in 17-hydroxyprogesterone
b. exaggerated increase in 17-hydroxypregnenolone with no change in 17-hydroxyprogesterone
c. exaggerated increase in corticosterone
d. exaggerated increase in 17-hydroxyprogesterone with no change in 11-deoxycortisol
e. exaggerated increase in 11-deoxycortisol with no change in cortisol

16. 3β-hydroxysteroid dehydrogenase deficiency

17. 21α-hydroxylase deficiency

18. 11β-hydroxylase deficiency

19. 17α-hydroxylase deficiency

20. Aldosterone synthase deficiency

Choose the single best answer to each of the following questions.

21. At *steady state*, which of the following would most likely be found in a patient with partial 11β-hydroxylase deficiency?
a. very low portal venous CRH concentration
b. very low pituitary venous ACTH concentration
c. elevated adrenal venous cortisol concentration
d. elevated adrenal venous 11-deoxycortisol concentration
e. elevated insulin concentration in the pancreatic vein

22. You examine a patient with a history of gradual weight gain, hyperglycemia, facial plethora, easy bruisability, thin skin, hypertension, and hypokalemia. The patient works as a nurse in an allergist's office. You measure plasma ACTH and cortisol, both of which are very low. Which of the following is the most likely diagnosis?
a. a pituitary tumor secreting ACTH
b. a lung tumor with a derepressed proopiomelanocortin (POMC) oncogene

c. 11β-hydroxylase deficiency
d. surreptitious dexamethasone use
e. surreptitious cortisol (hydrocortisone) use

23. You examine a patient with a history of gradual weight loss, hypoglycemia, hypotension, and increased skin darkening even in the winter in Wisconsin. You suspect primary adrenal insufficiency and measure plasma cortisol, which is very low. What is the *best* measurement to prove that the patient has primary adrenal insufficiency?
a. elevated plasma vasopressin
b. elevated 11-deoxycortisol
c. elevated plasma ACTH
d. elevated plasma glucagon
e. attenuated ACTH response to CRH

24. Which of the following is *not* consistent with hypopituitarism?
a. plasma ACTH within the normal (reference) range
b. plasma TSH within the normal (reference) range
c. plasma LH within the normal (reference) range
d. plasma GH within the normal (reference) range
e. exaggerated ACTH response to CRH

25. Which of the following will increase the secretion of aldosterone?
a. infusion of losartan, an angiotensin II antagonist
b. infusion of captopril, an angiotensin-converting enzyme inhibitor
c. eating a potassium-rich meal
d. ACTH-dependent Cushing's syndrome of 3 years' duration
e. infusion of atrial natriuretic peptide

26. Which of the following would be most likely to increase radioactive iodide uptake in the thyroid gland?
a. increase in TSH due to total thyroidectomy
b. chronic administration of thyroxine
c. administration of short-acting T_3
d. administration of competitive antagonist of the T_4 receptor
e. administration of a drug that accelerates the monodeiodination of T_4 to T_3

27. Which of the following occurs in the follicular lumen (colloid) of the thyroid gland?
a. iodide pump
b. iodination of thyroglobulin
c. storage of T_4 bound to thyroid binding globulin
d. proteolysis of thyroglobulin
e. deiodination of diodotyrosine (DIT)

28. Which of the following is *not* a typical sign or symptoms of Graves' disease?
a. increased alveolar ventilation
b. increased heart rate
c. increased thermogenesis
d. increase in body weight
e. increase in appetite

29. Which of the following leads to a decrease in free T_4 concentration in the plasma in the steady state?
a. pregnancy
b. TSH-secreting tumor

c. Graves' disease
d. hypoalbuminemia
e. hypopituitarism

For questions 30–34, match the following injection with the corresponding GH response. Each answer will be used only once.

a. injection of somatostatin analog
b. injection of somatostatin analog and GHRH receptor antagonist
c. injection of somatostatin analog with GHRH receptor agonist
d. injection of somatostatin antagonist and GHRH receptor agonist
e. injection of GHRH receptor agonist

30. GH increases from 5 ng/mL to 100 ng/mL.

31. GH increases from 5 ng/mL to 10 ng/mL.

32. GH does not change from 5 ng/mL.

33. GH decreases from 5 ng/mL to 2 ng/mL.

34. GH decreases from 5 ng/mL to undetectably low levels.

Choose the single best answer to the following question.

35. Which of the following directly or indirectly leads to an increase in insulin secretion?

a. glucocorticoid therapy
b. somatostatin analog
c. starvation
d. hypoaminoacidemia
e. β-adrenergic blockade

For questions 36–40, match the clinical or biochemical findings below with the appropriate diagnosis. Assume each patient is *not* currently under treatment for the disorder listed.

a. hypoglycemia, hyperinsulinemia
b. hypoglycemia, hypoinsulinemia
c. hyperglycemia, hyperinsulinemia, normal urine free cortisol
d. hyperglycemia, hyperinsulinemia, elevated urine free cortisol
e. hyperglycemia, hypoinsulinemia

36. Diabetes mellitus type I

37. Diabetes mellitus type II

38. Insulinoma (pancreatic insulin-secreting tumor)

39. Cushing's syndrome

40. Adrenal insufficiency

For questions 41–44, select the correct answer from the five choices below. Answers can be used more than once.

a. calcitonin
b. parathyroid hormone

c. $1,25(OH)_2D$
d. 25(OH)D
e. ingestion of cholecalciferol

41. Increased GI calcium absorption is induced by:

42 Increased renal calcium reabsorption is induced by:

43. Increased endogenous production of 25(OH)D is induced by:

44. Increased osteoclastic calcium resorption is induced by:

Choose the single best answer to the following question.

45. A patient presents with hypocalcemia and an elevated parathyroid hormone (PTH) level. Of the following, which would be the first diagnosis you would consider?
a. parathyroid adenoma
b. parathyroid carcinoma
c. GI malabsorption
d. vitamin D intoxication
e. tumor secreting PTHrp

46. Which statement best describes the *major* difference between the control of LH secretion and the control of ACTH secretion?
a. Hypothalamic hormonal controller of LH is mainly inhibitory.
b. LH is not controlled by negative feedback.
c. LH is primarily controlled by inhibin, a nonsteroid.
d. LH can be stimulated by a steroid hormone.
e. LH is a peptide while ACTH is a glycoprotein.

47. Which of the following is *not* true of a typical menstrual cycle?
a. Menses is induced by an increase in estrogen and progesterone.
b. The increase in FSH on day 28 is induced by loss of steroid negative feedback.
c. Nondominant follicles undergo atresia due to a decrease in FSH.
d. The ratio of LH to FSH increases before ovulation.
e. Corpus luteum secretion of progesterone is dependent on low (but adequate) LH levels.

48. Which of the following is true about circulating sex steroids in the male?
a. Most of the circulating testosterone is from peripheral conversion of dehydroepiandrosterone (DHEA).
b. Most of the circulating estrogen is from peripheral conversion of androgens.
c. Most of the circulating dihydrotestosterone (DHT) is secreted by the testes.
d. Most of the circulating DHEA is secreted by the testes.
e. Human males do not normally have measurable plasma estrogen levels.

49. Which of the following will lead to an increase in GnRH pulses in the adult male hypothalamic-pituitary portal vein?
a. decrease in free testosterone in the plasma despite no change in total testosterone
b. DHT administration
c. FSH administration
d. LH administration
e. estrogen administration

50. Which of the following statements about male development is true?
 a. Gonadal androgens are not necessary for normal fetal development.
 b. DHT is not necessary for normal puberty.
 c. Like menopause in women, the typical man develops hypergonadotropic hypogonadism after the age of 50 (male climacteric).
 d. Adrenal androgens can produce subtle masculinization before puberty.
 e. Synthetic (nonaromatizable) androgens increase androgen binding protein release.

51. Which of the following statements about hypogonadotropic hypogonadism in males is true?
 a. 5α-Reductase expression in the Leydig cell is increased.
 b. Hypogonadotropic hypogonadism can be due to hyperprolactinemia.
 c. LH levels are not frankly elevated because of loss of negative feedback.
 d. Hypospermia occurs due to loss of sex hormone–binding globulin (SHBG) secretion by the Sertoli cells.
 e. Hypogonadotropic hypogonadism never occurs in hypopituitary men.

ANSWER KEY

1. b
2. d
3. c
4. a
5. b
6. d
7. c
8. a
9. d
10. e
11. c
12. b
13. a
14. d
15. e
16. b
17. d
18. e
19. a
20. c
21. d
22. d
23. c
24. e
25. c
26. d
27. b
28. d
29. e
30. d
31. e
32. c
33. a
34. b
35. a
36. e
37. c
38. a
39. d
40. b
41. c
42. b
43. e
44. b
45. c
46. d
47. a
48. b
49. a
50. d
51. b

FINAL EXAM: BONE PHYSIOLOGY

Choose the single best answer to each of the following questions or incomplete statements. Answer key at end.

1. **The process of deposition of calcium and phosphate in adult bone is called:**
   a. resorption
   b. osteocytic entrapment
   c. remodeling
   d. mineralization
   e. ossification

2. **Which of the following is *not* true about bone remodeling?**
   a. Approximately 20% of the trabecular surface is remodeling at any one time.
   b. Bone remodeling helps to repair fatigue damage.
   c. Osteoblasts tunnel into bones to mediate bone resorption.
   d. Osteoblasts surrounded by mineralized bone transform into osteocytes.
   e. Bone resorption and formation are normally coupled.

3. **Bone mass is:**
   a. normally highest during puberty
   b. not determined by genetic background
   c. not determined by amount of weight-bearing exercise a person does
   d. increased by normal secretion of gonadal steroids
   e. highest at the beginning of the menopause in women

4. **Which is true about osteoporosis?**
   a. Peak bone mass is unrelated to the development of osteoporosis.
   b. Osteoporosis cannot be prevented.
   c. Risk for osteoporosis is increased with the use of tobacco and excess alcohol.
   d. Osteoporosis usually precedes the development of osteopenia.
   e. Osteoporosis is caused by a failure to adequately mineralize osteoid.

ANSWER KEY

1. d
2. c
3. d
4. c

FINAL EXAM: ENDOCRINE–METABOLIC INTEGRATION

Choose the single best answer to each of the following questions or incomplete statements. Answer key at end.

1. **Which of the following statements about human obesity is true?**
   a. Obesity is commonly caused by mutations in the leptin receptor.
   b. Obesity is commonly caused by mutations in the proopiomelanocortin (POMC) gene.
   c. Obesity is defined as a body mass index between 25 and 29 kg/m^2.
   d. Obesity does not affect life expectancy.
   e. Obesity is affected by multiple genes and environmental factors.

2. **Genetic mutations that impair β_3-adrenergic receptor function might be associated with:**
   a. increased body fat
   b. increased lipolysis
   c. increased thermogenesis
   d. no effect, because β_3-adrenergic receptors are specific to brown fat, which is not present in significant amounts in adult humans
   e. increased leptin sensitivity

3. **Meal size is controlled largely at the level of the:**
   a. hypothalamus
   b. gastrointestinal tract
   c. pituitary
   d. brainstem
   e. spinal cord

4. **If all other factors remain unchanged, which of the following is *least* likely to affect body weight over an extended period of time?**
   a. intestinal malabsorption of nutrients
   b. decreased meal size
   c. diarrhea
   d. increased exercise
   e. decreased total food intake

5. **If all other factors remain unchanged, which of the following is *most* likely to affect body weight over an extended period of time?**
   a. amino acid intake
   b. cholecystokinin (CCK)
   c. meal timing
   d. gastric distention
   e. types of carbohydrates in the diet

6. **Which of the following statements is correct?**
   a. Leptin decreases uncoupling protein-1 (UCP-1) expression.
   b. Leptin stimulates hypothalamic neuropeptide Y (NPY) expression.
   c. Leptin stimulates hypothalamic POMC expression.

d. Leptin decreases energy expenditure.
e. Leptin deficiency is the most common cause of obesity and excess weight in humans.

7. Which of the following is *least* likely to be associated with an increase in energy expenditure?
a. genetic deficiency of the leptin receptor
b. increased activity of uncoupling proteins
c. increased food intake
d. increased β_3-adrenergic receptor activity
e. increased muscle mass

8. Which POMC-derived peptide in the brain is thought to be important for control of appetite and body weight?
a. melanocortin-4
b. leptin
c. adrenocorticotropic hormone (ACTH)
d. β-lipotropic pituitary hormone (β-LPH)
e. α-melanocyte-stimulating hormone (α-MSH)

9. Which receptor type is thought to be important for the effects of the molecule in question 8 on food intake?
a. melanocortin-1 receptor
b. melanocortin-2 receptor
c. melanocortin-4 receptor
d. melanocortin-5 receptor
e. long form of the leptin receptor

10. Which of the following would increase during prolonged starvation?
a. leptin
b. NPY
c. metabolic rate
d. hypothalamic POMC
e. CCK

11. Which of the following statements is true about thermogenesis?
a. Thermogenesis is stimulated by CCK (cholecystokinin).
b. Thermogenesis is increased during prolonged fasting.
c. Thermogenesis is increased by stimulating β-adrenergic receptors on fat cells.
d. Thermogenesis is the largest component of total energy expenditure.
e. Thermogenesis is decreased by leptin.

For questions 12–18, select the correct answer from the five choices below. Answers may be used more than once.
a. increased total food intake
b. increased meal size
c. decreased gonadal steroid levels
d. reduced somatic growth
e. increased thermogenesis

12. Effect of interrupting vagal afferents to the nucleus of the solitary tract.

13. Typical behavioral result of decreasing meal number.

14. Effect of leptin treatment during food deprivation.

15. Endocrine result of chronic reductions in food intake in the adult.

16. Effect of CCK receptor antagonists.

17. Endocrine effect of chronic reductions in food intake in children.

18. Behavioral effect of Agouti-related peptide (AgRP), an endogenous antagonist of α-MSH.

19. Which of the following conditions typifies euthyroid sick syndrome?
   a. decreased triiodothyronine (T_3), increased thyroid-stimulating hormone (TSH)
   b. decreased T_3, unchanged TSH
   c. increased T_3, increased TSH
   d. increased T_3, unchanged TSH
   e. decreased T_3, decreased TSH

20. Which of the following gene mutations has *not* been found in an obese human?
   a. UCP-1
   b. leptin
   c. POMC
   d. melanocortin-4 receptor
   e. long form of the leptin receptor

ANSWER KEY

1. e
2. a
3. d
4. b
5. a
6. c
7. a
8. e
9. c
10. b
11. c
12. b
13. b
14. e
15. c
16. b
17. d
18. a
19. b
20. a

FINAL EXAM: ENDOCRINE–IMMUNE INTEGRATION

Choose the single best answer to each of the following questions or incomplete statements. Answer key at end.

1. **During systemic infection, which of the following is *not* likely to be caused by cytokines?**
   a. decreased metabolic rate
   b. decreased insulin-like growth factor-1 (IGF-1) secretion
   c. increased glucocorticoid secretion
   d. fever
   e. decreased gonadal steroid secretion

2. **What feature occurs in *both* prolonged starvation (> 3 days) and systemic infection?**
   a. increased metabolic rate
   b. increased catecholamine secretion
   c. decreased triiodothyronine (T_3) levels
   d. acute phase protein production
   e. increased appetite

3. **Cytokines are most likely to affect neuroendocrine neurons in the hypothalamus by:**
   a. crossing the blood-brain barrier
   b. inducing acute phase proteins
   c. affecting peripheral hormone secretion
   d. acting at circumventricular organs such as the median eminence
   e. causing edema

4. **Which of the following will *not* cause symptoms of malnutrition?**
   a. systemic infection
   b. anorexia nervosa
   c. adequate caloric intake in the form of carbohydrates and fats
   d. untreated type 1 diabetes mellitus
   e. a balanced vegetarian diet

5. **What is an important effect of glucocorticoids on the response to inflammatory or immune challenge?**
   a. They inhibit cytokine production.
   b. They increase interleukin-6 (IL-6) production.
   c. They decrease acute phase protein synthesis.
   d. They increase fever.
   e. They stimulate T-lymphocyte proliferation.

6. **Cachexia (wasting) occurs in severe infection or injury because:**
   a. IGF-1 is inhibited
   b. energy expenditure is elevated relative to food intake
   c. glucocorticoids are increased
   d. glucagon is increased
   e. all of the above

7. Which of the following is *true* of the acute phase response?

a. It is usually initiated by decreases in IL-1 and tumor necrosis factor (TNF).
b. It is a defense against infection.
c. It inhibits resting energy expenditure.
d. It is not affected by glucocorticoid levels.
e. Its endocrine and metabolic effects are identical to those of starvation.

8. Which of the following is most likely to account for the levels of luteinizing hormone (LH) and follicle-stimulating hormone (FSH) during severe infection or injury?

a. inhibition of gonadal steroid secretion
b. stimulation of gonadal steroid secretion
c. inhibition of gonadotropin-releasing hormone (GnRH)
d. inhibition of thyroid hormone secretion.
e. inhibition of insulin secretion

9. Which of the following is *not* true of cytokines?

a. They function like hormones.
b. They can stimulate production of other cytokines.
c. They act as growth and chemotactic factors for immune cells.
d. They include interferons.
e. They only act in localized sites of infection or injury.

10. Insulin sensitivity is decreased in severe injury or infection because:

a. TNF is increased
b. glucocorticoids are increased
c. growth hormone is increased
d. glucagon is increased
e. all of the above

ANSWER KEY

1. a
2. c
3. d
4. e
5. a
6. e
7. b
8. c
9. e
10. e

FINAL EXAM: MATERNAL-FETAL PHYSIOLOGY

Choose the single best answer to each of the following questions or incomplete statements. Answer key at end.

1. **Which of the following cell layers is *not* a component of the human placenta?**
   a. cytotrophoblasts
   b. syncytiotrophoblasts
   c. maternal capillary endothelium
   d. fetal capillary endothelium
   e. all are components of the placenta

2. **Which of the following hormones is *not* synthesized by human placenta?**
   a. corticotropin-releasing hormone
   b. lactogen
   c. gonadotropin
   d. cortisol
   e. 1,25$(OH)_2$ vitamin D_3

3. **Which of the following estrogenic compounds is most directly associated with fetal well-being?**
   a. maternal 17α-estradiol
   b. maternal 17β-estradiol
   c. maternal estriol
   d. maternal estrone
   e. fetal 17β-estradiol

4. **Which one of the following changes in respiratory physiology does *not* occur during pregnancy?**
   a. increased tidal volume
   b. increased respiratory rate
   c. increased functional reserve capacity
   d. respiratory alkalosis

5. **Which of the following are stimulated by estrogen during pregnancy?**
   a. increased volume, secondary to increased angiotensin II and aldosterone
   b. decreased vascular resistance, particularly in the uterine vasculature
   c. lobuloalveolar development of the breast
   d. increased hepatic production of thyroxine-binding globulin
   e. all of the above

6. **Which of the following best describes the relationship between maternal and fetal thyroid hormone levels?**
   a. Most of maternal T_3 freely crosses the placenta to the fetus.
   b. No maternal T_3 or T_4 crosses the placenta to the fetus.
   c. Most of the maternal T_3 and T_4 reaching the placenta is inactivated by placental monodeiodinase.
   d. Maternal T_3 is transformed to T_4 by the fetal brain.
   e. All of the above describe the relationship.

7. Which of the following changes in metabolism occurs during pregnancy?

a. decreased insulin sensitivity caused by increased cortisol and growth hormones
b. increased basal metabolic rate caused by increased thyroid hormones
c. increased calcium absorption caused by $1,25(OH)_2$ vitamin D_3
d. increased triglyceride levels caused by increased growth hormone
e. all of the above

8. Which of the following describes the factors responsible for increasing uterine excitability during early labor?

a. increased estrogen to progesterone ratio increases prostaglandin $F_{2\alpha}$ ($PGF_{2\alpha}$) production, which stimulates myometrial contractions
b. increased estrogen to progesterone ratio increases gap junction formation between myometrial cells
c. increased sensitivity to oxytocin, which directly stimulates contraction and increases $PGF_{2\alpha}$ production
d. all of the above

9. Injection of dexamethasone into the maternal circulation would do what to the *maternal* plasma concentrations of cortisol and estriol?

a. increase cortisol and decrease estriol
b. increase cortisol and increase estriol
c. decrease cortisol and decrease estriol
d. decrease cortisol and increase estriol
e. no change in either cortisol or estriol

10. At 80% of gestation in the human, ablation of which of the following organs would be expected to induce premature labor?

a. fetal pituitary
b. maternal pituitary
c. fetal ovary (bilateral)
d. maternal ovary (bilateral)
e. none of the above

11. In sheep, induction of which enzyme in the placenta is critical for induction of parturition?

a. 11β-hydroxysteroid dehydrogenase
b. cytochrome $P450_{c17}$
c. 3β-hydroxysteroid dehydrogenase
d. cytochrome $P450_{arom}$
e. none of the above

12. Women in premature labor are sometimes treated with which steroid?

a. testosterone
b. estradiol
c. progesterone
d. dexamethasone
e. mifepristone

13. Which enzyme decreases the transfer of cortisol from mother to fetus?

a. 11β-hydroxysteroid dehydrogenase
b. cytochrome $P450_{c17}$
c. 3β-hydroxysteroid dehydrogenase
d. cytochrome $P450_{arom}$
e. none of the above

14. Which shunt within the fetal circulation carries blood from the umbilical vein to the vena cava?

a. ductus arteriosus
b. ductus venosus
c. foramen ovale
d. rete mirabile
e. ductus umbilicus

15. Which shunt within the fetal circulation is most important for allowing relatively low pulmonary blood flow, expressed as a percentage of combined ventricular output?

a. ductus arteriosus
b. ductus venosus
c. foramen ovale
d. rete mirabile
e. ductus umbilicus

16. Which of the following does *not* describe the fetal lung?

a. It serves a gas exchange function.
b. It is an endocrine organ.
c. It is a vascular bed.
d. It is a source of amniotic fluid.
e. It contains pulmonary surfactant.

17. The production of which surfactant protein increases most dramatically in the peripartum period?

a. SP-A
b. SP-B
c. SP-C
d. SP-D
e. SP-E

18. Which is the most abundant surfactant protein in fetal lung?

a. SP-A
b. SP-B
c. SP-C
d. SP-D
e. SP-E

19. Which drug would be most effective at accelerating the *closure* of a patent ductus arteriosus?

a. PGE_2
b. PGI_2
c. dexamethasone
d. estriol
e. indomethacin

20. Which drug would be most effective at *maintaining* a patent ductus arteriosus?

a. PGE_2
b. PGI_2
c. dexamethasone
d. estriol
e. indomethacin

21. In the human fetus, which steroid is the major secretory product of the fetal zone of the fetal adrenal?

a. cortisol
b. corticosterone
c. aldosterone
d. androstenedione
e. dehydroepiandrosterone

22. In the human placenta, 16-hydroxydehydroepiandrosterone is converted to which steroid?

a. estrone
b. estradiol
c. estriol
d. testosterone
e. androstenedione

23. Which substance causes contraction of myometrial cells during labor?

a. PGE_2
b. PGI_2
c. $PGF_{2\alpha}$
d. nitric oxide
e. endothelin

24. Which of the following is the most important factor influencing the rate of fetal growth?

a. maternal plasma growth hormone concentration
b. fetal plasma growth hormone concentration
c. maternal plasma insulin concentration
d. fetal plasma insulin concentration
e. nutrient supply to the fetus

ANSWER KEY

1. c
2. d
3. c
4. c
5. e
6. c
7. e
8. d
9. c
10. e
11. b
12. d
13. a
14. b
15. a
16. a
17. a
18. a
19. e
20. a
21. e
22. c
23. c
24. e

FINAL EXAM: EXERCISE PHYSIOLOGY

Choose the single best answer to each of the following questions or incomplete statements. Answer key at end.

1. **After completion of an endurance training program (3–5 times/wk, 30–60 min/day for 3 months at 60% of $\dot{V}O_2$max), all of the following will occur in skeletal muscle *except:***
   a. an increase in biceps muscle cross-sectional area
   b. an increase in mitochondrial density
   c. angiogenesis
   d. an increase in myoglobin
   e. an increased utilization of fats

2. **The physiologic adaptations that you can expect to see in the skeletal muscle of an immobilized or bedridden patient are the opposite of those seen during aerobic training and include all of the following *except:***
   a. rarefaction
   b. decreased myoglobin
   c. decreased pyruvate dehydrogenase activity
   d. increased resting heart rate
   e. increased density of mitochondria

3. **Which of the following are the appropriate hemodynamic responses during a graded exercise test on a treadmill?**
   a. Heart rate, respiratory rate, systolic pressure, diastolic pressure, and pulse pressure increase as work increases.
   b. Heart rate, respiratory rate, systolic pressure, diastolic pressure, and pulse pressure decrease as work increases.
   c. Systolic pressure decreases; diastolic pressure, heart rate, and respiratory rate increase as work increases.
   d. Diastolic pressure decreases or is unchanged; systolic pressure, heart rate, and respiratory rate increase as work increases.
   e. None of the above are normal responses to a graded exercise test.

4. **Which is *not* a good marker for monitoring the intensity of training?**
   a. the perceived exertion score
   b. the 15-second heart rate
   c. the 1-minute postexercise heart rate
   d. body weight
   e. lactate concentration

For questions 5–11, select from the three choices below the answer that *best* describes the effect that a 12-week aerobic training program consisting of 30–60 minutes of aerobic exercise 5 days/week would have on each variable in a healthy adult.

a. increases
b. decreases
c. no change

5. **Heart rate at rest.**

6. **Morbidity and mortality rate from all causes.**

7. **Capillary density in lower leg skeletal muscle.**

8. **Mitochondrial size, number, and oxidative phosphorylation following a period of exercise training.**

9. **Oxygen uptake during an incremental exercise test.**

10. **Total blood flow to skeletal muscle during exercise compared with rest.**

11. **Double product following a 12-week moderate intensity walking program.**

12. **Which statement about the effects of endurance training on skeletal muscle is false?**
    a. Endurance training results in an increase in the size and number of mitochondria.
    b. Endurance training results in less lactic acid formed at a given level of exercise.
    c. Endurance training results in an increase in myoglobin content in the muscle.
    d. Endurance training results in an increase in the number of muscle fibers within the muscle.
    e. Endurance training results in an increase in the intramuscular triglyceride content and fat utilization.

13. **In response to a 12-week endurance exercise training program, all of the following would occur except:**
    a. increased efficiency of the cardiovascular and pulmonary systems
    b. increased efficiency of oxygen utilization by skeletal muscle
    c. decreased diastolic and systolic pressures during exercise
    d. angiogenesis in skeletal muscle
    e. increased myocardial oxygen consumption during exercise

14. **Select the appropriate hemodynamic response to an increase in submaximal exercise intensity.**
    a. an increase in systolic and diastolic blood pressure
    b. a decrease in systolic and diastolic blood pressure
    c. an increase in systolic blood pressure as diastolic blood pressure stays the same or decreases
    d. an increase in diastolic blood pressure as systolic blood pressure stays the same or decreases
    e. none of the above

15. **The primary energy system(s) used for the 100-meter dash is:**
    a. aerobic glycolysis
    b. anaerobic glycolysis
    c. Krebs cycle
    d. ATP-CP system
    e. 50% aerobic and 50% anaerobic glycolysis

For questions 16–20, determine whether each statement is true or false.

16. **At higher altitudes or in hypoxic conditions, cardiac output is decreased.**

17. **During exercise, the unloading of oxygen from hemoglobin is facilitated by metabolic waste products.**

18. The oxyhemoglobin dissociation curve shifts to the right with a rise in body temperature and/or a decrease in pH.

19. The major effect of endurance training is to increase skeletal muscle myoglobin, mitochondria, and metabolic enzymes so that the overall aerobic efficiency of the muscle is increased.

20. A kilocalorie is equal to 1000 calories and can also be written as 1 kCal or 1 C.

ANSWER KEY

1. a	6. b	11. b	16. false
2. e	7. a	12. d	17. true
3. d	8. a	13. e	18. true
4. d	9. a	14. c	19. true
5. b	10. a	15. d	20. false

FINAL EXAM: TEMPERATURE REGULATION

Choose the single best answer to each of the following questions or incomplete statements. Answer key at end.

1. **Which of the following is *not* a physiologic adaptation to heat?**
   a. Sweating is initiated earlier.
   b. One sweats more for a given exposure.
   c. Heart rate is elevated at a given exposure.
   d. Plasma volume increases
   e. Sweat rate is maintained.

For questions 2–6, select the correct answer from the three choices below. Each answer may be used more than once.

a. increases above basal state
b. decreases from basal state
c. does not change from basal state

2. **Resistance to blood flow in the cutaneous circulation during heat exposure.**

3. **Sympathetic cholinergic nerve activity to sweat glands during heat exposure.**

4. **Sympathetic nerve activity to hair follicles during cold exposure.**

5. **Metabolic activity of brown fat during cold exposure.**

6. **Hypothalamic thermostat set-point following bacterial infection and pyrogen release.**

For questions 7–11, select the correct answer from the four choices below. Each answer may be used more than once.

a. heat stroke
b. heat exhaustion
c. heat fatigue
d. none of the above

7. **A medical emergency requiring immediate intervention.**

8. **A precursor to heat stroke.**

9. **A precursor to circulatory shock.**

10. **Appropriately treated with monitoring for progression.**

11. **Associated with a rapid drop in core temperature.**

Choose the single best answer to each of the following questions or incomplete statements.

12. Which of the following are *not* correct regarding radiation and conduction?

a. Radiation and conduction account for 75% of heat loss at rest.
b. Radiation and conduction are the primary heat loss systems during exercise
c. Radiation and conduction are ineffective when external air temperature is greater than skin temperature.
d. Radiation and conduction are the primary heat loss systems in a patient with a fever.
e. Both b and d are not correct.

13. All of the following are common symptoms of heat stress *except:*

a. muscle cramps
b. profuse sweating
c. dizziness
d. angina
e. nausea

ANSWER KEY

1. c
2. b
3. a
4. a
5. a
6. a
7. a
8. b
9. a
10. d
11. d
12. e
13. d

FINAL EXAM: AGING

From the choices below, select the answer that best describes the normal aging process on each variable in a healthy adult. Answer key at end.

a. increased
b. decreased
c. not changed

1. **amount of sleep**

2. **resting heart rate**

3. **total blood volume**

4. **circulating angiotensin II concentration**

Indicate whether the following statements are true or false with respect to normal aging.

5. **Resting EKG changes include a prolongation of the T wave and a depressed j point.**

6. **Resting cardiac output is not changed in physically active elderly adults.**

7. **Number of glomeruli in the kidney is decreased.**

8. **Ventilation/perfusion matching in the lungs is decreased.**

9. **Glucose intolerance results from an atrophied pancreas.**

10. **Adrenal production of both DHEA and growth hormone is decreased.**

11. **Osteopenia and osteoporosis are equivalent processes in the aging population.**

Choose the single best answer to each of the following questions or incomplete statements.

12. **Select the correct statement that describes the changes that occur with normal aging in the lung.**
    a. Vital capacity and physiologic dead space are increased
    b. Costovertebral stiffness and chest wall rigidity are decreased
    c. Elastic recoil is decreased and residual volume is increased
    d. Alveolar surface area is decreased and oxygen diffusing capacity is increased

13. **All of the following are typical aging changes observed in skeletal muscle except:**
    a. sarcopenia
    b. rarefaction
    c. decreased force production capability

d. increase in skeletal muscle elasticity
e. homogeneity of fiber types

14. Which of the following is/are decreased with aging?

a. estrogen (women)
b. free testosterone (men)
c. DHEA
d. IGF1
e. all of the above

ANSWER KEY

1. b
2. a
3. b
4. c
5. False
6. True
7. True
8. True
9. False
10. True
11. False
12. c
13. d
14. e

INDEX

Page numbers in **boldface type** indicate complete chapters.